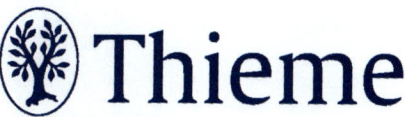

Endoscopic Transsphenoidal Surgery

A Practical Guide

Editors-in-Chief

Nishit Shah, MS (ENT), DNB, DORL
Honorary Consultant,
Department of ENT,
Bombay Hospital and Medical Research Centre;
Breach Candy Hospital,
Mumbai, Maharashtra, India

C. E. Deopujari, MS, MCh, MSc (Neurosurgery)
Professor and Head,
Department of Neurosurgery,
Bombay Hospital and Medical Research Centre,
Mumbai, Maharashtra, India

Associate Editor

Sai Spoorthi Nayak, MS, DNB (ENT)
Consultant,
Department of ENT,
Bombay Hospital,
Indore, Madhya Pradesh, India

Thieme
Delhi • Stuttgart • New York • Rio de Janeiro

Publishing Director: Ritu Sharma
Development Editor: Dr Gurvinder Kaur
Director-Editorial Services: Rachna Sinha
Project Manager: Arindam Banerjee
Vice President Sales and Marketing: Arun Kumar Majji
Managing Director & CEO: Ajit Kohli

Thieme Medical and Scientific Publishers Private Limited.
A - 12, Second Floor, Sector - 2, Noida - 201 301, Uttar Pradesh, India, +911204556600
Email: customerservice@thieme.in
www.thieme.in

Cover design: Thieme Publishing Group
Typesetting by RECTO Graphics, India

Printed in India by Nutech Print Services - India

5 4 3 2 1

ISBN: 978-93-88257-23-7
eISBN: 978-93-88257-24-4

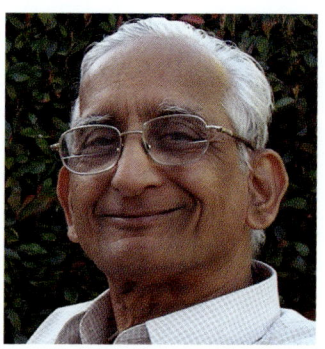

Dr Jawaharlal T. Shah
1932–2018

I would like to dedicate this book to the memory of my father, Dr Jawaharlal T. Shah. My father was the sole inspiration for me to pursue ENT as a career, and become the third-generation ENT surgeon in the family. He passed his MS ENT from KEM Hospital in the footsteps of his father, Dr T. O. Shah, who founded the department of ENT at KEM Hospital. He was the first person to introduce me to the world of nasal endoscopy in 1989, and I did my first uncinectomy under his supervision. Much later, even after his retirement, he would attend our workshops to see the advances in endoscopic sinus and skull base surgery. He was a skilled ENT surgeon and pioneered the use of lasers for laryngeal surgery in India. He was also an avid yoga practitioner and teacher. His book on therapeutic yoga has been internationally acclaimed. He was a thorough gentleman, who always had a twinkle in his eyes and the warmest of smiles. He was much loved and respected by his family, peers, students, friends, and patients alike. He will always be in our hearts and fondly remembered and missed.

Dr Nishit Shah

Contents

Foreword

"The beginning is the most important part of the work."
                                                              Plato

I have been conferred the privilege to write a foreword for *Endoscopic Transsphenoidal Surgery: A Practical Guide.* This is a source of great personal pleasure and professional honor, as I have witnessed the professional development of the authors, from their inception as a skull base surgery team to their becoming of a world-renowned skull base surgery center.

The beginning of any enterprise often filters who will continue trying to perform and learn and who will quit and move on to other endeavors. Therefore, it is of utmost importance to facilitate the launching of novice surgeons into new procedures and strategies. As a relatively young group, it seems fitting that the authors have organised and edited a book dedicated to facilitate the entry, and enhance the surgical competency, of developing skull base surgeons with interest in learning endoscopic techniques.

This book includes 11 chapters that guide the reader from fundamentals, such as anatomy, peri-operative assessment, and basic surgical techniques, to advanced concepts and techniques, including extended approaches, management of complications, and decision-making. The final chapter offers case examples where the authors apply all the concepts in context. The book offers detailed and precise conceptual and technical descriptions that are complemented by equally explicit, high-definition photographs and illustrations. Readers will benefit greatly from the approach and perspective offered by the authors. Undoubtedly, the exchange of ideas among all interested specialties have produced a solid foundation that should be emulated.

Though this book is targeted to newcomers in endoscopic skull base surgery and organised as a "beginner's guide," it will also serve as a comprehensive yet practical reference to anyone with interest in this field. I commend the authors for their commitment to education and patient care and welcome *Endoscopic Transsphenoidal Surgery: A Practical Guide* to the collection of important references in skull base surgery.

Ricardo L. Carrau, MD, FACS
Professor,
Department of Otolaryngology-Head and Neck Surgery;
Director,
The Comprehensive Skull Base Surgery Program,
The Ohio State University Medical Center,
Columbus, Ohio, United States

Foreword

It is a distinct pleasure to write a foreword for this outstanding publication of Dr Shah and Dr Deopujari. I have known them for over a decade, and their commitment to patient care, innovation, and education is unparalleled. I consider them to be among the global leaders in the field of skull base surgery. I have watched them evolve in their technique as pioneers in the field of skull base surgery, adding critical technology founded on an unwavering principle of anatomy.

This book represents a distinct body of work that is both practical and nuanced. It covers a range of fundamental topics that incorporate the entire continuum of care, rather than just surgical technique. The reader is carefully counseled in peri-operative imaging, surgical decision-making, patient selection, technical considerations, and post-operative complications and their management. The topics covered are foundational, beginning with pituitary tumors, and then the text systematically extends through the variety of expanded approaches.

A critical feature of the book is its ability to be patient-centric while simultaneously being surgeon-centric. The book provides a step-by-step approach that can take the surgeon from "nares-to-the-nares" not from a theoretical, but rather from a truly practical perspective that provides the patient with the best possible outcome.

What I love about the book is that it is written for the "real-world" surgeon, rather than a purely academic pursuit. The book provides practical considerations based on the available resources in a given environment: as an example, the equipment chapter discusses the use of instrumentation that is readily available in most institutions, as opposed to expensive and difficult-to-access technology. It has been one of the distinct honors of my career to have operated shoulder-to-shoulder with Dr Shah and Dr Deopujari, who always prefer to put the team first before any individual surgeon. There were several nuances that I learned from them.

The work is shared in the spirit of education and is a must read for young skull base surgeons as well as experienced veterans.

Thank you, Dr Shah, Dr Deopujari, and Dr Nayak.

Amin B. Kassam, MD
Chair of Department of Neurosurgery V;
Vice President of Neurosciences System Clinical Program,
Department of Neurosurgery,
Aurora Neurosciences Innovation Institute,
Aurora St. Luke's Medical Center,
Milwaukee, Wisconsin, United States

Preface

When I first joined the senior authors for fellowship in Endoscopic Sinus and Skull Base Surgery, my knowledge in skull base surgery was limited. It was only under their guidance and mentorship that the doors of skull base were open to me and I realised that these surgeries, despite being so complicated, intricate, and ever evolving, could be demystified and explained in a simple language. This is when the idea struck me to help other beginners to venture a step further beyond routine sinus surgeries.

A surgeon who has limited exposure to advanced endoscopic surgeries could also benefit from this book covering practical aspects of peri-operative management of skull base surgeries. The content is easy to read and comprehend with a lot of intra-operative pictures for better reader orientation, and is written with a point of view of a young budding ENT/neuro skull base surgeon. Much of the theory is avoided, making the book a light and easy-to-assimilate read, in terms of surgical aspects.

Although the book does not aim at making an exhaustive list of all the possible lesions or surgeries of anterior/middle/posterior skull base, it will act as a quick reference guide, making basic concepts clear and simultaneously evoking interest of young surgeons in this field.

Sai Spoorthi Nayak

I must congratulate Sai for her enthusiasm to convince and push us to contribute to this book. The book introduces the concept of "endoscopic pituitary surgery" quite well for beginners and also introduces the possibilities of extended approaches to the midline skull base.

For a neurosurgeon, the challenge of understanding the endonasal as well as paranasal sinus anatomy has become essential to practice skull base surgeries. The book describes this well and prepares the neurosurgeon to operate on pituitary in a more confident and elaborate manner. The advantages of tumor resection, functional preservation, and avoidance of complications are well described.

I hope our effort to familiarize the ENT/neuro skull base surgeon will encourage them to take up this surgery in a proper manner, which is now close to becoming the standard of care.

C. E. Deopujari

Since many books address endoscopic skull base surgery in a great degree of detail, our idea was to keep this book completely practical with an emphasis on surgery and instrumentation and for it to be used as a quick reference.

We started as a team in December 1999 and now, after almost 20 years, with the help of new concepts and modern instruments we have tried to modify the present technique to make it as simple as possible and easily replicable. This has, of course, been shaped by the numerous visiting international and national experts who have been faculties for our annual workshop (since 2004). We are in great debt to everyone who has contributed to our understanding and development. We hope this book will be useful to the future generation.

Nishit Shah

Acknowledgements

The completion of this book could not have been accomplished without the support of numerous people who have contributed to this book in ways more than one.

At the outset, we are extremely grateful to all the world renowned neuro as well as ENT surgeons who have graced all our annual skull base workshops and have been kind enough to share their knowledge and skills and helped us grow and strengthen our comprehension in the subject. We would like to extend our special gratitude to Dr Amin Kassam and Dr Riccardo Carrau who have been our mentors and guides, and they are the reason we have reached this far. We would also like to thank them for taking time out of their busy schedule and writing forewords for this book.

We cannot proceed further without thanking Dr Milind Kirtane, who has been our teacher, inspiration, and constant support ever since we started as an Endoskullbase team. No book would ever be complete without duly extending our sincere gratitude towards him.

We would also like to thank the entire administrative department of Bombay Hospital and Medical Research Centre for their support extended to the departments of ENT and Neurosurgery. Shri B. K. Taparia (Chairman Bombay Hospital) and Dr R. V. Patil (Medical Director Bombay Hospital) have been extremely supportive throughout the last two decades in developing both the departments and procuring state-of-art equipments. We would like to thank Mrs Maria D'Souza, secretary to Dr Nishit Shah, for managing the patients and their records at the outpatient basis.

A special thank you to all the fellows/clinical assistants of Dr Nishit Shah and Dr C. E. Deopujari who have toiled for months together in assisting all the endoscopic skull base cases, and helped in assimilating and organising all the patient data ever since we began our journey in 2004. It was only because of their efforts that we could use the best cases and pictures for this book. We would especially like to mention the names of Dr Salman Shaikh, Dr Anamika Rathore, Dr Viraj Kaluskar, Dr Radhika Shree, Dr Vyshnavi Jajee, Dr Danish Andrabi, Dr Janhavi Bhati, Dr Darshan Jhaveri, Dr Saumya, Dr Anupriya Hajela, Dr V. K. Anand, Dr Varun Malu, Dr Sujata Gawai, Dr Vivek Sasindran, Dr Ajay Shegde, Dr Jyotirmay Hegde, Dr Rahul Tejankar, Dr Rashmi Shukla, Dr Sudarshan

Ahire, Dr Prashant, Dr Rajesh Kumar, and Dr Baisakhi Bakat for their extensive efforts.

Dr Sujata Muranjan and Dr Vikram Karmarkar have been greatly instrumental in all the Endoskullbase workshops and has always been a constant source of support and help.

We would like to thank Dr Varsha Joshi, Radiologist, for providing us the image of conchal pneumatisation of sphenoid.

The entire neurosurgery OT staff, ICU staff, and the anaesthetists of Bombay Hospital deserve due acknowledgement for co-operating and assisting in all endoscopic skull base cases.

We must not forget the entire team of Thieme Publishers who have accepted the book, gone through our proofs umpteen number of times, made endless corrections, and were even kind to accommodate last moment changes in the book, in order to deliver the best product.

This book would not have been possible without the constant support, patience, and love from our respective families who have always put our careers in the forefront and all other household hassles in the back seat. We would like to thank Dr Nishit Shah's mother, Mrs Smita Shah and his wife Mrs Rachana Shah; Dr C. E. Deopujari's wife, Dr Mrs Rajashree Deopujari; and Dr Sai Spoorthi Nayak's husband, Dr Archan Naik, her parents, Mr Ramesh Nayak and Mrs Geeta Nayak, and her in-laws Mr Devidas Naik and Mrs Roshan Naik.

Contributors

Nishit Shah, MS (ENT), DNB, DORL
Honorary Consultant,
Department of ENT,
Bombay Hospital and Medical Research
Centre;
Breach Candy Hospital,
Mumbai, Maharashtra, India

**C. E. Deopujari, MS, MCh,
MSc (Neurosurgery)**
Professor and Head,
Department of Neurosurgery,
Bombay Hospital and Medical Research
Centre,
Mumbai, Maharashtra, India

Sai Spoorthi Nayak, MS, DNB (ENT)
Consultant,
Department of ENT,
Bombay Hospital,
Indore, Madhya Pradesh, India

Sonali Shah, DNB, DMRD
Assistant Professor,
Department of CT and MRI,
Bombay Hospital and Medical Research
Centre,
Mumbai, Maharashtra, India

Introduction

Nishit Shah and Sai Spoorthi Nayak

In the last 15 years or so, endoscopic skull base surgery has increasingly gained popularity and importance over conventional open transcranial surgery. In this era of minimally invasive surgery, open surgeries are being rapidly replaced by endoscopic surgeries. Initially, endoscopic endonasal surgeries were restricted to paranasal sinus surgeries, but now with the advent of newer imaging techniques, improved three-dimensional understanding of the endonasal, skull base, and intracranial anatomy, and intra-operative neuro-navigation and imaging system, surgeons have realised the potential of the nose as a vital corridor to access most of the central skull base lesions. Endoscopic endonasal surgery is not only less invasive, but gives a magnified and yet panoramic view of the intra-operative field. Post-operatively, the patient encounters no facial sutures or scars; there is no brain retraction or bone flap involved, and the recovery period is less stormy with decreased neurological sequelae and complications. The hospital stay is also reduced as the patient faces less post-operative morbidity and may get back to his or her routine activities much quicker.

In experienced hands, the surgical outcome with endoscopic surgery is comparable and sometimes even better than conventional transcranial surgery or transcranial microsurgery.[1]

The important factors to keep in mind for endoscopic surgery are proper understanding of the endonasal and intracranial anatomy, improved ability to read computed tomography (CT) and magnetic resonance imaging (MRI) images, and correct case selection. Before venturing into skull base surgeries, the practising otolaryngologist must have enough proficiency over endoscopic sinus surgeries and must be confident enough to handle intra-operative as well as post-operative complications encountered during sinus surgeries. Secondly, in order to gain enough familiarity of the endonasal skull base anatomy, it would be immensely beneficial for both the ENT and the neurosurgeon to participate/ attend cadaveric dissection courses together. Remember, there is no substitute to cadaveric dissection in understanding anatomy. Participating in cadaveric dissection courses helps both the surgeons to develop a comfort zone to work around each other. Both the surgeons develop a unified vision and mutual respect and trust towards each other.

There is a certain protocol or a learning curve that a beginner must follow when considering endoscopic skull base surgeries. We would like to mention here a modified level of complexity for endoscopic skull base surgeries (**Table 1.1**).

Endoscopic skull base surgery is a joint venture. A healthy partnership and integrated approach towards the patient are the key to a successful practise. This partnership should sustain over years and should progress from level I to level V and not just over a few cases. The aim should be to work together and graduate from simple to difficult cases. Unless you work together for simple cases, it is rather difficult to co-operate and co-ordinate for the more complex ones. There is some overlap in the roles of the ENT surgeon and the neurosurgeon. Before posting a patient for surgery, the entire team should sit down and discuss as to which would be the best surgical approach for the patient, devise a roadmap, and follow it for the concerned pathology. It is not necessary that endoscopic route has to be chosen just because it is an option. If the morbidity of endoscopic approach is more than transcranial, then an appropriate approach should be chosen in unison. Intra-operatively too, the roles of the ENT surgeon and the neurosurgeon should be complementary. As the neurosurgeon is completely focused on the tumour and its removal, the ENT surgeon can keep an eye on the surrounding vital structures and warn the neurosurgeon of any impending/ avoidable injury. Also, each of them can have different outlook or technique when it comes to tumour removal and when one faces a roadblock, the other can come to the rescue with his or her inputs or surgical assistance.

Table 1.1 The learning curve; level of complexity of endoscopic endonasal skull base surgeries

Level I	• Sinonasal surgery (sphenoidal and frontal) • Small sellar (pituitary) tumours • Small CSF leaks	
Level II	• Large CSF leaks • Optic nerve decompression • Larger pituitary tumours (including parasellar extension)	

Level III	• Extradural	• Sagittal
		  ○ Transcribriform
		  ○ Transplanum
		  ○ Transclival
		  ○ Transodontoid
		• Coronal
		  ○ Transpterygoid
		  ○ Transorbital

Level IV	• Intradural	• Without cortical cuff
		  ○ Sagittal
		    ▪ Transplanum
		    ▪ Transcribriform
		    ▪ Pre-infundibular craniopharyngiomas
		  ○ Coronal
		    ▪ Petrous apex lesions
		    ▪ Meckel's cave lesions
		• With cortical cuff
		  ○ Transplanum
		  ○ Transcribriform
		  ○ Infundibular craniopharyngiomas
		  ○ Retro-infundibular craniopharyngiomas
		  ○ Transclival

Level V	• Cerebrovascular surgery	• AVM, aneurysm

Abbreviations: AVM, arteriovenous malformation; CSF, cerebrospinal fluid.
Source: Modified from Prevedello et al.[2]

3

Endoscopic skull base surgery is only possible with a team approach. In fact, a successful endoscopic neurosurgery revolves around a team comprising of a myriad of specialists and not confined to just the neurosurgeon and the ENT surgeon. The following specialities constitute a team for any endoscopic skull base surgery.

- Endocrinologist.
- Radiologist and interventional radiologist.
- Ophthalmologist.
- Pathologist.
- Neuroanaesthetist.
- Intensivist.
- Medical oncologist.
- Nursing staff.

It should be emphasised that endoscopic skull base surgery should be performed in a multi-speciality hospital with a fully functional ICU set-up and well-trained nursing staff. The OT should be equipped with good quality straight as well as angled endoscopes with HD camera system and intra-operative neuro-imaging system and surgical Doppler systems.

References

1. Verillaud B, Bresson D, Sauvaget E, et al. Endoscopic endonasal skull base surgery. Eur Ann Otorhinolaryngol Head Neck Dis 2012;129(4):190–196

2. Prevedello DM, Kassam AB, Snyderman C, et al. Endoscopic cranial base surgery: ready for prime time? Clin Neurosurg 2007;54:48–57

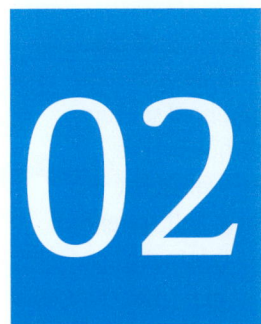

Surgical Anatomy

Sai Spoorthi Nayak

Sphenoid Sinus

The sphenoid bone is a bat wing–shaped bone divided into the body centrally, pterygoid processes inferiorly, and greater and lesser wings laterally. The lesser wing and planum sphenoidale (sphenoid sinus roof) form the medial anterior cranial fossa. The medial portion of the middle cranial base is formed by the sphenoid body, tuberculum sella, sella turcica, middle and posterior clinoid processes, and dorsum sellae. The lateral portion of the middle cranial base is formed by the lesser and greater wings of the sphenoid bone which house the temporal lobe.[1] The posterior limit of the middle cranial fossa is formed by the clivus, which is in turn formed by the sphenoid and the occipital bones.

The sphenoid sinus is a centrally located paired paranasal sinus divided into the right and left side by an intersphenoid septum. This septum usually deviates towards one side thus dividing the sinus into a dominant sinus and a smaller sinus. More often than not, the septum localises on the internal carotid artery (ICA), or the optic nerve or the optic-carotid recess (OCR). In a cadaveric study, only 13% of the specimens had an isolated midline septum, 89% of the cadavers had one septum, and 48% had two septations inserted on the ICA (**Fig. 2.1**).[2]

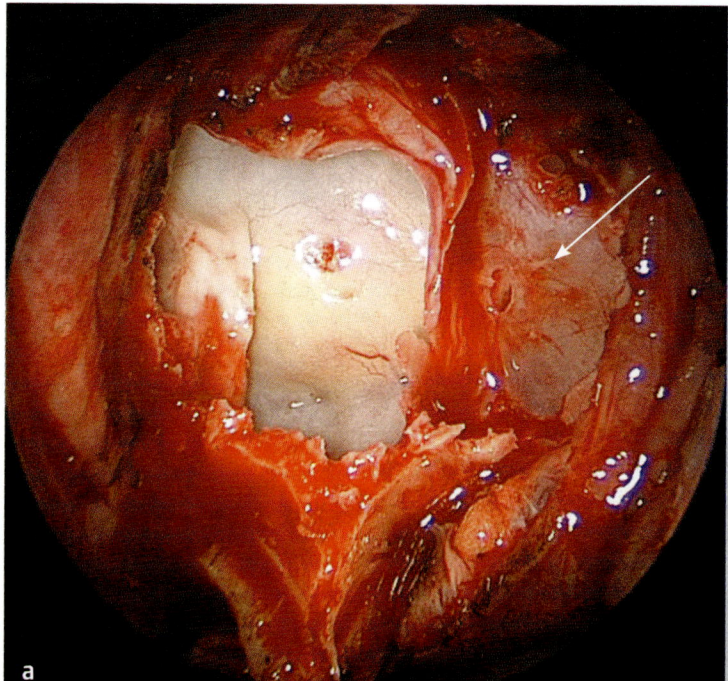

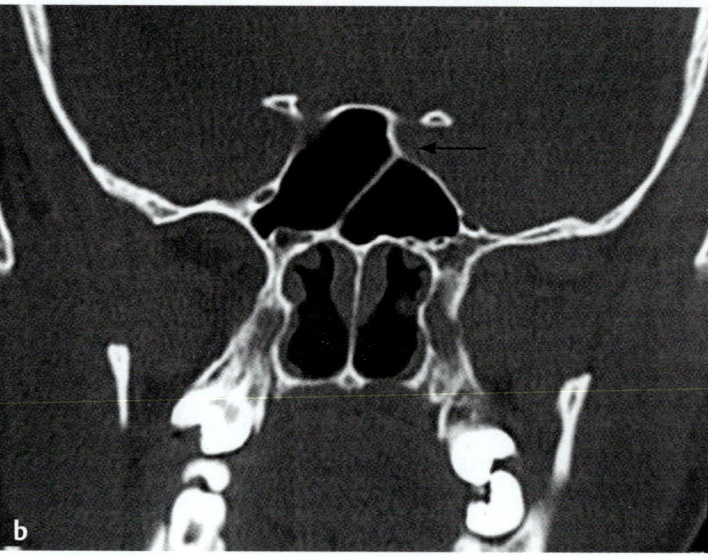

Fig. 2.1 **(a)** Intra-operative view of the sphenoid sinus and the intersphenoid septum after removing the anterior wall of the sphenoid. Left sphenoid mucosa is intact (*white arrow*). **(b)** CT scan image showing intersphenoid septum ending on left ICA (*black arrow*).

The sphenoid sinus ostium is located 1.5 cm above the choana (**Fig. 2.2**). It is located at the level of the lower one-third of the superior turbinate and is visualised by a slight lateralisation of the superior turbinate.

The sphenoid sinus varies according to its pneumatisation. The degree of pneumatisation varies with age. There are three major pneumatisation patterns: conchal (3%), pre-sellar (17%), and sellar (80%).[3]

Conchal type of sphenoid is a virtually non-pneumatised sphenoid (**Fig. 2.3**). A conchal sphenoid poses an anatomical challenge to the skull base surgeons.

There are no landmarks visualised on its walls. Hence, it is dangerous to drill on such a sphenoid without the use of navigation.

Pre-sellar pneumatisation of sphenoid is pneumatisation up to the plane of the tuberculum sella or the anterior face of sella (**Fig. 2.4**). An experienced surgeon may go below the sella and drill without the use of an image guidance system, but for a beginner, intra-operative navigation is a must in this type of sphenoid.

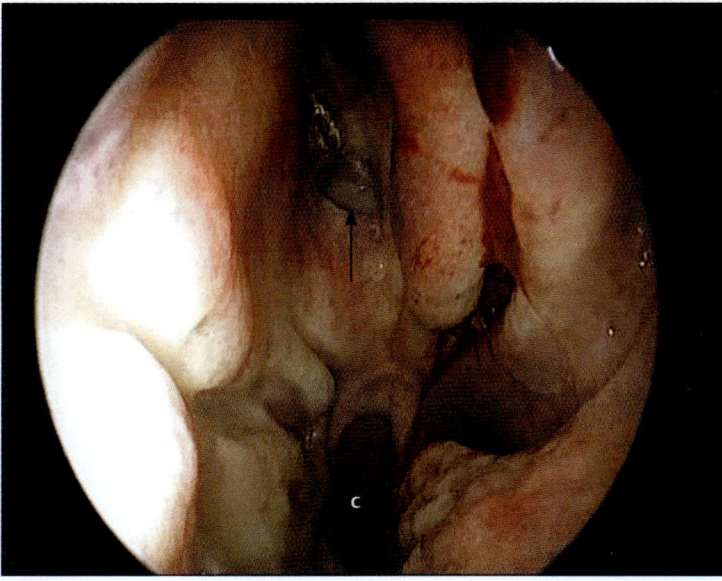

Fig. 2.2 Intra-operative view of the left sphenoid natural ostium (marked by a *black arrow*) around 1.5 cm above the choana **(c)**. The left middle and the inferior turbinates have been lateralised.

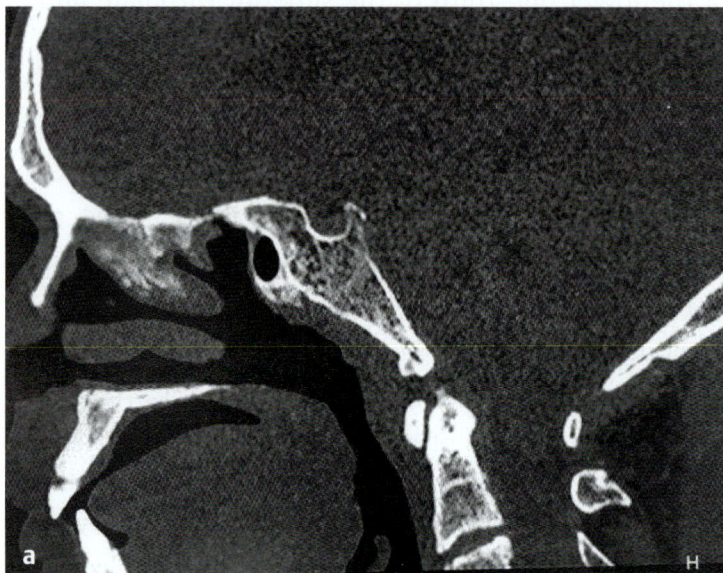

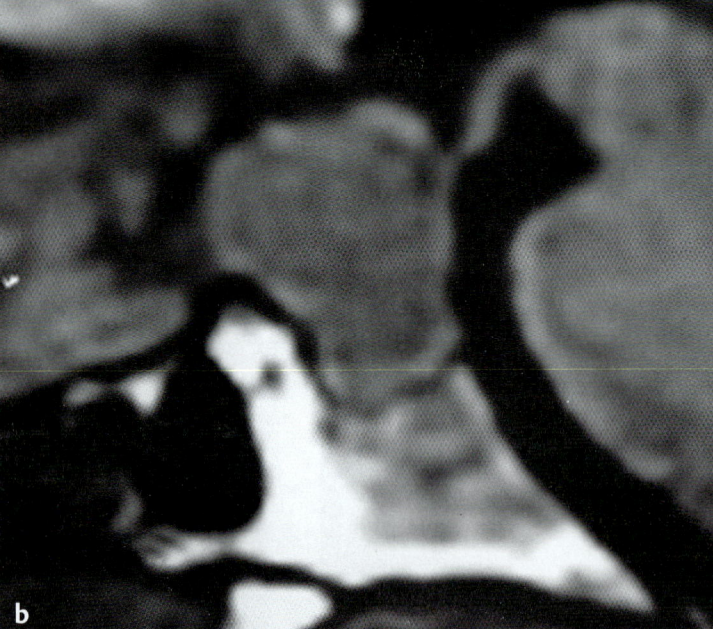

Fig. 2.3 **(a)** Sagittal CT bone window showing conchal type of sphenoid. The sphenoid in this patient is virtually absent (This image is provided courtesy of Dr Varsha Joshi). **(b)** T1 sagittal MRI picture of a different patient showing conchal type of sphenoid pneumatisation. Note the thick bone that needs to be drilled in order to reach up to the sella which is occupied by a pituitary tumour.

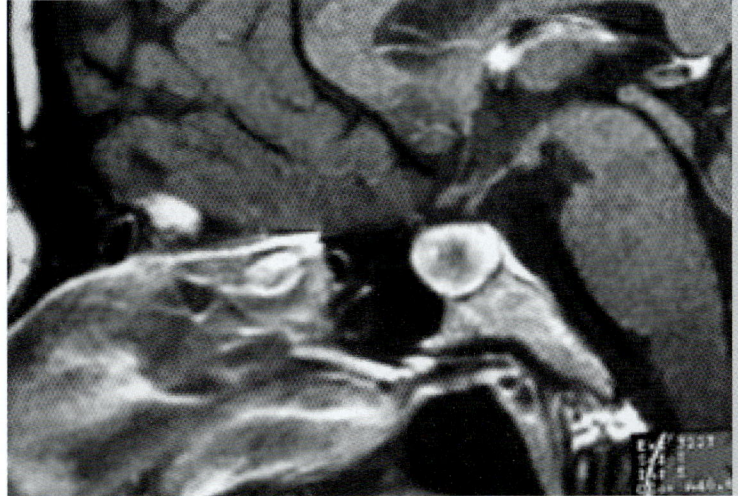

Fig. 2.4 T1 sagittal MRI image of pre-sellar type of sphenoid pneumatisation. The sphenoid is pneumatised up to the anterior wall of the sella. The sella shows a presence of a pituitary tumour.

Sella type of pneumatisation is the most common type (**Fig. 2.5**). It extends beyond the floor of the sella. The pneumatisation may be complete or incomplete, involving just the body or going right up to the clivus.

The reason behind classifying the types of pneumatisation is that they are recognised early during the reading of the scans and neuro-navigation system can be arranged to delineate the important structures during drilling of the sphenoid. Sagittal cuts in a computed tomography (CT) scan are useful to classify and recognise the type of pneumatisation of the sphenoid. CT scan images, used for intra-operative navigation, not only aid in drilling of the sphenoid/clivus, but also help in predicting the level of difficulty during the surgery.

With greater pneumatisation, the sphenoid landmarks become more and more obvious. Superiorly and anteriorly, is the planum sphenoidale or the roof of the sphenoid which forms the floor of the medial anterior cranial fossa. The planum and the sella are divided by a thick ridge of bone called the tuberculum which corresponds to the optic chiasmatic sulcus intracranially. The landmarks on the lateral wall of a well-pneumatised sphenoid sinus from superior to inferior, are, optic nerve prominence, the lateral OCR, the parasellar and clival ICA, the maxillary division of the trigeminal nerve (V2), and the vidian nerve (**Figs. 2.6, 2.9**).

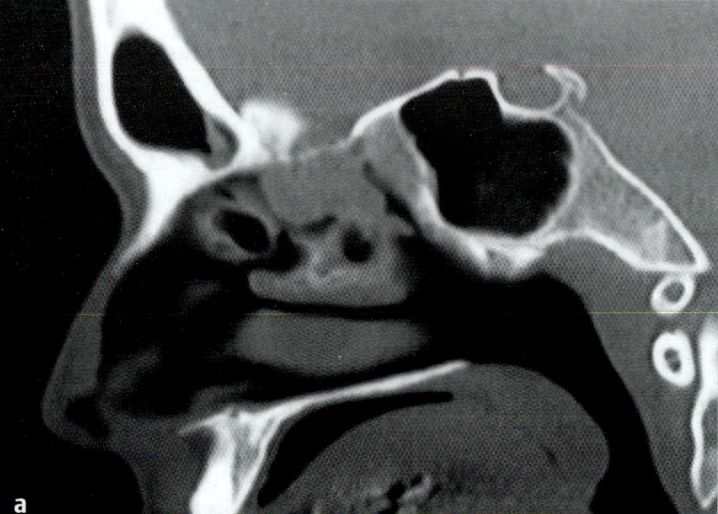

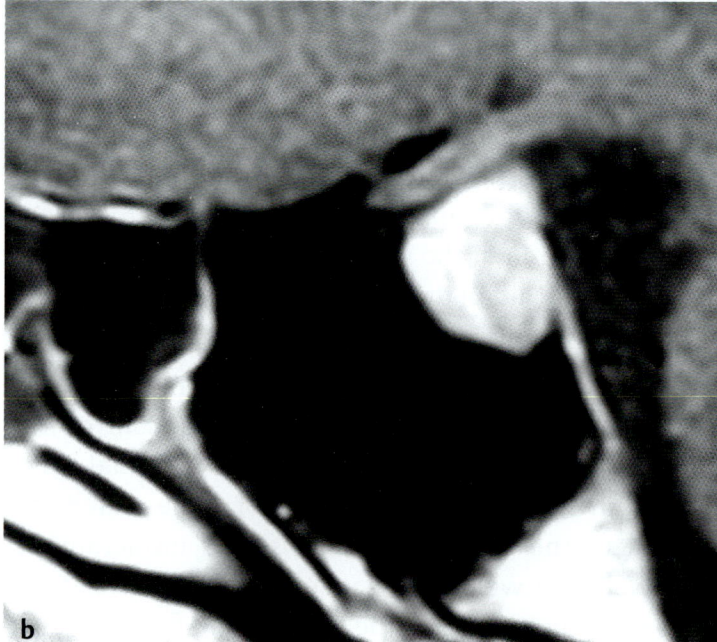

Fig. 2.5 **(a)** Sagittal CT bone window showing a sella type of sphenoid pneumatisation. **(b)** T1 sagittal MRI picture of a different patient showing complete sellar type of sphenoid pneumatisation in which the entire sphenoid floor is included in the sphenoid sinus. There is very thin bone of the clivus under the sella.

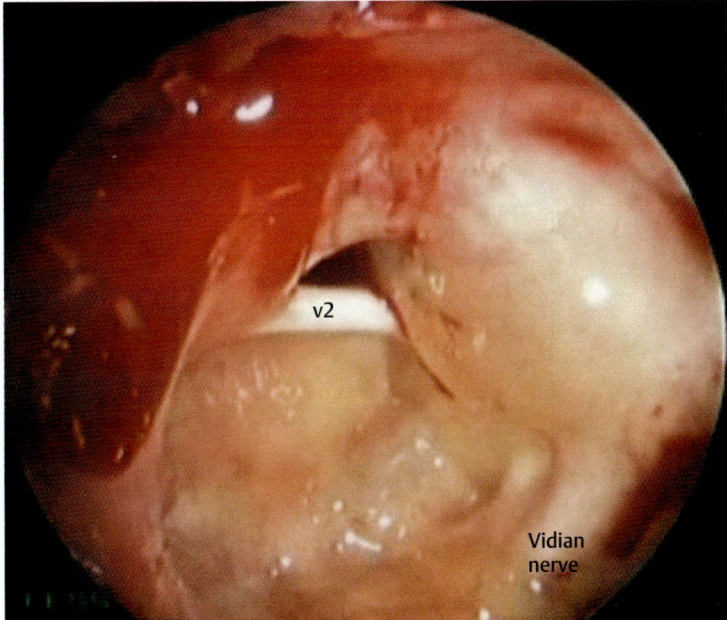

v2

Vidian nerve

Fig. 2.6 Intra-operative image showing lateral recess in a hyper-pneumatised, right sphenoid sinus showing maxillary division of trigeminal nerve (v2) superolaterally (dehiscent in this case), and vidian nerve on the floor of the sphenoid.

After the **internal carotid artery** exits the foramen lacerum in its subpetrous part, it climbs along the mid part of the clivus to become the paraclival carotid. The paraclival carotid runs superiorly to become the cavernous carotid beside the sella. It turns and runs in a horizontal plane and then turns anteriorly and superiorly to loop back on itself. The cavernous carotids form a prominence on either side of the sella. Superiorly above the cavernous carotid portion where it loops back posteriorly, it forms the paraclinoid carotid. The paraclinoid carotid is the portion of the carotid between the proximal and the distal dural rings. It is the most prominent portion and often dehiscent (**Fig. 2.7**). Above the paraclinoid, carotid prominence runs the optic nerve prominence. The depression between the carotid and the optic nerve is called the lateral OCR and is formed by the pneumatisation of the optic strut (**Fig. 2.8**). The pneumatisation of the middle clinoid process forms the medial OCR. This represents the area near the lateral tubercular strut where the ICA and the optic nerve are at their closest.

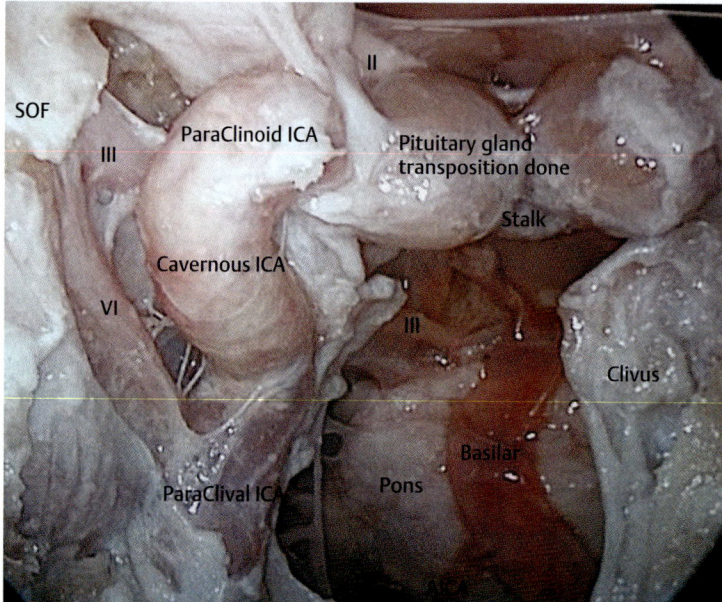

Fig. 2.7 Cadaveric image showing sphenoid portion of the ICA on the right side. The pituitary gland is seen surrounded by important neurovascular structures. II, optic nerve; III, oculomotor nerve; VI, abducens nerve; SOF, superior orbital fissure; AICA, anteroinferior cerebellar artery; ICA, internal carotid artery

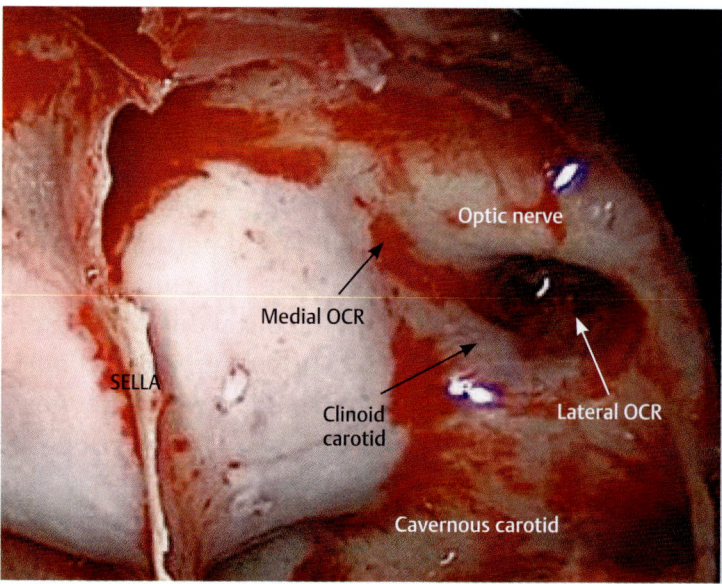

Fig. 2.8 Intra-operative image showing left lateral optic-carotid recess (OCR) and medial OCR. The bone separating the paraclinoid carotid and the optic nerve is the optic strut.

Keeping the sella in the centre and considering the sphenoid as a dial of a clock, the following structures are noted. At 12 o'clock is the tuberculum sellae. At 1 and 11 o'clock positions are the optic nerves. At 2 and 10 o'clock positions are the left and right paraclinoid carotids, respectively. From 2 to 4 o'clock position on the left and from 10 to 8 o'clock position on the right are the cavernous carotids. At 5 and 7 o'clock positions are the left and right paraclival carotids, respectively. At 6 o'clock position lies the clivus (**Fig. 2.9**).

On the floor of a well pneumatised sphenoid, one can also delineate the prominence of vidian nerve medially (**Fig. 2.6**). In case of a non-pneumatised sphenoid, one can identify it at the junction of medial pterygoid and the floor of the sphenoid. Identification of the vidian nerve occasionally requires the opening of the pterygopalatine fossa. It is an important marker because when it is followed posteriorly, it leads towards the junction between the subpetrous portion and the paraclival portion of the carotids. It is mostly useful in cases where the pathology fills the sphenoid, or surrounds the carotid or even in cases with a non-pneumatised sphenoid.

Superolaterally to the vidian nerve lies the prominence of the maxillary division of the trigeminal (V2) nerve (**Fig. 2.6**). V2 nerve is often encountered in cases which require transpterygoid approaches and may be damaged in such cases. When traced behind, it leads to clival part of the ICA.

Rostrum of sphenoid defines the midline. It is removed to open the anterior face of sphenoid (**Fig. 2.10**).

Keel of the sphenoid is another structure which defines the midline and helps us keep our orientation intact intra-operatively (**Fig. 2.11**). It is formed by the vomer alae and so called because it is shaped like a keel of a boat. Even after removing the rostrum, the keel is maintained in order to keep track of the landmarks, unless one is going transclival. In cases where there is lot of nasal pathology, and other nasal landmarks are lost, the keel acts as a guide. It also helps the otolaryngologist orient the endoscope in the centre, keeping the keel at 6'o clock position. However, the keel needs to be drilled down or flattened completely so that the nasoseptal flap (for reconstruction) can sit properly over it, or when pathology extends to the floor of the sphenoid.

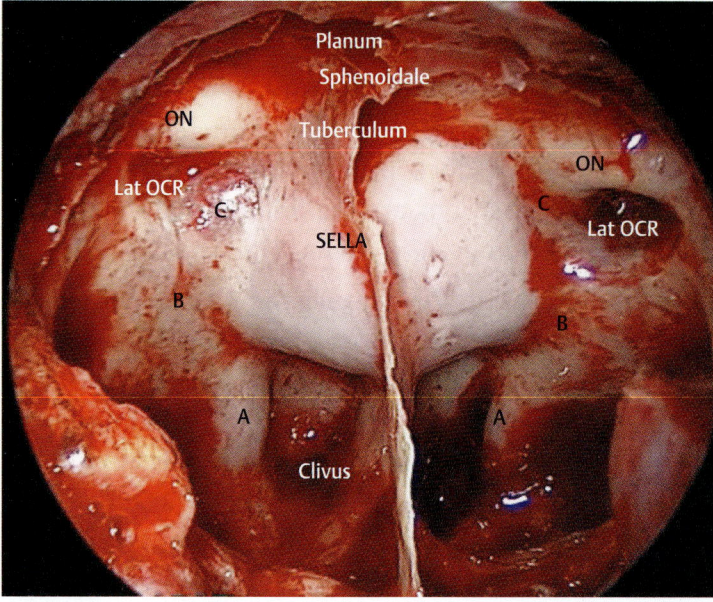

Fig. 2.9 Intra-operative image showing the important landmarks around the sella, keeping the sella in the centre as a dial of a clock. A, paraclival carotid; B, cavernous carotid; C, paraclinoid carotid; OCR, optic-carotid recess; ON, optic nerve.

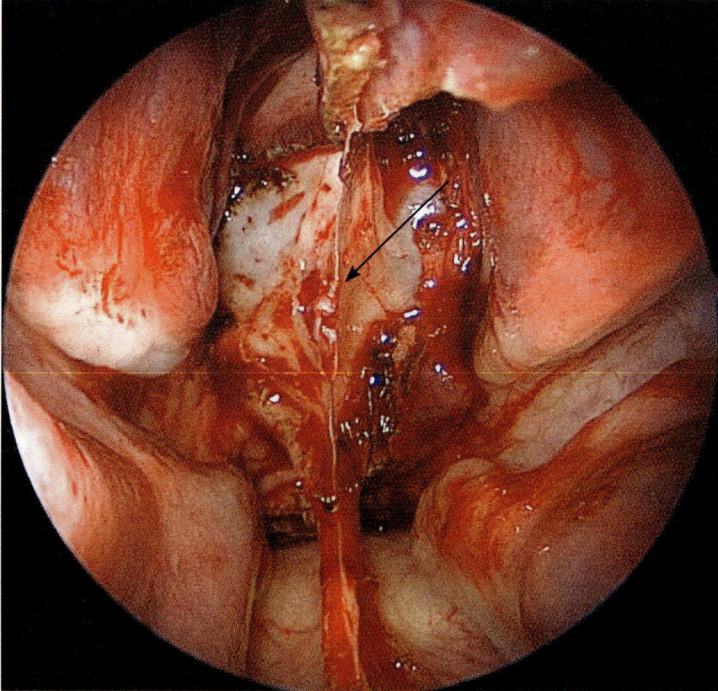

Fig. 2.10 Intra-operative binostril image of the sphenoid rostrum seen after posterior septectomy. The rostrum of the sphenoid (*thin black arrow*) defines the midline. It keeps the endoscopic orientation intact.

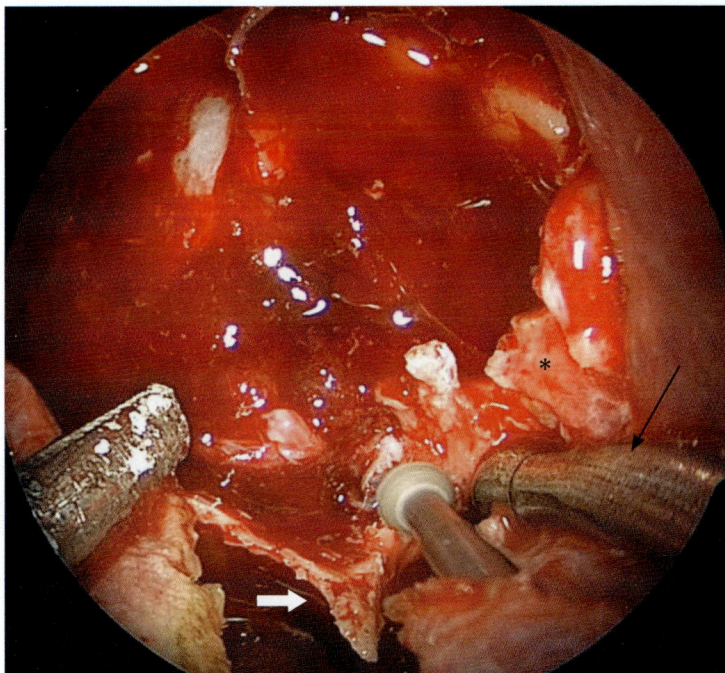

Fig. 2. 11 The keel of the sphenoid seen (*white block arrow*) after opening anterior wall of the sphenoid sinus (*). The curved suction cannula (*thin black arrow*) (See **Fig. 10.17** in chapter 10), held by the ENT surgeon, helps in irrigation while also affording to retract the rescue flaps (described in detail in chapter 5).

Intersphenoid septum, as the name suggests, divides the septum into right and left sphenoid. More often than not, this intersphenoid septum ends on important structures like the carotid or the optic nerve (**Fig. 2.1b**). It is important to know the position of this septum beforehand, from the scan, because it needs to be drilled down or flattened for complete exposure of the sphenoid.

Onodi cell is a posterior ethmoidal cell which pneumatises posterior, lateral, and superior to the sphenoid sinus (**Fig. 2.12**). It can pneumatise posteriorly up to the posterior clinoids. This sphenoethmoidal cell is intimately related to the optic nerve. Sometimes, the ICA bulge can be seen prominently in its posterior wall. Onodi cell has to be identified pre-operatively on the CT scans in order to avoid damage to these vital structures intra-operatively and also for complete exposure of the sella, and its landmarks.

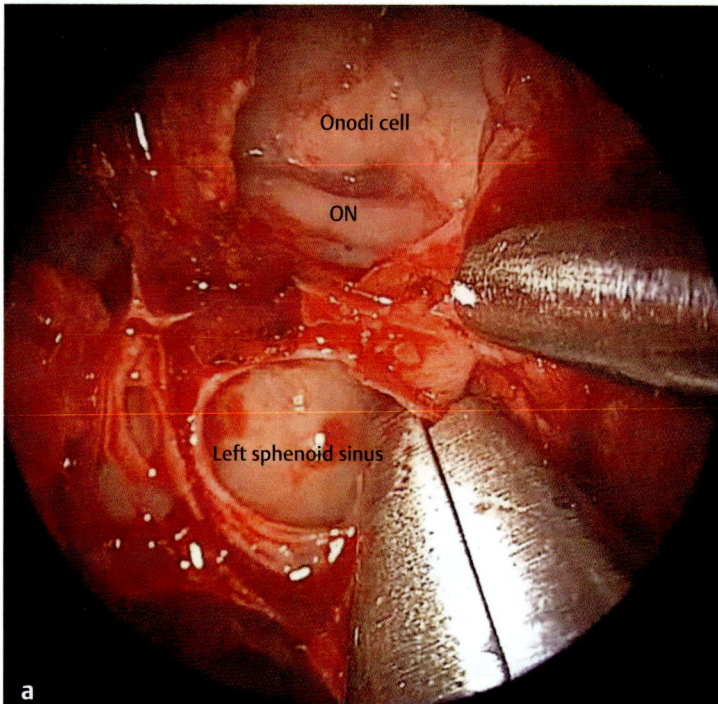

Onodi cell

ON

Left sphenoid sinus

a

Fig. 2.12 **(a)** Intraoperative image showing Onodi cell on the left side, posterosuperior to the sphenoid, indicated by a straight suction (See **Fig. 10.12** in chapter 10). The Kerrison's punch (See **Fig. 10.13** in chapter 10) is seen to punch out the anterior wall of the left sphenoid sinus. Left optic nerve bulge is seen on the wall of the Onodi cell. ON, optic nerve. **(b)** Coronal CT bone window of the patient in **Fig. 2.11a**. The left Onodi cell is indicated by single *white arrow*.

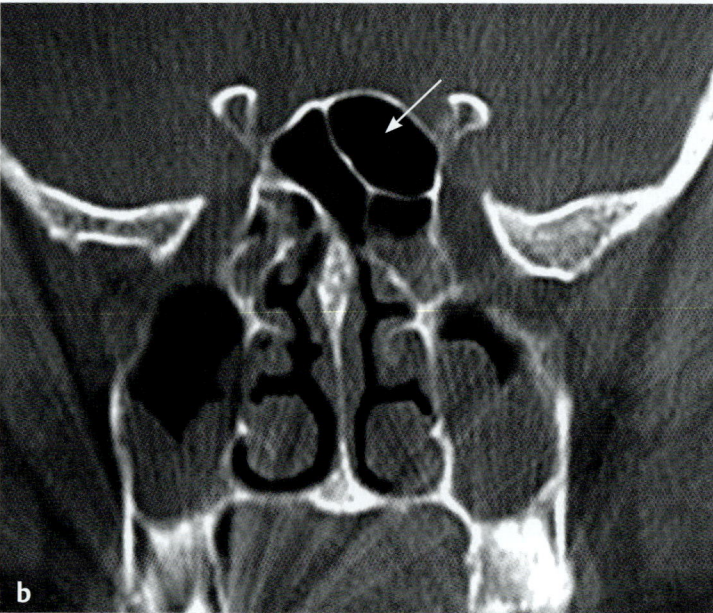

b

Clivus

The clivus separates the nasopharynx from the posterior cranial fossa. It is formed by the basi-sphenoid and the basi-occiput. It is further divided into upper, middle, and lower clivus. The upper clivus is formed by the basi-sphenoid limited by the dorsum sellae anteriorly and the floor of the sella posteriorly. The middle clivus is formed by the rostral part of the basi-occiput, forming part of the posterior wall of the sphenoid sinus. The inferior limit of the middle clivus roughly corresponds to the floor of the sphenoid (**Fig. 2.13**). The lower clivus is formed by caudal part of the basi-occiput superiorly and the foramen magnum inferiorly (**Fig. 2.13**).

The upper two-thirds of the clivus faces the pons intracranially, whereas the lower clivus faces the medulla. The basilar venous plexus lies between the periosteal layer and the inner meningeal layer of the dura, opposite the middle

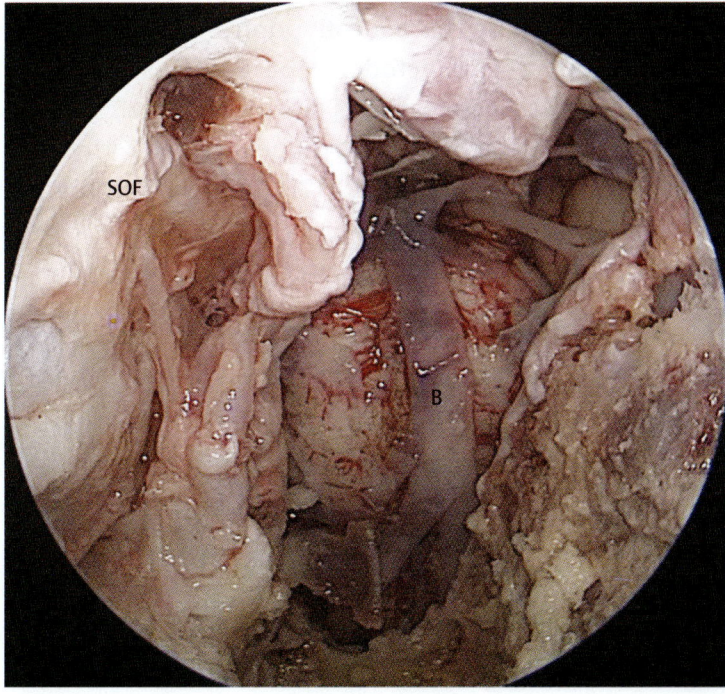

Fig. 2.13 Cadaveric view, after drilling of the entire clivus. The basilar artery (**B**) is seen posteriorly. SOF, superior orbital fissure.

and the lower clivus. This venous plexus bleeds continuously with clival drilling and needs to be controlled by continuous irrigation and by application of bone wax.

In order to approach the posterior cranial fossa through the upper and middle clivus, one needs to go trans-sphenoid. Lower clival drilling would require one to go below the sphenoid sinus, either transnasally or transorally.[4]

Pituitary Gland

The pituitary gland, located in the sella turcica is surrounded by a variety of important neurovascular structures, including the optic nerve, optic chiasm, and the anterior circulation superiorly; the cavernous sinuses, the internal carotid arteries, and multiple cranial nerves laterally; the brainstem and the posterior circulation posteriorly (**Figs. 2.7, 2.14**).

The pituitary gland is composed of a larger anterior lobe or the adeno-hypophysis and a smaller posterior lobe or the neurohypophysis. The anterior lobe develops from an invagination of oral ectoderm or Rathke's pouch. It is responsible for production and release of various hormones, viz., growth hormone (GH), prolactin, adrenocorticotrophic hormone (ACTH), thyroid-stimulating hormone (TSH), leuteinising hormone (LH), follicle-stimulating hormone (FSH).

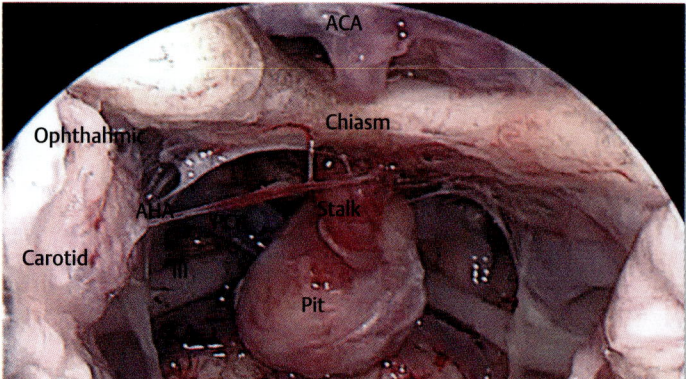

Fig. 2.14 Cadaveric view of the pituitary gland (Pit) with surrounding neurovascular structures. ACA, anterior cerebral artery; PCA, posterior cerebral artery; AHA, anterior hypophyseal artery; SCA, superior cerebellar artery.

The posterior lobe is a direct extension of the neural ectoderm from the floor of the third ventricle. It is more vascular than the anterior lobe. It is the posterior lobe which picks up contrast and appears in a post-contrast magnetic resonance (MR) study. It is not a glandular structure like the anterior lobe and it stores and releases oxytocin and vasopressin.

Most of the pituitary gland is covered by two layers of dura: the outer periosteal layer and the inner meningeal layer. These two layers split laterally to form part of the cavernous sinuses. Between these two dural layers run the superior and the inferior intercavernous sinuses.

The cavernous sinuses are located on the lateral aspects of the sphenoid sinus, sella, and pituitary gland. They extend from the superior orbital fissure anteriorly to the petrous apex posteriorly. The medial cavernous sinus walls abut the lateral walls of the pituitary gland, usually separated by a single layer of dura (**Fig. 2.15**). The internal carotid artery is the most medial structure in the cavernous sinus. A number of venous channels called intercavernous sinuses

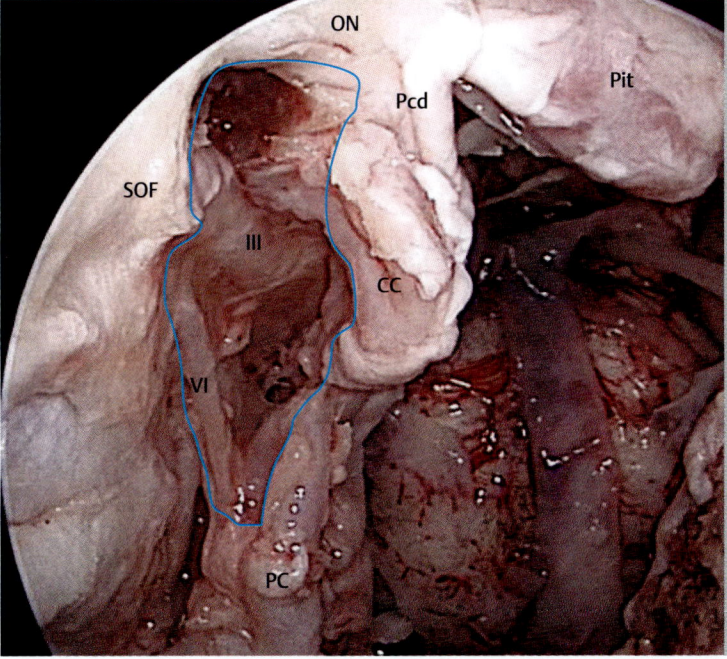

Fig. 2.15 Right cavernous sinus (*outlined in blue*) in a cadaver. ON, optic nerve; SOF, superior orbital fissure; Pc, paraclival carotid; CC, cavernous carotid; Pcd, paraclinoid carotid; Pit, pituitary gland transpositioned; III, oculomotor nerve; VI, abducens nerve.

connect the bilateral cavernous sinuses. These sinuses are located anterior, posterior, and inferior to the pituitary gland.[1] Each cavernous sinus is a venous lake which communicates with multiple venous tributaries and spaces such as, basilar plexus, superior and inferior petrosal sinuses, superior and inferior ophthalmic veins, veins of foramen rotundum, ovale and spinosum, foramen of Vesalius, deep middle cerebral vein, superficial sylvian vein, and contralateral cavernous sinus via the intercavernous sinuses.

The carotid artery divides the cavernous sinus into multiple venous compartments, such as the superior, inferior, lateral, and posterior compartments. These compartments can be selectively occupied by pituitary adenomas.[5] The superior compartment is formed between the paraclinoid part of the carotid and the roof of the cavernous sinus. The inferior part of the oculomotor nerve sits in the posterolateral aspect of this compartment. The inferior compartment is formed below the horizontal part of the cavernous carotid and the paraclival carotid. The venous gulf is formed in this area which is formed by the confluence of the cavernous sinus, the petrosal sinus, and the basilar sinus. The abducens nerve and the sympathetic plexus lie in this compartment. Overzealous packing in this venous gulf can result in post-operative abducens nerve palsy. The posterior compartment lies behind the junction between the paraclival and the cavernous carotid. The abducens nerve enters from the inferior aspect of this compartment. Finally, the lateral compartment lies lateral to the cavernous carotid. All the cranial nerves lie in this compartment and travel towards the superior orbital fissure.[5]

The suprasellar space extends from the diaphragma sellae inferiorly to the floor of the third ventricle superiorly. It can be accessed by drilling the tuberculum sella, and the planum sphenoidale. The anterior wall is formed by the tuberculum, anterior optic chiasm, lamina terminalis, anterior cerebral arteries, and their communicating branches. The lateral walls are composed of the internal carotid arteries, optic tracts, anterior choroidal vessels, and posterior cerebral arteries. The posterior wall consists of the posterior perforated substance and the cerebral peduncles. The optic nerves traverse through the suprasellar space[6] (**Fig. 2.16**).

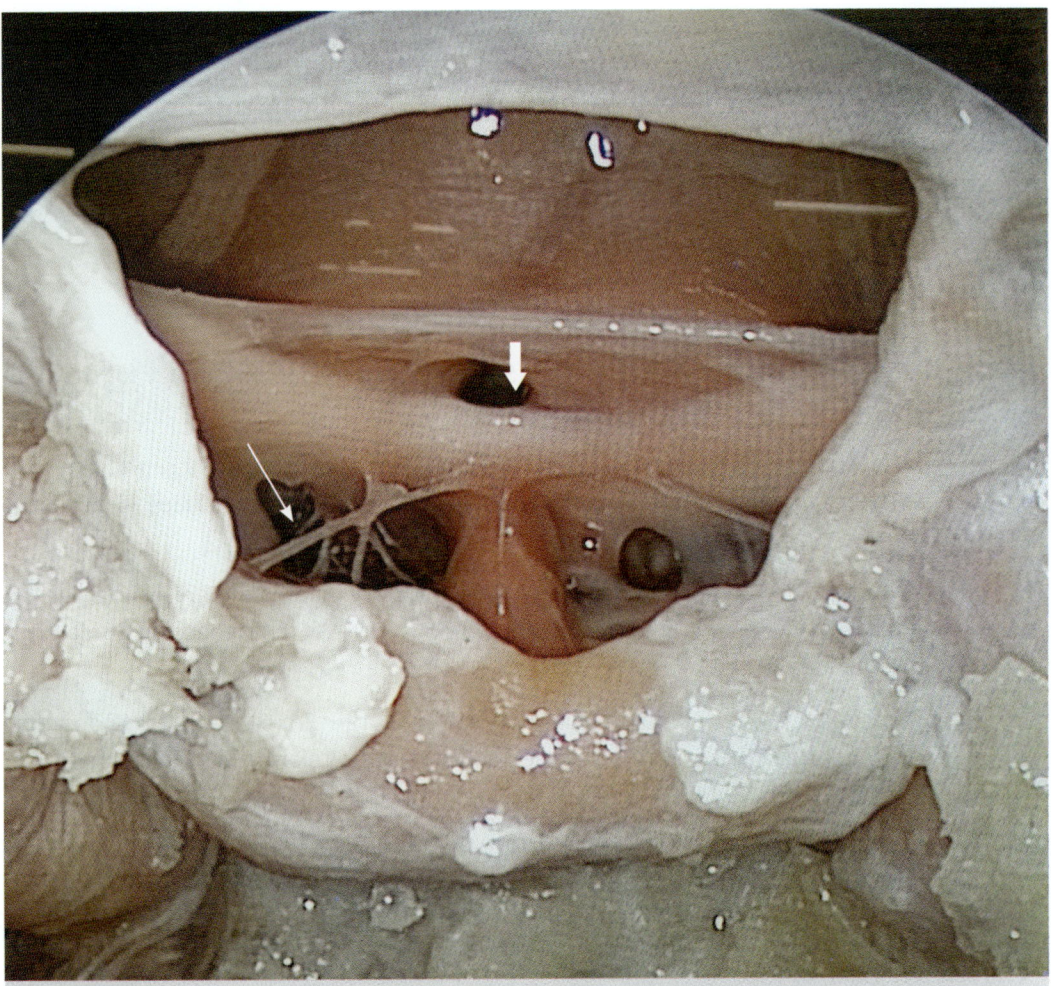

Fig. 2.16 Cadaveric image showing suprasellar space. The optic chiasm (*thick white arrow*) is seen dividing the space into suprachiasmatic and infrachiasmatic space. Hypophyseal artery (*single white arrow*) is seen supplying the stalk and the chiasm.

The optic chiasm is located at the junction of the anterior wall and floor of the third ventricle. The optic chiasm divides the suprasellar space into suprachiasmatic, infrachiasmatic, and retrochiasmatic spaces. Structures situated superior to the optic chiasm are the anterior cerebral and anterior communicating arteries, lamina terminalis, and third ventricle. Inferior to the optic chiasm lie diaphragma sellae and pituitary gland, laterally lie the internal carotid arteries and posteriorly lies the infundibulum. The infundibular recess lies at the base of pituitary stalk behind the chiasm.[5]

References

1. Singh A, Wessell A, Anand VK, Schwartz T. Surgical anatomy and physiology for the skull base surgeon. Otolaryngology 2011;22:184–193

2. Fernandez-Miranda JC, Prevedello DM, Madhok R, et al. Sphenoid septations and their relationship with internal carotid arteries: anatomical and radiological study. Laryngoscope 2009;119(10):1893–1896

3. Singh A, Roth J, Anand VK, et al. Anatomy of the pituitary gland and parasellar areas. In: Schwartz TH, Anand VK, eds. Endoscopic Pituitary Surgery—A Comprehensive Guide. New York, NY: Thieme; 2011

4. Mangussi-Gomes J, Beer-Furlan A, Balsalobre L, Vellutini EA, Stamm AC. Endoscopic Endonasal management of skull base chordomas. Otolaryngol Clin North Am 2016;49(1):167–182

5. Patel CR, Fernandez-Miranda JC, Wang WH, Wang EW. Skull base anatomy. Otolaryngol Clin North Am 2016;49(1):9–20

6. Perneczky A, Tschabitscher M, Resch KDM. Endoscopic Anatomy for Neurosurgery. New York, NY: Thieme; 1993

Pre-operative Assessment for Surgery

C. E. Deopujari and Sai Spoorthi Nayak

Signs and Symptoms

Presenting History of the Patient

The patient may present with any one or a combination of the following major symptoms:

- Headache.
- Visual symptoms.
- Hormonal dysfunction.
- Rare presentations viz. infection/meningitis, fatigue, electrolyte disturbances, and seizures.

Headache

Often the patient complains of mild headaches, usually retro-orbital and of a stretching kind. Onset of headache may be insidious and gradually progressing due to the slow growth of the tumour in the suprasellar direction and causing tenting of the diaphragm. It is the most common and important symptom in early stages. Sometimes it may be the only symptom. If the tumour is unde-tected and continues to grow, the diaphragm may occasionally give way and the headache may stop, as now the stretch on the diaphragm is relieved. This is a latent period wherein the patient may be asymptomatic and may actually start ignoring his or her symptoms, or delay his or her visit to the doctor.

The tumour, obviously undetected at this stage, may continue to grow and ultimately result in raised intracranial tension. This is when the patient again presents with headache. However, now the headache is of a different character and becomes more of a throbbing kind. It may be associated with other signs of raised intracranial tension like projectile vomiting, blurring of vision, etc.

Acute severe headache with onset of new neurological signs is a hallmark of pituitary apoplexy and may occur with bleeding or necrosis within the tumour.

Visual Symptoms

Usually, the onset of visual symptoms is gradual. Patients may have visual field defects, deterioration in visual acuity in one or both eyes or double vision (diplopia).

Visual field cut is the first to occur due to tenting of the optic chiasm. The progress is so insidious that the patient sometimes may be unaware of peripheral field defects. Perimetry, if performed at this stage will typically show a superior quadrantic defect either in one or both temporal fields. Multiple visits to ophthalmic clinics may make the patient go for new prescription glasses, steroid injections, and even cataract surgery. Depending on the size, location, and type of lesion, visual disturbances will vary in patients. Pituitary and suprasellar lesions will cause field defects and gradual vision loss, mostly bitemporal hemianopia. In other tumours, such as craniopharyngiomas, the field defect may be asymmetrical.

Visual acuity is not commonly affected except in tumours which infiltrate into the nerve sheath, for example, in meningiomas. Asymmetrical or large pituitary tumours may cause severe vision loss. In neglected cases or apoplexy, we still see an occasional patient with unilateral/bilateral blindness.

Cavernous sinus lesions will cause diplopia by affecting eye movement most commonly due to sixth nerve paresis. Malignancies and invasive pathologies will involve cranial nerves and vessels earlier. When the lesion extends lateral to the cavernous sinus, the patient may present with varying degrees of ophthalmoplegia and diplopia due to the involvement of cranial nerves III, IV, and VI.

In tumours like chordoma, complains of diplopia are more common than visual loss.

In suprasellar tumours, the patient can sometimes present with nystagmus specially in children with a characteristic seesaw movement typical of optic chiasmal glioma. The postulated reasons are that a suprasellar lesion either compresses or invades the meso-diencephalic region, or visual deprivation in the presence of bitemporal hemianopia.[1]

Hormonal Dysfunction

Pituitary hyperfunction is easy to diagnose to an accustomed eye. Common amongst secretory tumours are prolactinomas, adrenocorticotropic hormone (ACTH) (Cushing's disease), and growth hormone (GH)-secreting (acromegaly/gigantism) tumours.

Prolactinomas are the most common hypersecreting pituitary tumours and are easily diagnosed in females as they present with primary amenorrhoea and/or lactation without pregnancy. Patients may present with infertility to the obstetric clinics (secondary amenorrhoea) and may be advised fertilisation procedures and medical treatment. Prolactinomas are, however, difficult to diagnose in males. This is because they usually have lack of libido, loss of facial hair and chest hair which many people fail to notice or may not wish to disclose.

Cushing's disease in children as well as adult patients present with increased body mass, hyperpigmentation, hirsutism, and moon face. Pituitary versus adrenal Cushing's may be difficult to diagnose and may need the expertise of an endocrinologist.

Adult patients with GH-secreting tumours present with acromegaly, enlargement of the palms and toes, coarse facial features, and enlargement of the tongue and nose. GH-secreting tumours in children will present with gigantism.

Pituitary hypofunction: In large tumours, the normal pituitary gland is compressed which may result in hypofunction. Since the growth of the tumour is insidious, the patient may present with vague non-specific clinical symptoms, like weight loss, fatigue, etc. In fact, many of these patients may not even be diagnosed with hypopituitarism unless properly investigated. Children suffering from GH deficiency may show features of stunting or lack of growth. Hormonal deficiency amounts to loss of target organ function.

Rare Presentation

1. **Meningitis**: Meningitis usually does not occur unless there is a cerebrospinal fluid (CSF) fistula or history of an earlier surgery. Malignancy eroding the skull base and dura can cause CSF leaks. Occasionally patients, post radiation or with sudden tumour shrinkage, as in medically treated prolactinomas, have presented with CSF leaks. Such patients carry the potential risk of meningitis.

2. **Fatigue**: Many patients with hyponatremia, hypocortisolemia may present with insidious onset of fatigue as the main symptom. This may also be seen in patients with hypothyroidism. There may also be growth hormone deficiency which can accentuate the symptoms.

3. **Electrolyte disturbances:** Hyponatremia may be the first presentation with pituitary tumour while diabetes insipidus may be the first presentation in germinomas/craniopharyngiomas.

4. **Seizures:** Seizures may occasionally happen from suprasellar extension of the tumour in subfrontal/subtemporal direction. They can also be due to hypo-/hypernatremia even without suprasellar extension.

Onset—Progress

Duration of the symptoms will depend on the severity and the patient's outlook to surgery. Insidious vision loss or headaches may be well tolerated and ignored for a long time. An apoplexy, however, will usually result in a quick diagnosis. Non-functional pituitary tumours which form the bulk of skull base lesions, are slow growing, and these do not require urgent surgery in most cases, so the patient may choose the time for intervention. Similar is the situation for meningiomas. Secretory adenomas on the other hand as well as most other lesions such as craniopharyngiomas, chordomas do need early intervention. Prolactinomas are usually amenable to medical therapy and require surgery only if medical therapy fails or in special circumstances such as intratumoural bleeds or cases with neurovascular involvement.

Examination

A general examination must be done to assess all systems and vital parameters. Systemic examination will include looking for signs of acromegaly or Cushing's as previously described. Hypertension is one of the hallmarks of a patient with Cushing's and acromegaly and needs to be controlled reasonably.

A complete neurological examination should include a detailed check of all cranial nerves. Assessment of eye movements, vision, perimetry, and fundoscopy are required. It is important to check the nasal cavity as well. An endoscopy will provide information on the septum, turbinates or presence of any infection. This allows for surgical planning as well as pre-operative antibiotic cover.

Pre-Operative Assessment of the Patient

Radiology

MR Scan

Magnetic resonance (MR) scanning is the gold standard for intracranial pathology and a good-quality scan is a prerequisite in all cases. When required, a contrast or an MR angiography study is added to the basic scan. Radiologists have several imaging options in MR to differentiate the pathology and arrive at a more accurate diagnosis, enabling a comprehensive discussion with the management team.

MR also allows excellent differentiation of lesion from normal tissue, being able to assess invasion or involvement of dura and orbit, separate tumour from sinusitis and cystic from solid lesions. In addition, we can study the relation of blood vessels to tumour, whether there is encasement or infiltration or mere pushing of the blood vessels, and thus, the inherent risks of surgery. We may be able to guess whether a tumour is likely to be soft and suckable, or firm and difficult to remove, from an MR study—though these interpretations may not be always correct.

CT scan

A computed tomography (CT) scan is a must in endonasal skull base surgery as it defines the route of access. A plain CT paranasal sinus study is enough; however, it is required in all three planes, viz. axial, coronal, and sagittal for proper planning. Areas of interest include deviations of the septum, concha bullosa, pneumatisation of sinuses (especially sphenoid), presence of inflammation, relation of posterior ethmoid cells to the sphenoid and optic nerve. Presence of deviated nasal septum or sharp spurs influences the side on which the Hadad flap is to be taken. Other areas of concern are the intersphenoid septum, which may deviate towards the internal carotid artery (ICA) or optic canal of one side, slope of the skull base and planum, areas of erosion if any, size of sella, etc.

In revision cases, one looks at the posterior septum for a prior septectomy, amputation of turbinates, synechiae, sella bone defects and sphenoid anterior wall relation to the sphenopalatine foramen to assess potential for a Hadad flap.

It is advisable to do a diagnostic nasal endoscopic examination in revision cases, to look for any synechiae or septal perforations that might be missed on the CT scan.

Details of imaging can be found in a separate chapter (see chapter 4).

Laboratory Investigations

Hormonal Assessment

Serum prolactin, cortisol and thyroid levels (**Table 3.1**) should be checked in all patients.

For prolactinomas, the prolactin levels less than 100 ng/mL are considered a manifestation of 'stalk effect'. Levels between 100 and 200 ng/mL are considered

Table 3.1 Featuring the normal hormonal values according to NABL guidelines

Sr Prolactin	Normal men: 1.5 to 19 ng/ml Normal women: 1.3 to 25 ng/ml Menopausal women: 0.7 to 19 ng/ml Pregnant women: 10-50ng/ml
Sr FSH	1.5 to 12.4 mlU/mL
Sr LH	1.7 to 8.6 mlU/mL
Sr Testosterone	2.8 to 3 nmol/L
Sr cortisol	07:00 -09:00am: 4.3 to 22.4 mcg/dl 03:00 -05:00pm: 3.09 to 16.66 mcg/dl
Free T3	1.4 to 3.48 pg/ml
Free T4	0.71 to 1.85 ng/dl
Free TSH	0.49 to 4.67 ulU/ml
Sr GH	<5ng/ml
Sr iGF	180 to 200 ng/ml

Abbreviations: FSH, follicular stimulating hormone; LH, leutinising hormone; TSH, thyroid stimulating hormone; GH, growth hormone; iGF: insulin like growth factor.

borderline. Levels greater than 200 ng/mL are pathognomonic of prolactinoma. Cabergoline (0.5 mg twice a week) is the first-line drug of choice for prolactinoma and has obviated the need for surgery to less than 15 to 20% cases.

Serum cortisol levels are checked diurnally, that is 8 am and 4 pm. Values differ according to age, sex, and laboratory calibration. Low cortisol levels need to be supplemented with hydrocortisone pre-operatively and is tapered rapidly in the immediate post-operative period. Long-term steroid replacement decision is based on repeat hormonal profile done at least 48 to 72 hours after stopping the last supplemental dose. Response of cortisol to oral glucose tolerance test is a good screening tool for differentiating Cushing's syndrome from pseudo-Cushing's state. Methods of differentiating between pituitary, that is Cushing's disease, and ectopic source of raised ACTH include magnetic resonance imaging (MRI) brain, corticotropin-releasing hormone (CRH) stimulation test, urinary cortisol levels, sonography of the abdomen, and high-dose dexamethasone suppression test, which is considered the primary non-invasive diagnostic test. Bilateral inferior petrosal sinus sampling should be performed when MRI brain yields equivocal results in the diagnosis of Cushing's disease.[2]

Growth hormone level greater than 10 ng/mL is a marker for secretory pituitary adenoma although raised levels are quite inconsistent in projecting the active status of the disease. Insulin-like growth factor 1(IGF-1) is a better marker for this purpose. Ideal surgical excision should result in fall of growth hormone to less than 2 ng/mL in the immediate post-operative period. IGF binding protein 3 (IGFBP-3) is a marker for malignancy.

Fundoscopy and Perimetry

Pre-operative visual field loss is assessed for each eye in each quadrant as well as the whole field. Both the eyes are compared for symmetry in visual field loss. The amount of field loss may be correlated to the degree of compression of the optic nerves and the chiasm. Pre-operative perimetry serves as a legal document showing the degree of field loss prior to the surgery. It can also serve as a tool to compare the post-operative recovery in the visual field.

Fundoscopy is done to assess the degree of optic nerve atrophy and also to detect the signs of early raised intracranial tension.

References

1. Moura FC, Gonçalves AC, Monteiro ML. Seesaw nystagmus caused by giant pituitary adenoma: case report. Arq Neuropsiquiatr 2006;64(1):139–141

2. Gross BA, Mindea SA, Pick AJ, Chandler JP, Batjer HH. Diagnostic approach to Cushing disease. Neurosurg Focus 2007;23(3):E1

04 | Radiological Investigations: A Prerequisite

Sonali Shah

Over the years endonasal endoscopic approaches for skull base lesions have rapidly developed and are being increasingly used. The endonasal procedures comprise of three basic components:

1. Creating a passage through the sinonasal cavities to reach the skull base.

2. Resection of the pathology which depends on the location, type, and extent of the lesion.

3. Reconstruction of the skull base to recreate the anatomical barrier between the nose and intracranial space to prevent cerebrospinal fluid (CSF) leak and its complications.

Pre-operative high-resolution imaging is essential in patients with skull base lesions to ensure adequate planning for the surgeries.

Magnetic resonance (MR) imaging is a gold standard modality for imaging of skull base and intracranial lesions. **Computed tomography (CT) imaging**, though thought of as a complementary tool, is an important adjunct to MR imaging as it helps in characterising the lesion by detection of calcium and depiction of type of bony involvement in the form of hyperostosis, permeative osteolytic erosion, and bone remodelling. CT imaging is indispensable for providing important information about normal anatomy and variants of the sinonasal cavity that has an impact on the surgical approach.

CT/MR angiography help in evaluating the major skull base and intracranial vessels, their relationship to the pathological lesions, and for detection of possible vascular abnormalities like an aneurysm.

A **dedicated sella protocol** is recommended[1,2] for optimal evaluation of central skull base lesions, which include the following:

- Thin-section T1 weighted, small field of view (FOV) coronal and sagittal images.

- Thin-section T2 weighted, small FOV, coronal images with fat saturation.

- Post-contrast thin section small FOV, T1 weighted coronal and sagittal images.

- Whole-brain fluid-attenuated inversion recovery (FLAIR), gradient, diffusion-weighted, and post-contrast images are acquired.

- Pre- and post-contrast thin-section axial images can be obtained but are not mandatory.

Dynamic contrast-enhanced MR in the coronal plane, using a power injector is a must when evaluating pituitary microadenomas and is routinely performed in some institutes for all sellar–suprasellar lesions.[3]

High-resolution 3D skull base MR imaging is suggested for pre-operative assessment of patients with skull base pathologies when the lesion is not clearly identified on conventional images, to define relationship to adjacent neurovascular structures, to evaluate segments of the cranial nerves, and for detection of subtle tumour extension. Blitz and colleagues[4] incorporate use of short tau inversion recovery (STIR), constructive interference in steady state (CISS), and pre- and post-contrast T1-weighted volumetric breath-hold examination (VIBE).

Multidetector CT imaging is used for volumetric acquisition of the skull base in axial plane with sub-millimetre slices, which is followed by reconstruction in all three planes with a slice thickness of up to 1 mm in soft and bone windows. Contrast should be used in all dedicated sella studies where MR has not been or cannot be performed.

Computer-guided neuro-navigation systems are useful for improving localisation in minimally invasive procedures. It can be done on the basis of CT or MRI images. Though MR images have higher spatial resolution, it provides lesser detailed information of the osseous structures, which are traditionally used as anatomic landmarks to guide for endoscopic surgery, hence CT neuro-navigation is preferred. During CT neuro-navigation, a series of contiguous 1.0-mm axial sections are acquired without a gantry tilt, from the symphysis menti to top of the head using a 512 × 512 pixel matrix. Contrast may or may not be given. This enables correlation of intra-operative registration with pre-operative CT images, giving a three-dimensional road map that provides position of surgical instruments in relation to the patient's anatomy. This correlation improves the surgeon's anatomical orientation, reduces complication, and improves efficacy[5] (**Fig. 4.1**).

Advanced neuro-navigation with CT angiography can be performed, which is especially useful in the trans-sphenoidal surgeries as critical vascular structures are seen at the skull base. The information for the neurosurgeon is further enhanced by the intra-operative screen display of three-dimensional reconstructions of the lesion, bones, and vessels.

Common Central Skull Base Lesions

Pituitary Adenomas

Pituitary adenomas are the commonest tumours of the sellar region, which are WHO grade 1 tumours with rare malignant transformation. These are classified according to the size as microadenoma (< 10 mm) and macroadenoma (> 10 mm) or as functioning and non-functioning tumours, the commonest functioning tumour being a prolactinoma.

The normal anterior lobe of the pituitary gland is isointense to grey matter on T1- and T2-weighted images, revealing moderate-to-intense homogenous

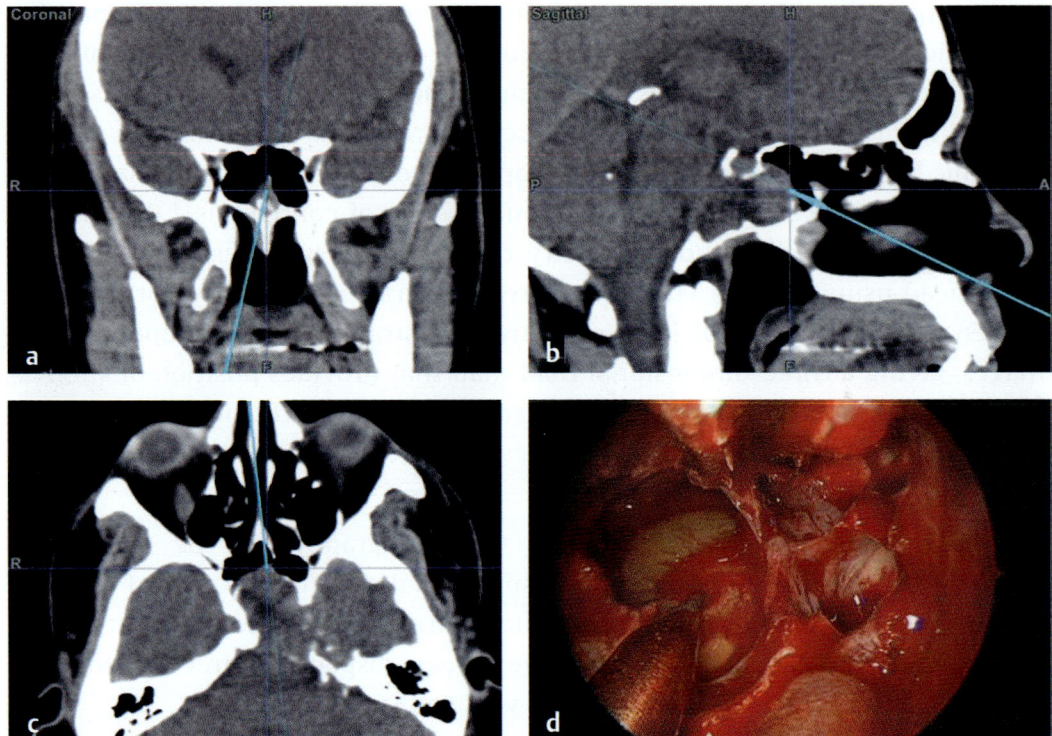

Fig. 4.1 **(a–d)** CT-guided surgical navigation system being used intra-operatively for a case of left petrous apex lesion. The navigation pointer (in *blue*) is pointing towards the lesion occupying the sphenoid sinus as seen in **a**, coronal; **b**, sagittal; **c**, axial planes, and **d**, endoscopically.

enhancement. On the dynamic images, the anterior lobe reveals progressive and rapid enhancement. The posterior pituitary appears hyperintense on T1-weighted and iso- to hypointense on T2-weighted images (**Fig. 4.2**).

The microadenomas may be incidentally detected on imaging or may present with endocrine dysfunction, commonly in young females with prolactinoma. On the plain study they may appear as a 3- to 4-mm-sized lesion with a more definitive diagnosis made during the dynamic post-contrast study, as the microadenomas reveal poor and delayed enhancement, and stand out amidst the avidly enhancing normal pituitary gland (**Figs. 4.3, 4.4**).

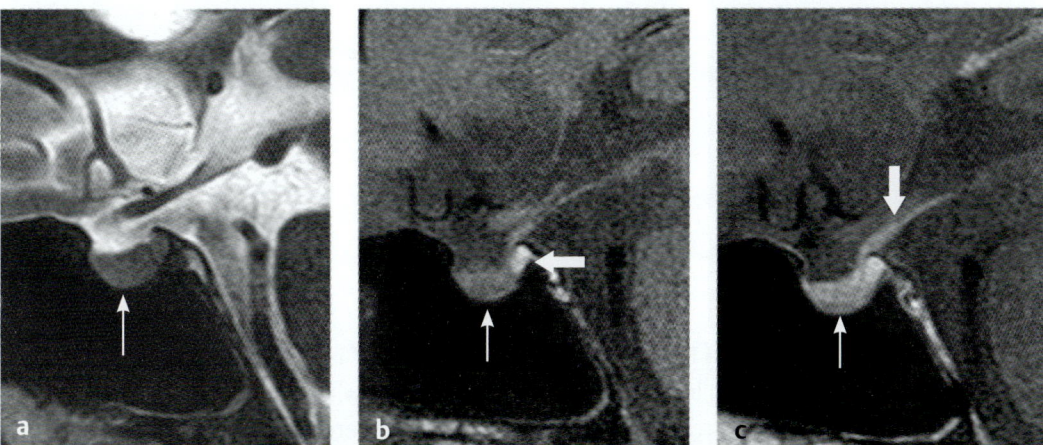

Fig. 4.2 Normal pituitary gland (*thin white arrow*). **(a)** T2-weighted sagittal. **(b)** Plain T1-weighted sagittal revealing hyperintense posterior pituitary gland (*short white arrow*). **(c)** Post-contrast T1-weighted MR images with the infundibulum (*white block arrow*).

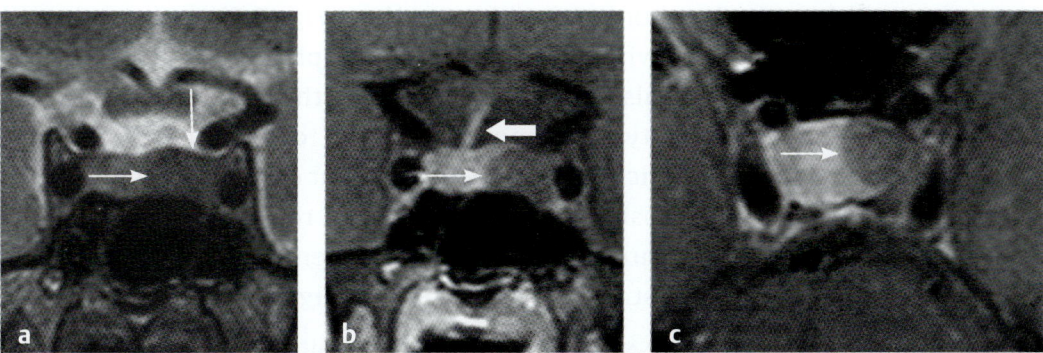

Fig. 4.3 **(a)** Coronal T2-weighted. **(b)** Coronal and **(c)** axial post-contrast T1-weighted MR images reveal a hypoenhancing pituitary microadenoma (*white thin arrows*) involving the left half, causing displacement of the stalk to the contralateral side (*short white block arrow*).

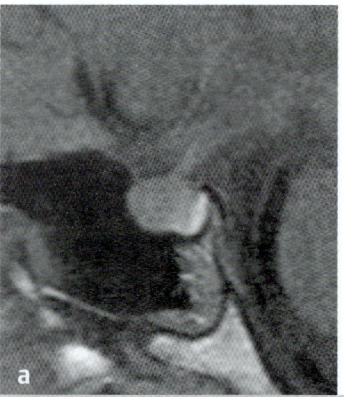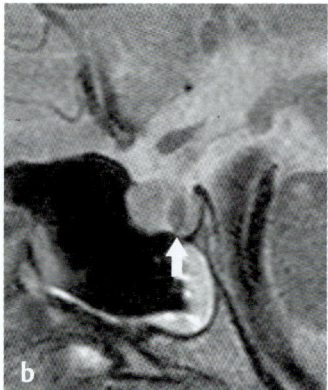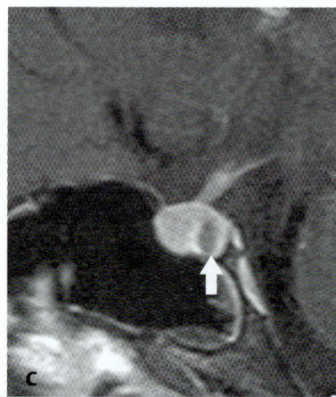

Fig. 4.4 (a) T1-weighted. **(b)** T2-weighted. **(c)** Post-contrast T1-weighted sagittal MR images reveal a small hypoenhancing lesion in the adenohypophysis with a blood-fluid level which is a microadenoma with haemorrhage (*white arrow*). A close differential is a Rathke cleft cyst.

The macroadenomas are larger lesions, commonly seen in the middle aged, presenting with headache, visual disturbance, or endocrine dysfunction. They are variable sized enhancing nodular sellar–suprasellar lesions (**Fig. 4.5**) appearing isointense to hypointense to the gland on T1-weighted images and isointense to brain cortex on T2-weighted images with heterogeneity seen often due to internal haemorrhage or cystic degeneration (**Fig. 4.6**). It expands and occasionally erodes the sella with extension into the sphenoid sinus (**Fig. 4.5**), while cranially it usually reveals suprasellar extension through the diaphragma sellae, occasionally giving a typical 'snowman/figure of 8' appearance with possible mass effect on the optic chiasm and A1 segment of the anterior cerebral artery (**Fig. 4.7**). Lateral extension into the parasellar region with or without encasement of the internal carotid artery and involvement of the cavernous sinus is often noted which must be analysed in detail (**Fig. 4.6**).

Pituitary apoplexy can be seen in an underlying pituitary macroadenoma, which is mostly haemorrhagic. Macroscopic haemorrhage is often detected on plain MRI study appearing hyperintense on T1-weighted images, deeply hypointense on T2 and gradient images with or without blood-fluid levels with post-contrast study revealing peripheral enhancement and large central areas of necrosis (**Fig. 4.8**).

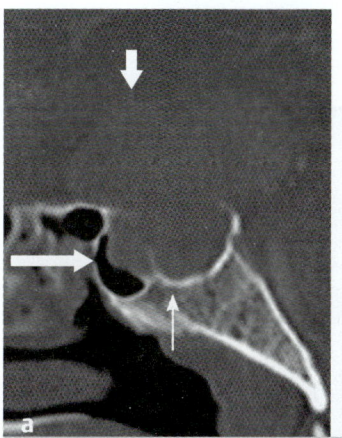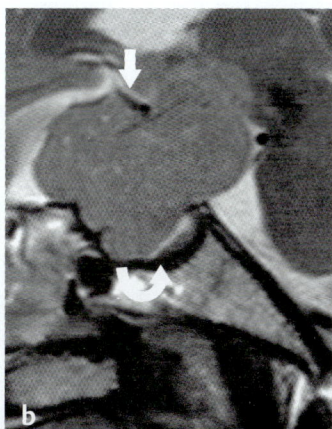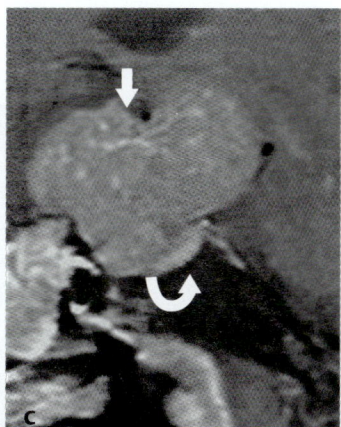

Fig. 4.5 **(a)** Sagittal CT bone window reveals a sellar–suprasellar mass (*short white block arrow*) causing expansion and erosion of the sella (*thin white arrow*) and extension into sphenoid sinus (*long white block arrow*). **(b)** T2-weighted sagittal and **(c)** post-contrast T1-weighted MR images reveal a large pituitary macroadenoma (*short white block arrow*) with normal pituitary gland seen compressed along sellar floor (*curved block arrow*) in **(b, c)**.

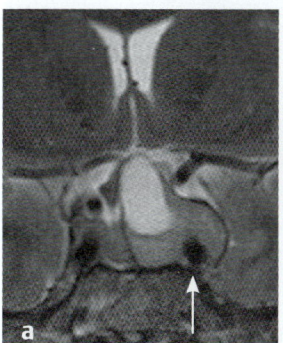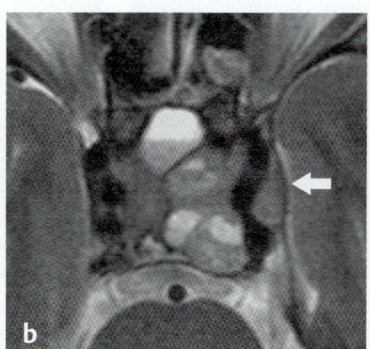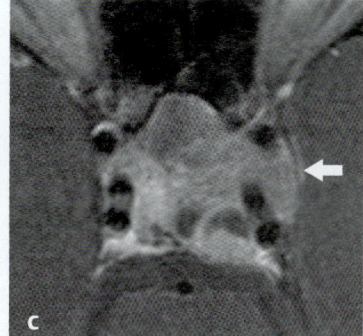

Fig. 4.6 **(a)** Coronal and **(b)** axial T2-weighted and **(c)** axial post-contrast T1-weighted MR images reveal a large macroadenoma with cystic degeneration. Left parasellar extension (*short white block arrow*) is seen which crosses the lateral intercarotid line and significantly encases the internal carotid artery (*thin white arrow*) with laterally bulging left cavernous sinus suggesting cavernous sinus invasion.

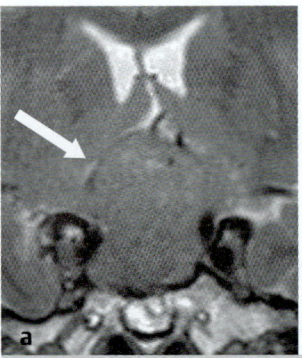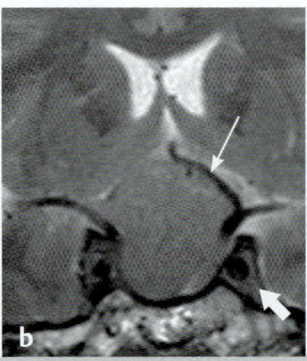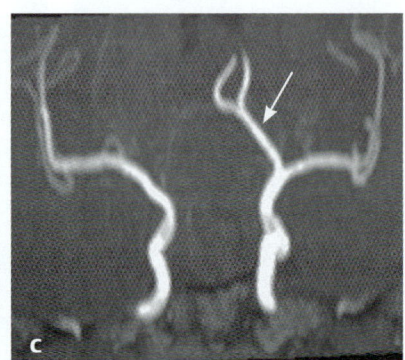

Fig. 4.7 **(a)** T2-weighted coronal MR images reveal a large pituitary macroadenoma causing superior displacement of right half optic chiasm (*long white block arrow*) **(b)** and of the A1 segment of the left anterior cerebral artery (*thin white arrow*). **(c)** MR angiography image reveals cranially displaced A1 segment with no luminal narrowing (*thin white arrow*).

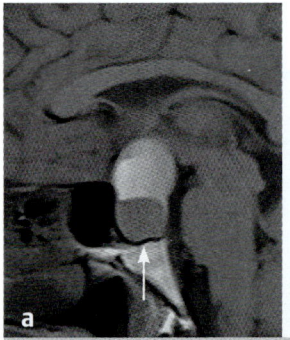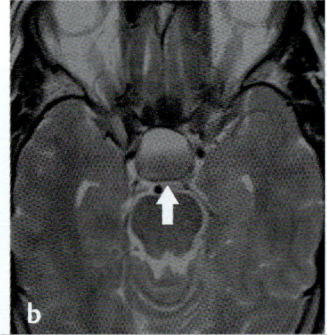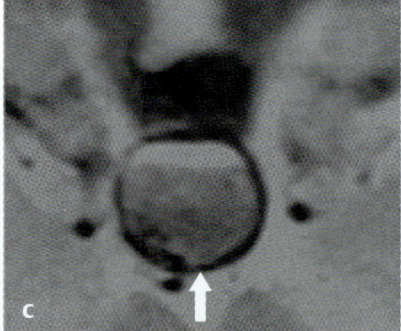

Fig. 4.8 **(a)** T1-weighted sagittal MR image reveals a sellar–suprasellar lesion (*white thin arrow*) with **(b)** T2 and **(c)** gradient axial images revealing a blood-fluid level (*white block arrow*), suggesting a pituitary macroadenoma with apoplexy.

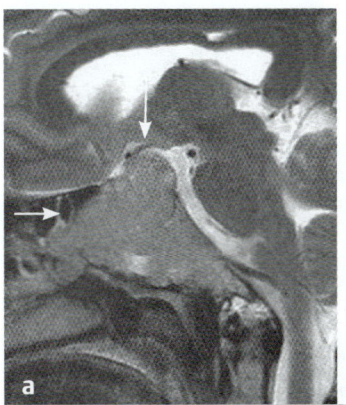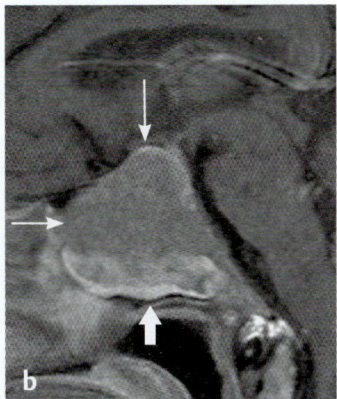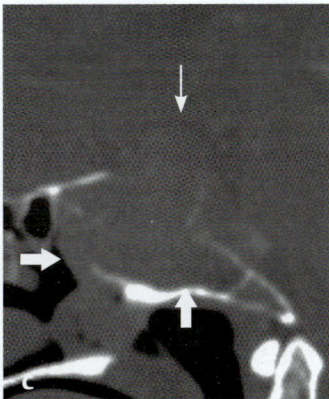

Fig. 4.9 **(a)** T2-weighted **(b)** T1-weighted MRI and **(c)** CT sagittal images reveal a sellar–suprasellar lesion (*white thin arrow*), eroding the sella and clivus and extending into the sphenoid sinus (*short white block arrow*), suggestive of an invasive pituitary macroadenoma.

Invasive pituitary macroadenomas with clival involvement is rare and often misdiagnosed as primary clival tumours or a meningioma. Clival invasion is seen more often with large tumour size and in null cell subtype, with associated higher rate of operative complications and recurrences (**Fig. 4.9**).

Meningioma

Meningiomas are the most common extra-axial intracranial tumours in adults, with 5 to 10% seen in the suprasellar and parasellar regions. These are named by their location, like planum sphenoidale, tuberculum sellae, and diaphragma sellae, parasellar or clival meningiomas (**Fig. 4.10**).

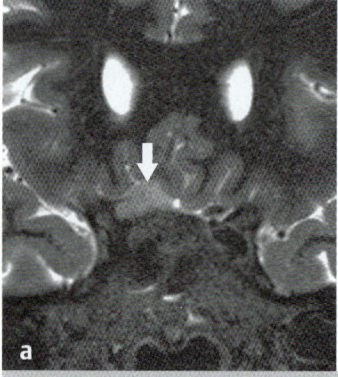
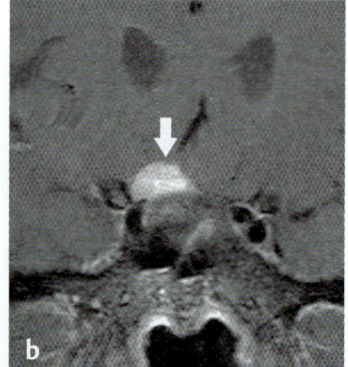
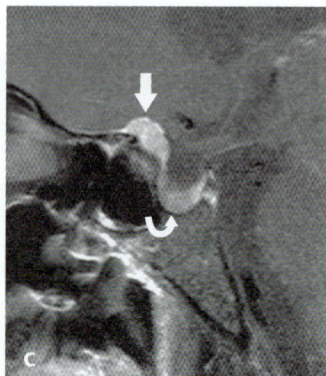

Fig. 4.10 **(a)** Coronal T2w **(b)** T1w and **(c)** post-contrast T1 weighted images reveal an intensely enhancing sulcus meningioma (*short block white arrow*) with minimal sellar extension but is seen separate from the normal pituitary gland (*curved white arrow*).

They appear hyperdense on plain CT images; nearly isointense to grey matter on T1- and T2-weighted images, revealing homogenous moderate-to-intense enhancement, with enhancing dural tails, restricted diffusion and calcification seen in many. Most planum meningiomas are seen superior to the sella, with the pituitary gland seen separately (**Fig. 4.10**). However, larger lesions extend into the sellar and parasellar regions mimicking a pituitary macroadenoma (**Fig. 4.11**). It is important to differentiate between the two, to decide the best surgical approach, with trans-sphenoidal approach used commonly for macroadenomas, while craniotomy may be preferred for a meningioma.[6]

The key to differentiate a meningioma from a pituitary macroadenoma is to look for a displaced and separate pituitary gland. Besides this, meningiomas are usually more homogenous, with associated bony hyperostosis/erosion and enhancing dural tails. They also tend to displace the internal carotid artery rather than encase it like a pituitary macroadenoma.

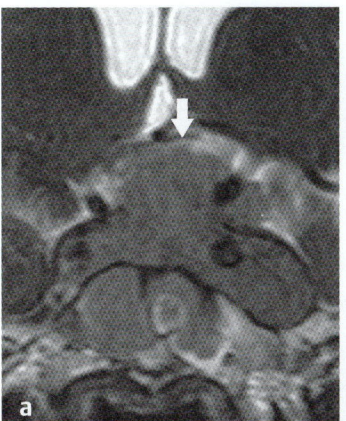 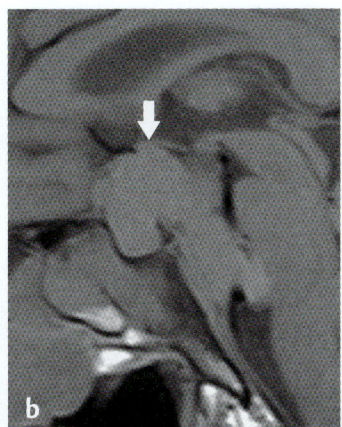 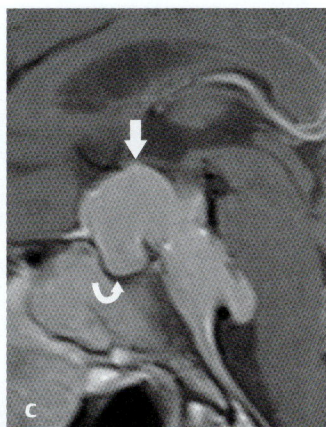

Fig. 4.11 **(a)** Coronal T2 **(b)** sagittal T1 and **(c)** post contrast MR images reveal an intensely enhancing sellar-suprasellar meningioma (*short block white arrow*) extending into retroclival region and sphenoid sinus, inseparable from the pituitary gland, mimics a pituitary macroadenoma.
Note: a normal sized sella (*curved white arrow*) suggesting possibilities other than a pituitary lesion.

Rathke's Cleft Cyst

These arise from the remnant of the Rathke pouch during development of the pituitary gland, which may be incidentally detected or present in the fifth decade with pituitary dysfunction, headache, or visual disturbance. These cysts are either seen in the sella, with or without suprasellar extension, or purely as a suprasellar cyst, but are always located below the optic chiasm.

On CT images, the cyst appears hypodense with wall calcification, while on MR images, the signal intensity varies due to the protein content, usually appearing hyperintense on T1-weighted images, hyperintense to hypointense on T2-weighted images with no internal enhancement. A non-enhancing intracystic nodule is seen at times (**Fig. 4.12**).

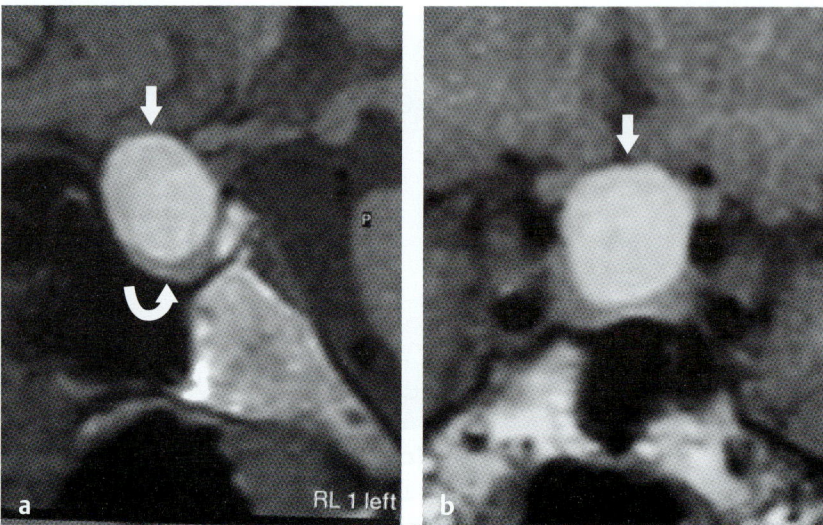

Fig. 4.12 **(a)** Sagittal T1 and **(b)** coronal T1 MR images reveal a sellar-suprasellar lesion (*short block white arrow*) appearing hyperintense on T1w images and separate from the pituitary gland (*curved white arrow*), suggesting a Rathke's cleft cyst.

The small intrasellar cyst may be confused with pituitary microadenomas (**Fig. 4.4**), while the larger suprasellar cyst have to be to differentiated from a cystic craniopharyngioma.

Craniopharyngioma

These are non-glial tumours, which are derived from the epithelium of the Rathke's pouch, with a bimodal peak of occurrence. The first peak is in child-hood (second decade), which on histopathology is commonly of the adaman-tinomatous type. These tend to be complex solid cystic lesions with the solid components revealing enhancement and calcification. The cystic components reveal variable signal intensity due to high protein contents appearing hypo- to hyperintense on T1-weighted and predominantly hyperintense on T2-weighted images (**Fig. 4.13**). Unlike Rathke's cyst, they reveal thick walls with enhancing solid component and calcification (**Fig. 4.14**).

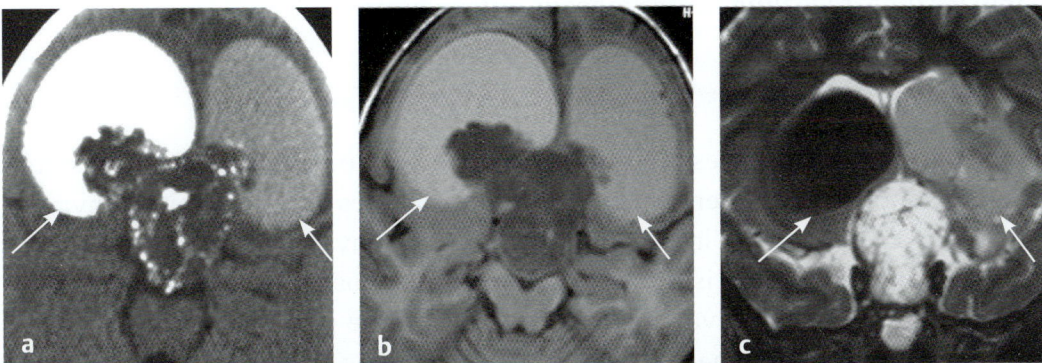

Fig. 4.13 **(a)** Axial CT. **(b)** Axial T1-weighted. **(c)** Coronal T2-weighted MR images reveal a multiloculated predominantly cystic sellar–suprasellar lesion (*white thin arrows*) of mixed density and calcification on CT images, appearing hyperintense on T1-weighted images and of mixed intensity on T2 images which is classical of a craniopharyngioma.

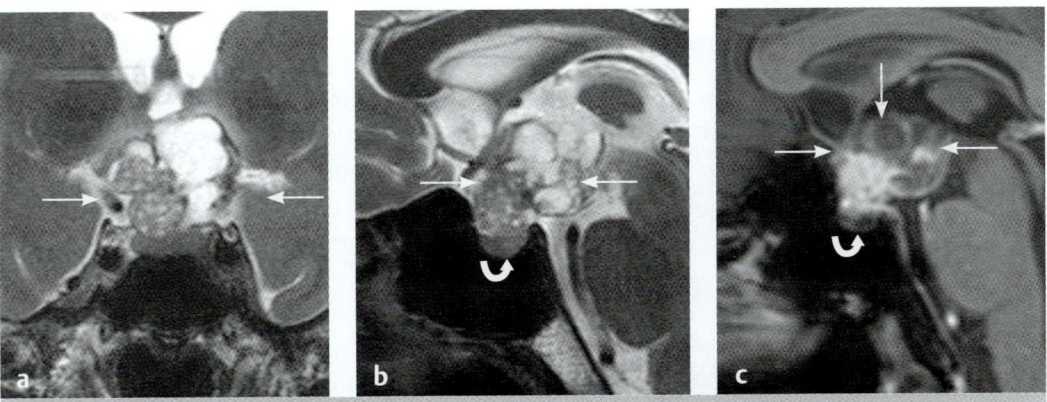

Fig. 4.14 **(a)** Coronal and **(b)** sagittal T2 and **(c)** sagittal post-contrast T1 MR images reveal a solid-cystic partially enhancing sellar-suprasellar lesion (*white thin arrow*) appearing inhomogenously hyperintense on T2w images is suggective of craniopharyngioma. The normal pituitary gland is separate and is seen compressed along the sella floor (*curved white arrow*).

The second peak is in the fourth to fifth decades, which are solid masses, of papillary type, revealing heterogeneous enhancement.

Hypophysitis

It is an autoimmune process commonly seen in post-partum women, and sometimes in middle-aged men presenting with diabetes insipidus or panhypopituitarism. It involves the infundibulum/stalk and may progress to the pituitary gland. On imaging, there is thickening of the stalk, loss of normal bright posterior pituitary signal, and variable enlargement of the pituitary gland, the latter resembling a pituitary macroadenoma. Hypophysitis may be accompanied by enhancement of the adjacent dura mater and sphenoid sinus (**Fig. 4.15**).

Granulomatous hypophysitis may be due to granulomatous involvement of the pituitary gland, especially of tubercular aetiology in our country, revealing inhomogeneous enhancement.

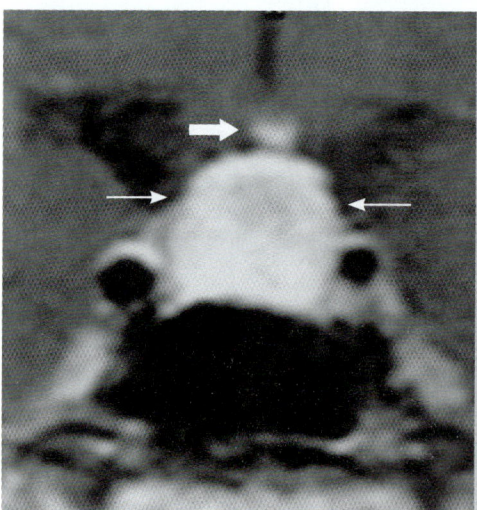

Fig. 4.15 Coronal post-contrast T1-weighted MR image reveals an enhancing sellar–suprasellar lesion (*white thin arrow*) with homogenous enhancement and a thick stalk raising a possibility of pituitary hypophysitis in the right clinical setting.

Chordoma

These are slow-growing, uncommon malignant tumours, originating from the notochordal remnants, with more than one-third of these tumours arising from the clivus at the spheno-occipital synchondrosis with an intracranial soft tissue component causing compression of the brainstem and cranial nerves. They usually present with headache or due to the mass effect on the brainstem or cranial nerves, seen at any age but commonly between 30 to 50 years.

CT imaging reveals a midline or paramedian area of osteolytic destruction of the clivus with radiodensities, which are likely to be remnants of destroyed bone rather than calcification. On MR imaging, this lesion appears of intermediate to profoundly hypointense signal on T1-weighted and markedly hyperintense on T2-weighted images with heterogeneous or mild enhancement (**Fig. 4.16**).

Chondrosarcoma

This lesion is a primary cartilage-based tumour, which in the skull base, is commonly seen off the midline, in the region of the petro-occipital synchondrosis.

They usually present in the middle aged, with headache and depending on its location and extent, with cranial nerve palsy.

It appears as an expansile osteolytic lesion with typical ring and arc-like chondral calcification on the CT images. On MR imaging, they reveal considerable T2 hyperintensity and enhancement like other chondroid tumours. It's off the midline location and presence of typical chondroid calcification helps to differentiate from the chordomas (**Fig. 4.17**).

Hypothalamic–Chiasmatic Glioma

Glial tumours involving the optic chiasm and optic nerves are commonly, pilo-cytic astrocytoma, presenting in children between 5 and 10 years and commonly seen in patients with neurofibromatosis type 1. This lesion often presents as a

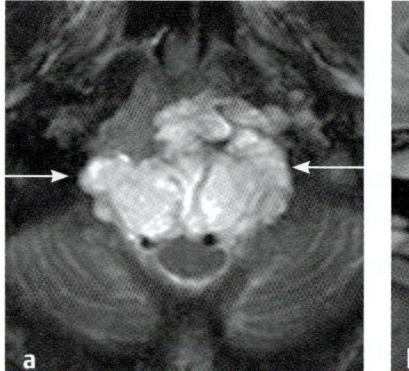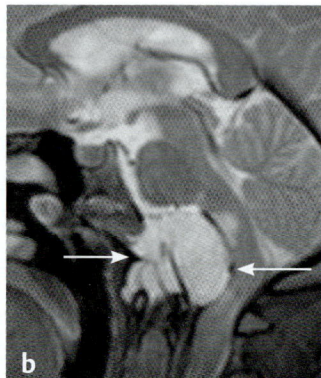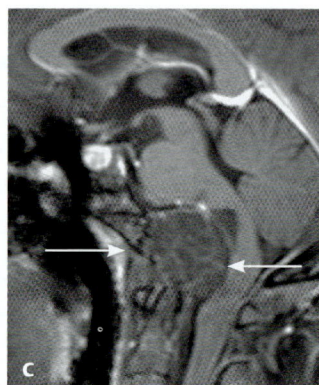

Fig. 4.16 **(a)** Axial and **(b)** sagittal T2 and **(c)** sagittal post-contrast T1 MR images reveal a large expansile midline central skull base mass (*white thin arrow*) involving the clivus, appearing intensely hyperintense on T2w images with mild post-contrast enhancement, suggesting a diagnosis of chordoma.

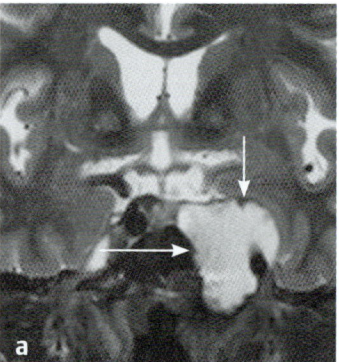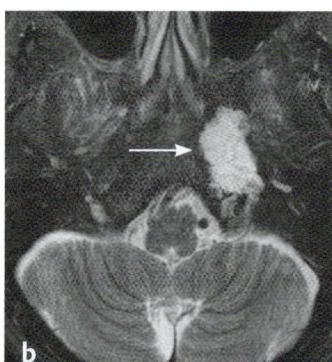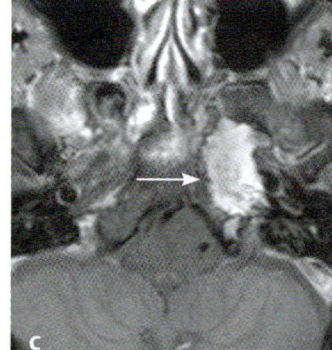

Fig. 4.17 **(a)** Coronal **(b)** axial T2w and **(c)** post-contrast T1w images reveals an expansile, left paramedian central skull base mass (*short thin arrow*) at the petro-clival synchondrosis, appearing intensely hyperintense on T2w images and homogeneously enhancing which is likely to be a chondrosarcoma rather than a chordoma due to its "off" the midline location.

suprasellar cyst with an enhancing mural nodule or as a completely solid mass revealing heterogeneous or homogeneous intense enhancement appearing inseparable from the optic chiasm. These lesions are WHO grade 1 type, though their aggressive appearances on imaging can be misleading (**Fig. 4.18**).

Aneurysm

Aneurysms in the sellar and parasellar regions arise from the intracranial segments of the internal carotid artery which may mimic a mass like a meningioma, appearing hyperdense on the plain CT studies; hence, it is mandatory to do a post-contrast study. On rare occasions, they may compress the pituitary gland and present with hyperprolactinemia. On MR imaging, an aneurysm appears profoundly dark due to large flow-related artefacts. The thrombus appears as an area of altered signal intensity with laminated appearance. CT, MR, or catheter angiography may be needed to fully characterise the aneurysm (**Fig. 4.19**).

Approach for Evaluation of Central Skull Base Tumours

- Identify the sella and pituitary gland.
- Decide whether lesion is sellar, suprasellar, parasellar, or infrasellar.
- Try to see if pituitary gland is separately visualised, and if yes, where is it located, so that it is not damaged while taking a dural incision in a transsphenoidal approach or while dissecting the mass.
- Identify the pituitary stalk, intracranial segments of internal carotid artery, optic chiasm, and hypothalamus.
- Then proceed to characterise whether lesion is solid, cystic, or solid cystic and if the lesion reveals calcification, haemorrhage, or necrosis.
- Often the signal intensity of the lesion on T1- and T2-weighted images help to narrow down the differential diagnosis.

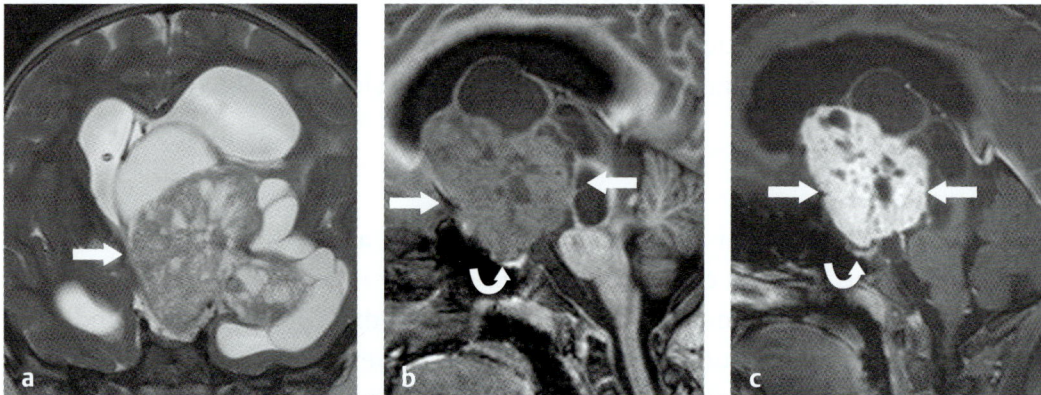

Fig. 4.18 **(a)** Coronal T2 **(b)** sagittal T1w plain and **(c)** post-contrast MR images reveal an intensely enhancing large suprasellar mass (*block white arrow*) in a middle aged child with mild sellar extension but appearing separate from the normal pituitary gland (*curved white arrow*), raising a possibility of an opticochiasmatic pilocytic astrocytoma.

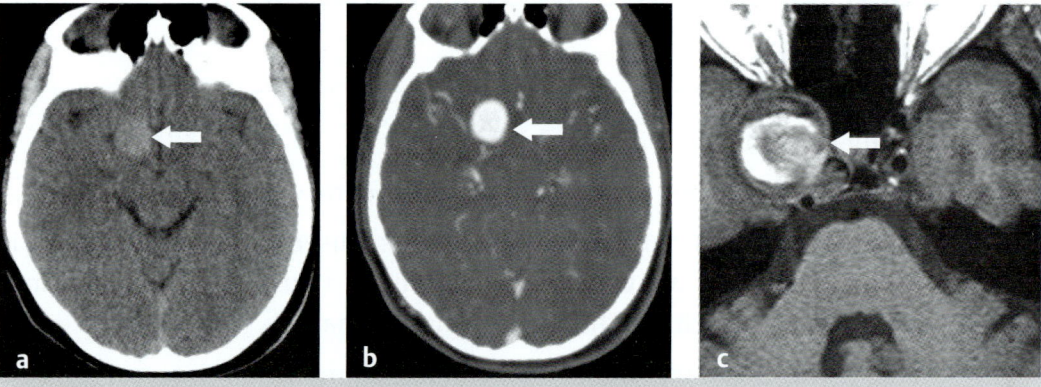

Fig. 4.19 **(a)** Plain and **(b)** post-contrast axial CT and **(c)** axial T1-weighted MR images reveal a right parasellar lesion (*white block arrow*) appearing hyperdense on the plain images and intensely enhancing on the contrast study, suggesting an aneurysm with T1 hyperintensity due to slow flow.

- Assess the exact extent of the lesion, involvement of the adjacent bone, neurovascular structures, dura mater, and the brain.

- Based on the above findings form a differential diagnosis.

- Look at other parameters, which help to decide on operability and surgical approach.

MR imaging is critical for pre-operative evaluation to **localise** the lesion, describe its extent, to assess its morphology, to **characterise** the lesion, and to form a **differential diagnosis**.

Identify the Pituitary Gland

The normal pituitary gland is very well visualised on the MR images especially in the sagittal plane. The adenohypophysis intensely enhances on the contrast study while the posterior pituitary typically appears as a hyperintense focus ('bright spot') on the plain T1-weighted images (**Fig. 4.2**).

The pituitary gland may be inseparable, flattened, or displaced to one side by pituitary macroadenomas and often appears clearly separate from non-pituitary masses (**Figs. 4.10, 4.12, 4.14, 4.18**). It is important to know the location of the normal gland so as to plan the dural incision safely without causing any damage and also to identify and preserve it during the dissection of the tumour.

Any injury to the pituitary stalk or the posterior pituitary carries a risk of hypopituitarism and diabetes insipidus. The pituitary stalk also carries the anterior hypophyseal artery, which supplies the optic chiasm.

Morphological Characterisation

The signal intensity of the lesions on T1- and T2-weighted MRI sequences, with the help of CT study often helps to narrow down the differential diagnosis.

The two Ms, meningioma and macroadenomas are usually isointense to grey matter on T2-weighted images. The macroadenomas often appear heterogeneous due to cystic degeneration or haemorrhage. Cystic areas reveal marked hyperintensity on T2-weighted images, while haemorrhage appears variably hyperintense on T1-weighted images, hypo- to hyperintense on T2-weighted images depending on the age of the blood products with blooming on the gradient sequence.

Meningiomas, generally appear homogeneous, may reveal restricted diffusion with detection of calcification and secondary bony changes often seen on CT images.

The two Cs, chordoma and chondrosarcoma are markedly hyperintense on T2-weighted images very similar to CSF signal intensity revealing variable degree of enhancement on the post-contrast study. Chordomas are generally seen in midline, while chondrosarcomas are off the midline and reveal characteristic ring and arc like chondroid calcification on CT images.

T1 hyperintense lesions are likely to be Rathke's cleft cyst, cranio-pharyngioma, pituitary apoplexy, or haemorrhage in pituitary adenomas. Presence of calcification on CT images tilts the diagnosis towards cranio-pharyngioma, while thin-walled cystic lesions are likely to be a Rathke cyst. Pituitary apoplexy is seen in an enlarged gland which is non-enhancing on contrast study due to necrosis.

Dural Involvement

Detection of dural invasion is important as a combined craniofacial approach is recommended. Dural thickening and enhancement may be present as an inflammatory reaction or due to dural invasion. Dural invasion is suspected when there is nodular or linear dural thickening of more than 5 mm.[7]

Vascular Involvement

Invasion of cavernous sinus by pituitary adenomas increases the morbidity and mortality associated with surgical procedures and suggests aggressive nature of the tumour regardless of the benign histology. Radiological diagnosis of cavernous sinus invasion is not easy, but several MRI criteria have been established to assist the diagnosis and pre-operative surgical planning.[8]

- Drawing of the intercarotid lines through the medial and lateral walls as well as the centre of the cavernous and supraclinoid segments of the ipsilateral internal carotid artery, on the coronal MR image, gives us the medial, lateral, and median intercarotid lines, respectively (**Fig. 4.20**). This formed the basis of Knosp et al's classification of cavernous sinus invasion.[9]

- To calculate the percentage of intracavernous carotid artery encasement by the tumour.

- To evaluate the venous compartments of the cavernous sinus (**Fig. 4.20**).

Absence of cavernous sinus invasion is suggested in case of the following:

- Normal pituitary gland is seen between the adenoma and cavernous sinus.

- Visualisation of normal medial venous compartment.

- When the median and medial intercarotid lines are not crossed by the tumour.

- Encasement of less than 25% of the intracavernous carotid artery.

Cavernous sinus invasion is suggested in case of the following:

- The lesion crosses the lateral intercarotid line.

- More than 67% encasement of the intracavernous carotid artery.

- Obliteration of carotid sulcus compartment.

- Asymmetry of the cavernous sinus.

- Lateral bulging of the cavernous sinus.

- Displacement of cavernous sinus.

Neural Involvement

As majority of patients with pituitary lesions come with visual complaints, MRI images help to locate the optic chiasm, and to decide whether it is compressed or infiltrated. The cisternal segments of other cranial nerves from third to eighth

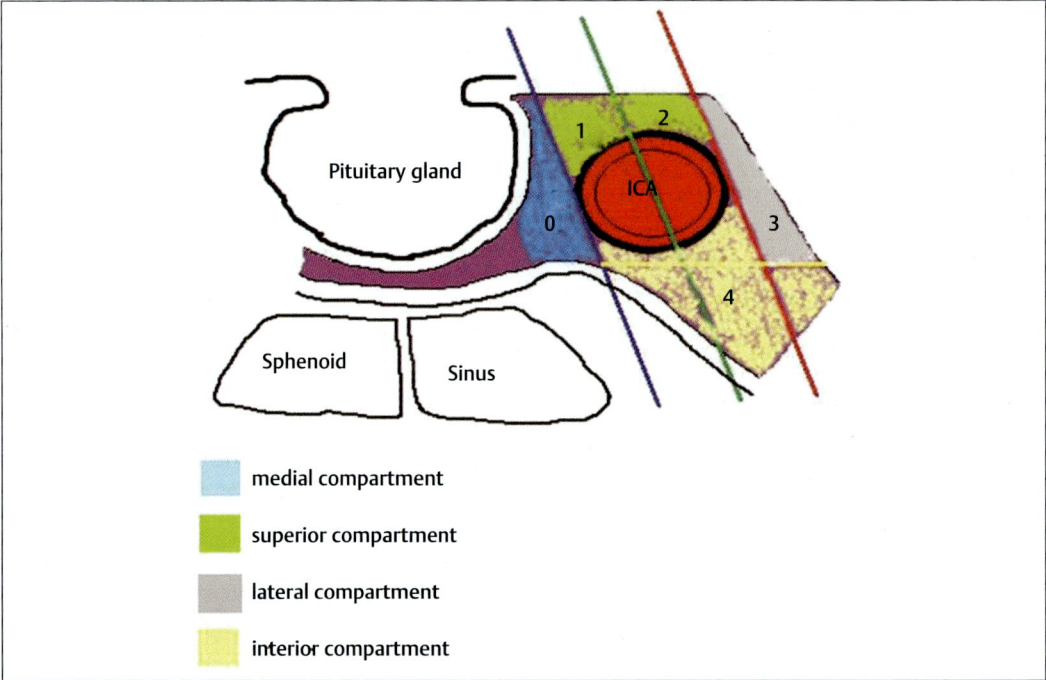

medial compartment

superior compartment

lateral compartment

interior compartment

Fig. 4.20 Grading of cavernous sinus invasion by pituitary macroadenoma according to Knosp et al's classification. The cavernous sinus is divided into four compartments by medial carotid line (*blue*), median carotid line (*green*), lateral carotid line (*red*). The invasion of the cavernous sinus is classified by the extension of the tumour beyond the intercarotid lines (Refer to **Table 4.1**). The cavernous sinus is also divided into medial, superior, inferior, and lateral venous compartments to assess invasion.

Table 4.1   Knosp et al's classification of cavernous sinus invasion[9]

Grade 0	Adenoma does not reach the medial carotid line
Grade 1	Adenoma extends beyond the medial carotid line but does not reach the median carotid line
Grade 2	Tumour extends beyond the median line but not beyond lateral line
Grade 3	Tumour extends beyond the lateral line
Grade 4	Tumour totally wraps around the intracavernous carotid artery

should also be assessed when lesions extend into the prepontine and cerebellopontine angle cisterns.

Normal and Variant Anatomy of Sinonasal Cavity on CT

CT imaging is an indispensable pre-operative imaging modality for assessment of the anatomy and variants of the sinonasal cavities. It also helps to characterise the lesion and is a modality of choice when MR imaging is contraindicated or unavailable.

It is pertinent to assess the normal and variant anatomy of the sinonasal cavity, as it forms the main passage for endoscopic access to the skull base.

Important structures and abnormality to look for are as follows:

Nasal Septum

The nasal septum may be commonly deviated and bony spurs are often seen. Gross septal deviation limits the access to the posterior nasal cavity and must be addressed to improve surgical exposure. It also determines the side from which the nasoseptal flap is to be taken. A narrow nasal route predisposes the nasal mucosa to trauma while introducing the endoscope and instruments.

Presence of a sharp bony spur may jeopardise the nasoseptal flap as it can cause a tear in the flap during its elevation (**Fig. 4.21**).

Concha Bullosa

The middle turbinates need to be lateralised in order to open the naso-sphenoid corridor. There may be variable pneumatisation seen of the middle turbinate. Pneumatisation of the inferior bulbous portion of the middle turbinate (concha bullosa) may prevent its lateralisation. Hence, conchoplasty would be required before lateralising the middle turbinates (**Fig. 4.22**).

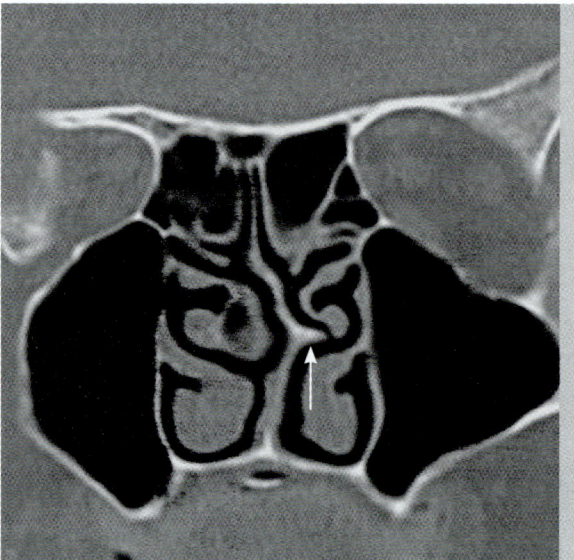

Fig. 4.21 Coronal high-resolution CT image (*bone window*) reveals a nasal septal spur directed to the left (*thin white arrow*).

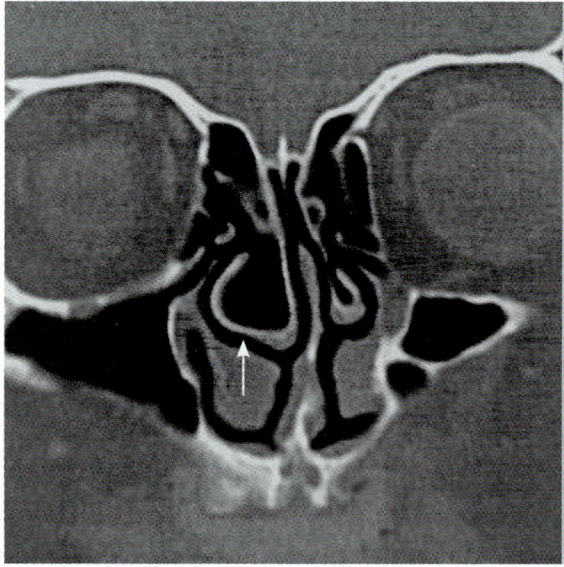

Fig. 4.22 Coronal high-resolution CT image (*bone window*) reveals a large right concha bullosa (*thin white arrow*).

Onodi Cells

Onodi/sphenoethmoidal cells are variant posterior ethmoid air cells that extend postero-superior to the sphenoid sinus. It is important to identify them as they lie close to the optic nerve and the carotid artery, with a risk of damage to these structures during surgery. They can be suspected if on coronal CT images a horizontal or obliquely traversing septum is seen or if there is cruciform septation noted in the sphenoid sinus at the level of the posterior choana[10] (**Fig. 4.23**).

Sphenoid Sinus

Type of Sphenoid Sinus

Depending on the degree of antero-posterior pneumatisation, the sphenoid sinus is classified as conchal, pre-sellar, and sellar, the latter is further divided as incomplete and complete sellar (**Fig. 4.24**).

A conchal sphenoid sinus reveals a minimal pneumatisation which doesn't reach up to the anterior wall of the sella turcica.

In a pre-sellar sphenoid sinus, the posterior sinus wall reaches up to the anterior wall of sella.

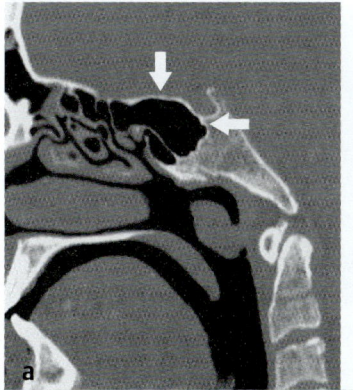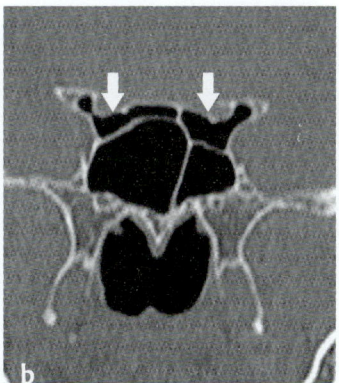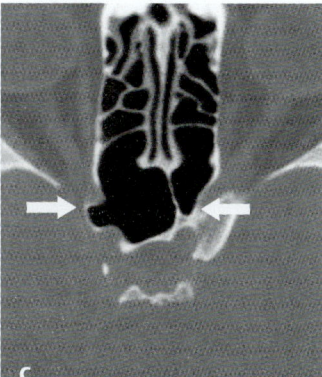

Fig. 4.23   (a) Sagittal. **(b)** Coronal. **(c)** Axial high-resolution CT images (*bone window*) reveal bilateral Onodi cells (*block white arrow*).

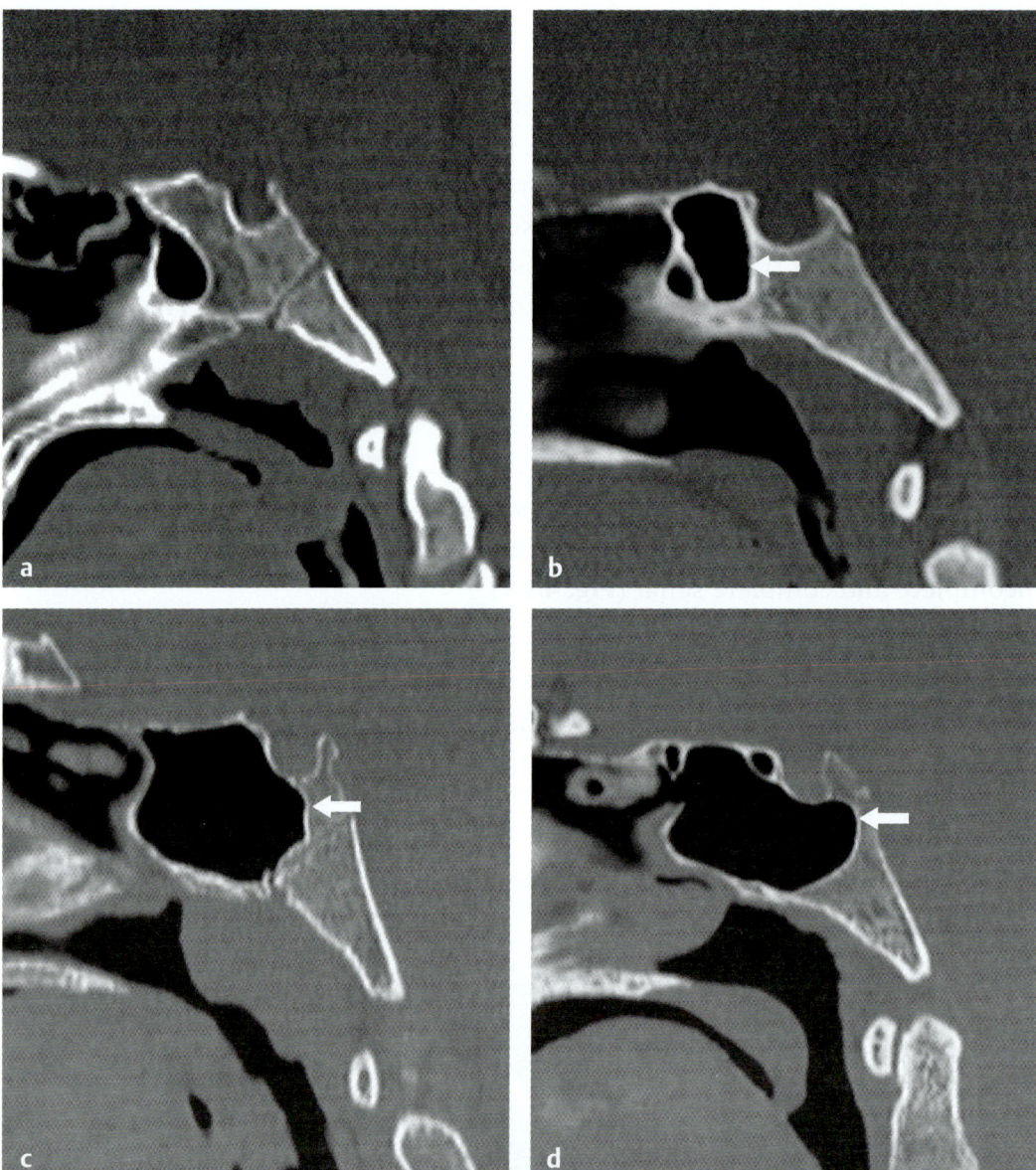

Fig. 4.24 Sagittal CT images reveal different types of sphenoid sinus depending on varying degree of anteroposterior pneumatisation. White block arrow shows posterior limit of the sphenoid sinus. **(a)** Conchal. **(b)** Presellar. **(c)** Sellar (incomplete). **(d)** Sellar (complete).

In sellar type, the pneumatisation extends beyond the anterior wall of the sella along the sellar floor which is either incomplete or complete involving the entire sphenoid body and reaching up to the clivus. The sellar type is commonly seen and favourable for trans-sphenoidal approach. On the contrary, a conchal or a pre-sellar sphenoid sinus is a challenge to skull base surgery, which would require drilling of the bone to access the sellar region.

Hyper-pneumatisation

The sphenoid sinus may be widely pneumatised extending laterally into the greater wing of sphenoid, superiorly into the anterior clinoid process, and inferolaterally into the pterygoid process. Hyper-pneumatisation of sphenoid sinus provides a natural passage for off-midline structures during a trans-sphenoidal surgery, but carries a higher risk of neurovascular injury,[11] due to dehiscence and intrasinus course of the neurovascular canals (**Fig. 4.25**).

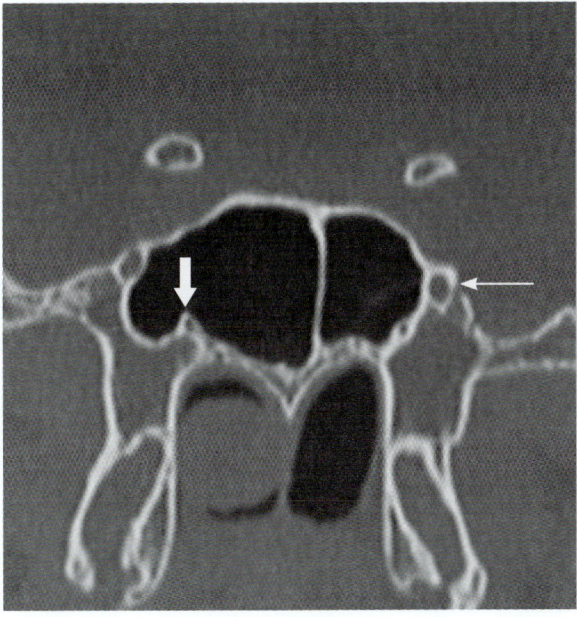

Fig. 4.25 Coronal high-resolution CT image (*bone window*) reveals a hyper-pneumatised sphenoid sinus with partial intrasinus course of the right vidian nerve at the junction of the floor of the sphenoid and the medial pterygoid plate (*white block arrow*). The V2 nerve/foramen rotundum is seen superolateral to the vidian canal (*thin white arrow*).

Sphenoid Septa

The intersphenoid or the accessory septa may insert into the bony walls of the carotid artery and optic nerve, which may be injured during surgery due to excessive traction. Pre-operative identification would be important to prevent catastrophic complications[11,12](**Fig. 4.26**).

Sella

The sella may be widened and descended into the sphenoid sinus. For a widened sella, it is necessary that the flap is broad anteriorly/caudally (**Fig. 4.27**).

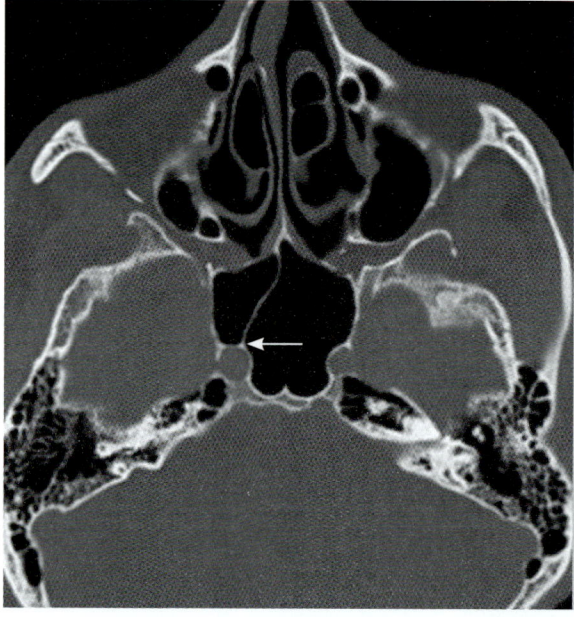

Fig. 4.26 Axial CT image reveals attachment of the intersphenoid septum to the right carotid canal (*white arrow*).

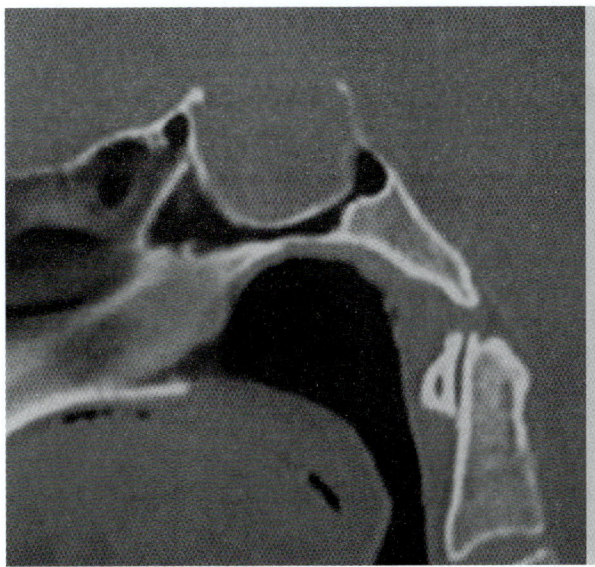

Fig. 4.27 Coronal CT image reveals an extensively widened sella descending into the sphenoid sinus.

Utility of Pre-operative Imaging

- To localise, characterise, and form a reasonable differential diagnosis.
- Assess extent of the lesion in each dimension and look for vascular, perineural, and dural/brain invasion, which helps to decide on operability/non-operability.
- To identify normal and variant anatomy which would affect the outcome of surgery.
- Guidance regarding type of surgical approach.
- Neuro-navigation greatly improves localisation of lesions in minimally invasive procedures with fewer complications.

To conclude, CT and MR imaging are complementary to each other and together can provide vital information to the surgeon regarding the possibility of resectability and best surgical approach.

References

1. Elster AD. Modern imaging of the pituitary. Radiology 1993;187(1):1–14

2. Go JL, Rajamohan AG. Imaging of the sella and parasellar region. Radiol Clin North Am 2017;55(1):83–101

3. Friedman TC, Zuckerbraun E, Lee ML, Kabil MS, Shahinian H. Dynamic pituitary MRI has high sensitivity and specificity for the diagnosis of mild Cushing's syndrome and should be part of the initial workup. Horm Metab Res 2007;39(6):451–456

4. Blitz AM, Aygun N, Herzka DA, Ishii M, Gallia GL. High-resolution three-dimensional MR imaging approach to the skull base: compartments, boundaries, and critical structures. Radiol Clin North Am 2017;55(1):17–30

5. Kacker A, Tabaee A, Anand V. Computer-assisted surgical navigation in revision endoscopic sinus surgery. Otolaryngol Clin North Am 2005;38(3):473–482, vi

6. Taylor SL, Barakos JA, Harsh GR IV, Wilson CB. Magnetic resonance imaging of tuberculum sellae meningiomas: preventing preoperative misdiagnosis as pituitary macroadenoma. Neurosurgery 1992;31(4):621–627, discussion 627

7. Parmar H, Gujar S, Shah G, Mukherji SK. Imaging of the anterior skull base. Neuroimaging Clin N Am 2009;19(3):427–439

8. Cottier JP, Destrieux C, Brunereau L, et al. Cavernous sinus invasion by pituitary adenoma: MR imaging. Radiology 2000;215(2):463–469

9. Knosp E, Steiner E, Kitz K, Matula C. Pituitary adenomas with invasion of the cavernous sinus space: a magnetic resonance imaging classification compared with surgical findings. Neurosurgery 1993;33(4):610–617, discussion 617–618

10. Vaid S, Vaid N. Normal anatomy and anatomic variants of the paranasal sinuses on computed tomography. Neuroimaging Clin N Am 2015;25(4):527–548

11. García-Garrigós E, Arenas-Jiménez JJ, Monjas-Cánovas I, et al. Transsphenoidal approach in endoscopic endonasal surgery for skull base lesions: what radiologists and surgeons need to know. Radiographics 2015;35(4):1170–1185

12. Mossa-Basha M, Blitz AM. Imaging of the paranasal sinuses. Semin Roentgenol 2013; 48(1):14–34

05 Pituitary Surgery: Basic Concepts

Nishit Shah and C. E. Deopujari

Pre-Operative Preparation

Antibiotics are required pre-operatively, in the full course, if there is any indication of nasal or sinus infection. If not, we usually start an oral antibiotic 2 days prior to surgery, to ensure there is no congestion from latent infection. Local decongestants in the form of oxymetazoline or xylometazoline nasal drops are started a day or two prior to surgery. It is a good practise to obtain a nasal swab prior to starting prophylactic antibiotics.

Surgeries are done under general anaesthesia. A lumbar drain is inserted in patients where a dural defect and reconstruction is expected, or when the suprasellar component is irregular in extended approach cases. The patient is given about 20–30 degrees head high, neck extension depends on the location of the lesion, with anterior lesions requiring more extension. The head is slightly angled so as to be 'looking' at the surgeon (**Fig. 5.1a**) on the right side, to enable ease of instrumentation, and reduce bending of operating surgeons. This works if both surgeons (ENT and neurosurgeon) are standing on the same side. If either surgeon is left handed, then the surgeons stand on opposite sides. This is also a routine position for some teams. The height of the table is adjusted for working comfort. A side Mayo Trolley is arranged for elbow support for the surgeon holding the endoscope. We prefer the lateral thigh as a donor site for fascia against the abdomen, unless the patient requests against a thigh scar (**Fig. 5.1a**).

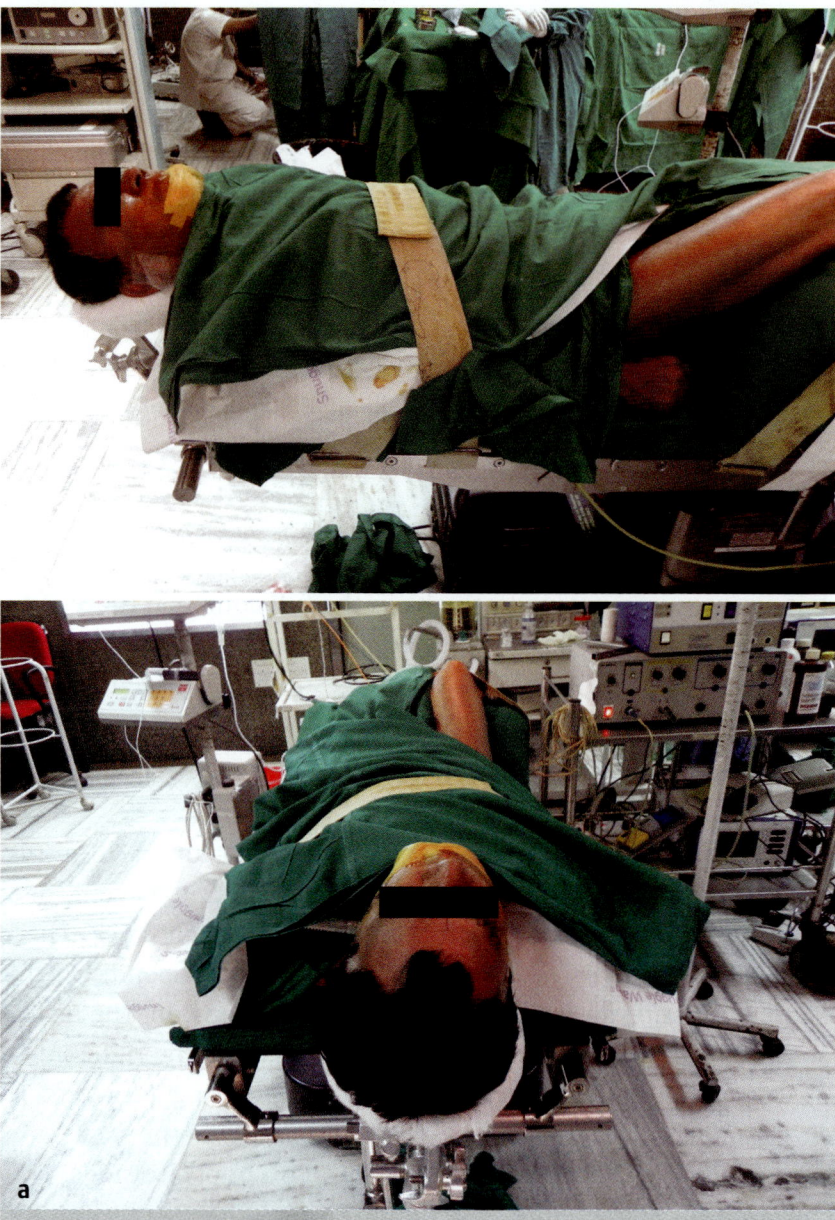

Fig. 5.1 **(a)** Preparation and position of the patient before the surgery. The head is tilted slightly, to be looking towards the surgeon. The lateral thigh is the preferred donor site for free fascia.

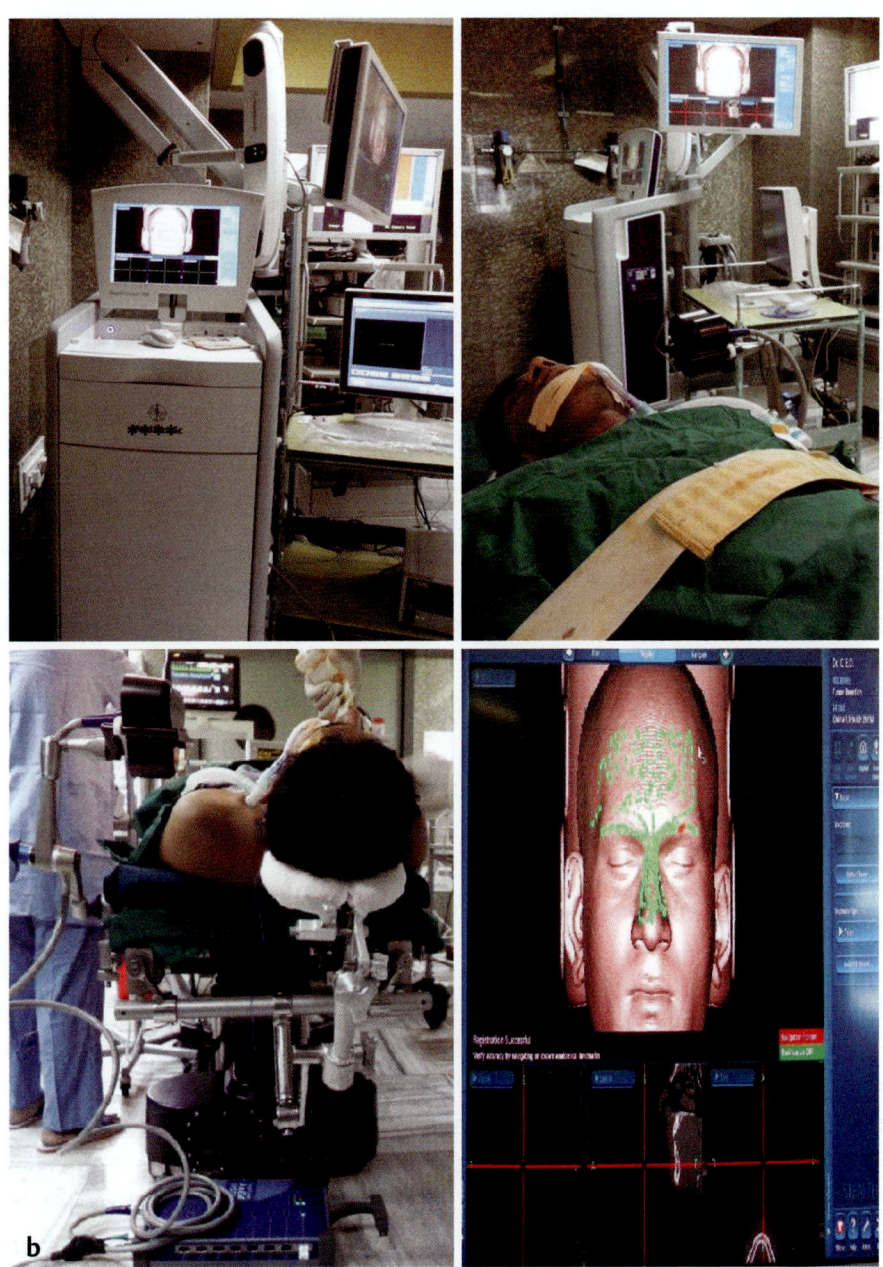

Fig. 5.1 **(b)** Position and preparation of the patient with electromagnetic navigation system.

The navigation system is used for all cases of extended approaches, re-do surgeries, and in patients with irregular suprasellar extensions of their pituitary tumours. The head fixation in Mayfield clamp is required for most of the optical systems of navigation. However, we have been using the face mask (pinless navigation system from Stryker) and the Electromagnetic (EM system of Medtronic) navigation successfully for these cases (**Fig. 5.1b**). This allows for intra-operative head movement should it be required. MRI and CT images are alternatively or collectively used for guidance with occasional need for CT angio.

A nasal probe of vascular Doppler (Mizuo corp. Japan) is kept ready for all extended approaches as well as cavernous sinus extensions.

The entire face and thigh are then prepared and draped for surgery.

The initial nasal packing is done using large cottonoids, soaked and squeezed dry, using 30 ml of 4% xylocaine with 3 ml of 1:10,000 adrenaline solution, using nasal packing forceps (See **Fig. 10.1** in chapter 10). Instruments, suctions, endoscope camera system, etc. are now neatly organised. Positions of nurses, assistants, and monitors are sorted and the checklist read out (**Fig. 5.2**).

Surgery

Nasal Stage

An initial diagnostic endoscopy is done to familiarise anatomy, check screen picture and navigation landmarks. The first step is to in-fracture the inferior turbinate by placing the shaft of the Freer's elevator (**Fig. 5.3a**) (See **Fig. 10.2** in chapter 10) in the inferior meatus. This allows subsequent out-fracture of the inferior turbinate without causing mucosal injury. This simple step is important to considerably increase the working space in the nose and make viewing of the middle turbinate and posterior structures better. Next, we lateralise the middle turbinate and the superior turbinate (**Fig. 5.3b**) to visualise the sphenoid sinus ostium. This may be aided by the insertion of cottonoids between the

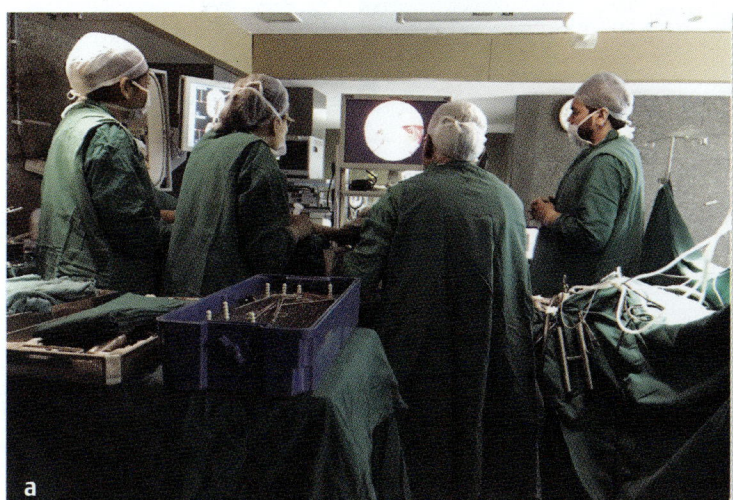

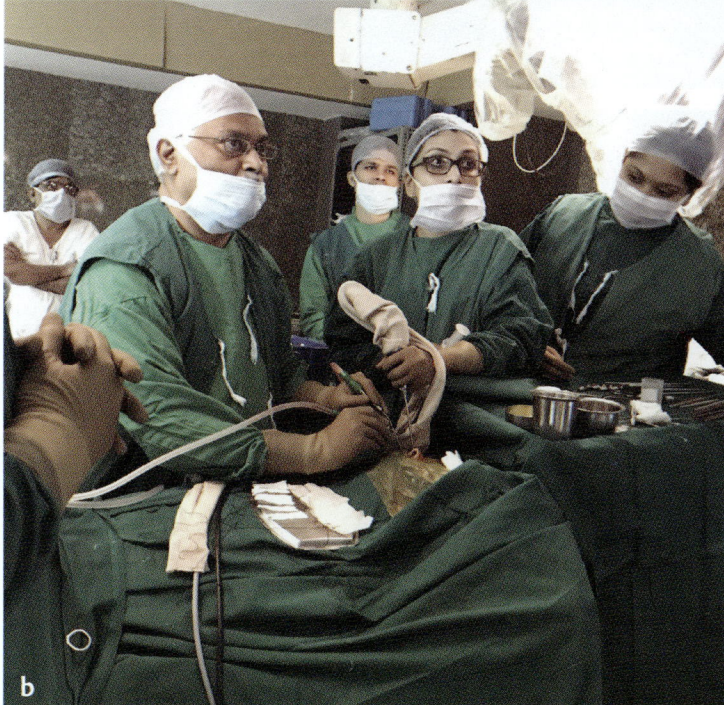

Fig. 5.2 **(a)** OT setup with position of the surgeons, assistants, nurses, and monitors. **(b)** The ENT surgeon stands close to the head end holding the scope and irrigation cannula, while the neurosurgeon uses two-handed technique for tumour removal.

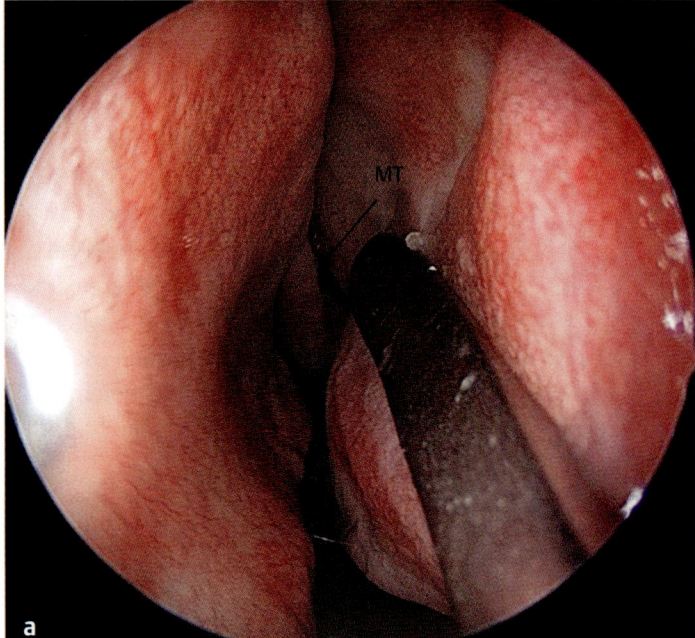

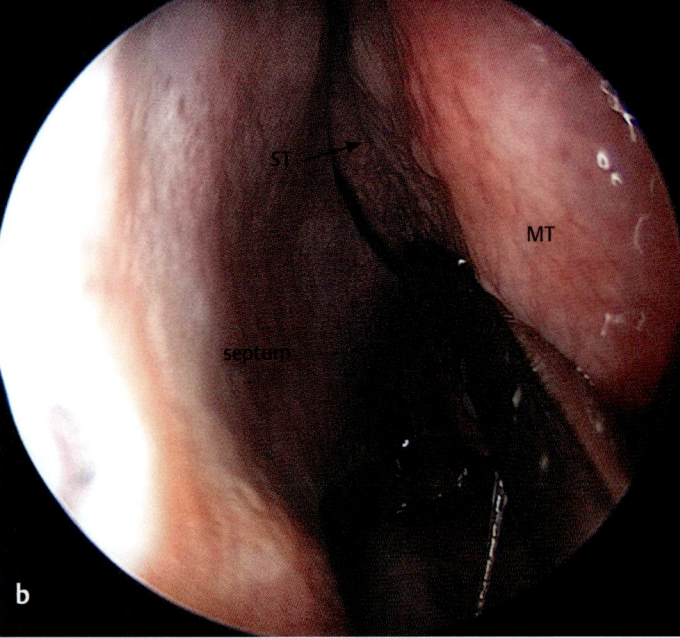

Fig. 5.3 **(a)** Lateralisation of left inferior turbinate using a Freer's elevator (See **Fig. 10.2** in chapter 10). The middle turbinate (MT) is seen above (*thin black arrow*). **(b)** Lateralisation of left middle turbinate. As the middle turbinate is lateralised, the superior turbinate is seen coming into view (*thin black arrow*). ST, superior turbinate; MT, middle turbinate.

septum and turbinates. The ostium is positioned about 1.5 cm above the superior choanal arch and if one is using a straight instrument, one will find it just behind the superior turbinate in its inferior half (**Fig. 5.4**). It is important to stay in the inferior half of the turbinates as going superior towards the skull base is hazardous in a number of ways. As you go higher, the space gets narrower, and the chance of mucosal trauma becomes higher. This leads to the blood trickling onto the scope, hindering vision, and potentially allowing for more trauma and hence bleeding. This will subsequently, lead to synechiae and olfactory disturbances. Also, as you go towards the skull base, the risk of a cerebrospinal fluid (CSF) leak also increases. One must clearly expose the sphenoid ostium and anterior sphenoid wall on both sides. This may occasionally be difficult if there is a severe deviation or septal spur. In these patients, it is advisable to finish one side first, and then do the septectomy. Post this step, it is easy to raise a flap on the opposite side.

In most cases of pituitary surgery, we take rescue flaps. A full nasoseptal or Hadad–Bassagasteguy (HB) flaps are only taken when anticipating a CSF leak. The middle turbinate is always preserved in pituitary cases, unless an extended approach is required. If there is a concha bullosa, a conchoplasty is done by removing the lateral part of the concha. The medial part can then be lateralised easily (**Fig. 5.5**) (See **Figs. 10.5, 10.10** in chapter 10). We do not excise the medial part as it is attached to the skull base and contains olfactory fibres.

In cases with large bulla ethmoidalis, bullectomy may be performed to facilitate lateralisation of the middle turbinate. Large non-pneumatised middle turbinate may be sacrificed to widen the nasosphenoid corridor.

Middle turbinectomy is performed for extended approaches to the lateral recess of sphenoid, pterygopalatine fossa, and infratemporal fossa. Large non-pneumatised middle turbinate which refuses to lateralise may be sacrificed. Cases with orbital or cavernous sinus pathology also warrant middle turbinectomy. The same applies in cases where a transcribriform or transplanum approach is required. For transsphenoid surgery, almost always, only the turbinate on the right side is amputated.

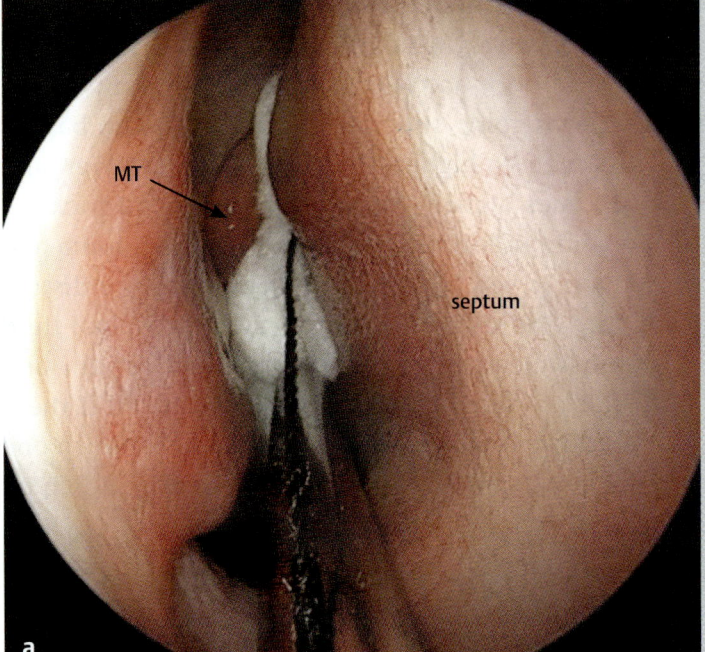

Fig. 5.4 Lateralisation of the turbinates being done in an atraumatic manner by pushing cottonoid patties between the septum and the turbinates **(a)**. Visualisation of the right sphenoid ostium after lateralising the middle turbinate (MT) **(b)** and the superior turbinate **(c)**. The sphenoid ostium (*thin black arrow*) lies around 1.5 cm above the choana (Ch) in the region of the lower one-third of the superior turbinate (ST) **(d)**.

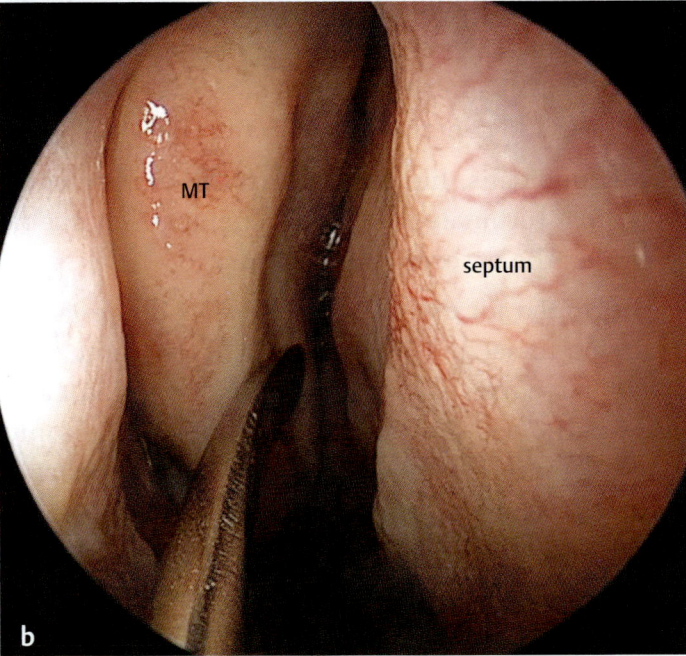

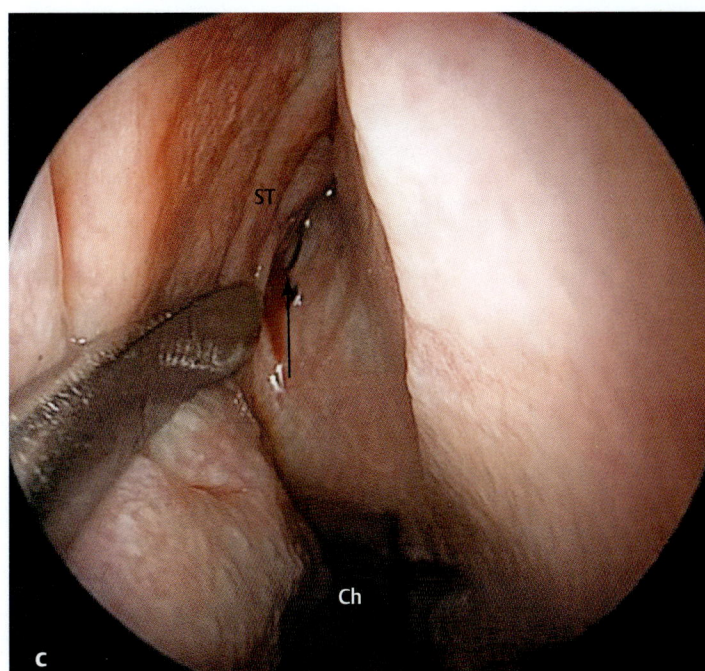

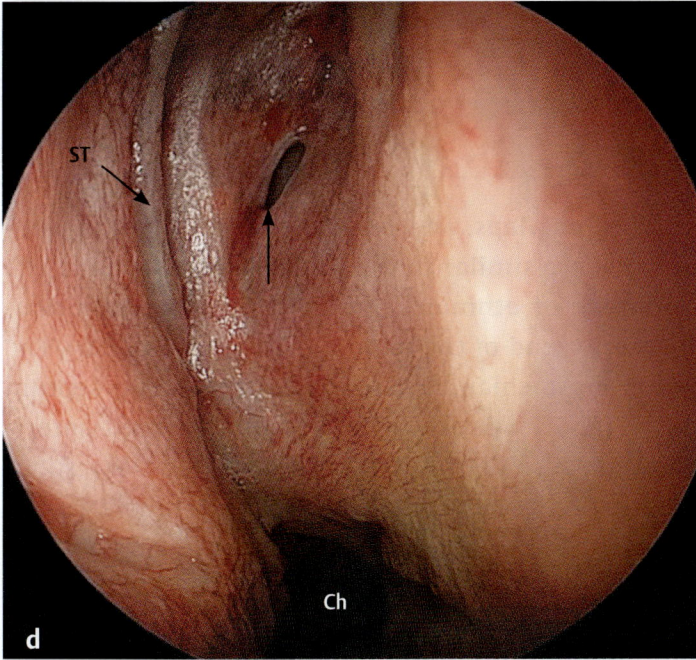

Fig. 5.4 Lateralisation of the turbinates being done in an atraumatic manner by pushing cottonoid patties between the septum and the turbinates **(a)**. Visualisation of the right sphenoid ostium after lateralising the middle turbinate (MT) **(b)** and the superior turbinate **(c)**. The sphenoid ostium (*thin black arrow*) lies around 1.5 cm above the choana (Ch) in the region of the lower one-third of the superior turbinate (ST) **(d)**.

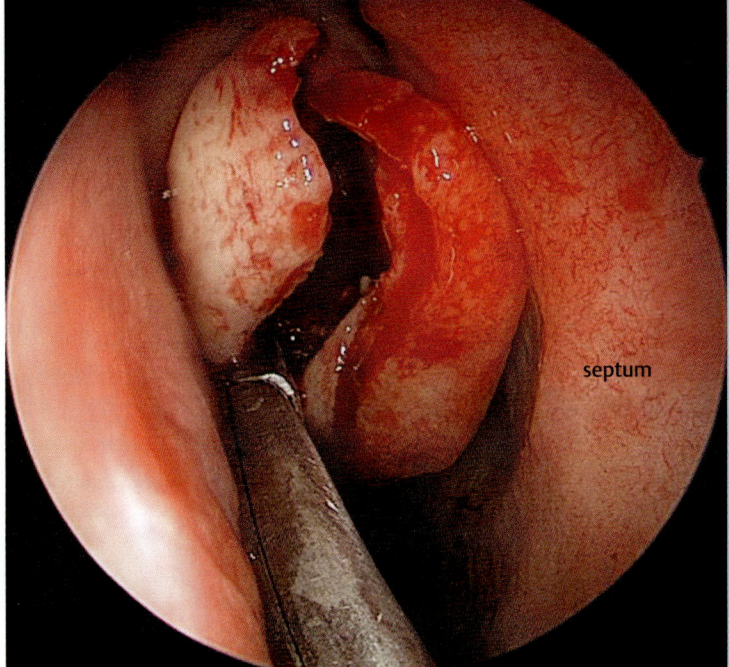

Fig. 5.5 Right conchoplasty is being done. The lateral half of the concha is excised.

septum

Rescue Flaps

Rescue flaps are incomplete nasoseptal flaps, which remain pedicled both posteriorly and anteriorly. The incisions are similar to the Hadad flap but end at the junction of the perpendicular plate of ethmoid and septal cartilage approximately corresponding to the anterior end of the middle turbinate (**Fig. 5.6**). The inferior incision starts above the eustachian tube, curves towards the septum staying just above the choana (**Fig. 5.7**). Once on the septum, proceed anteriorly staying low for a few centimetres. The upper incision starts at the sphenoid ostium, and comes anteriorly till the bone–cartilage junction, taking care to stay below the impressions of the olfactory fibres (**Fig. 5.8**). We use a monopolar cautery long needle (Colorado) with its tip bent to about 60 degrees (See **Fig. 10.3** in chapter 10). There is no vertical incision to join the two horizontal incisions.

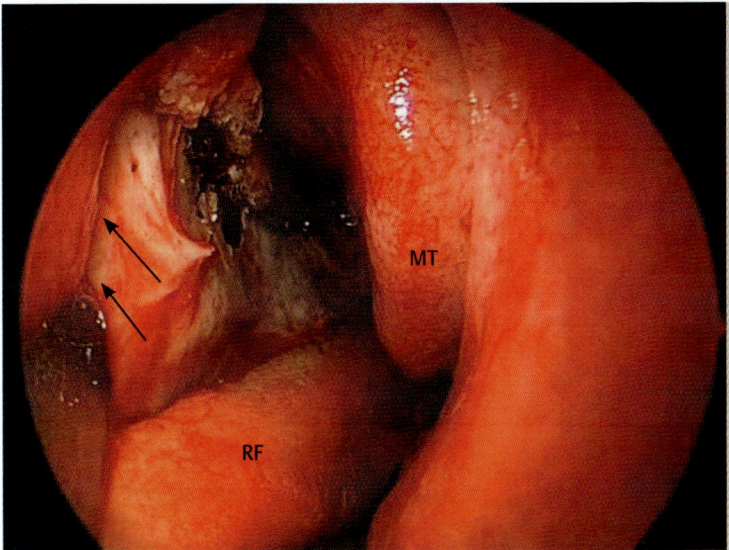

Fig. 5.6 Image of a rescue flap (RF) raised on the left side. The anterior limit of the incision is at the level of the bony cartilaginous junction of the septum (*thin black arrows*), which is marked roughly by the anterior end of the middle turbinate (MT).

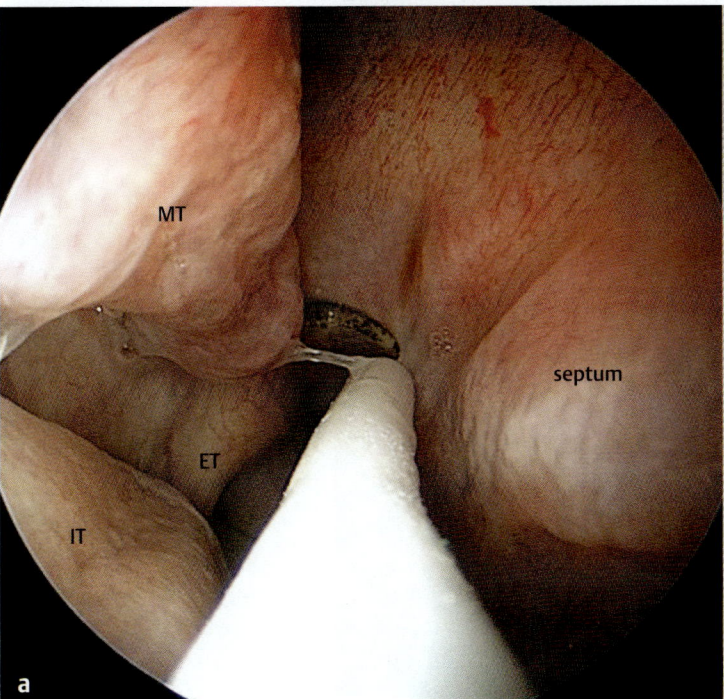

Fig. 5.7 (a-c) Image showing the beginning of inferior incision for rescue flaps and reverse flaps (on the right side). The inferior incision starts just above the eustachian tube (ET) along the arch of choana and along the inferior septum approximately till the bony cartilaginous junction. For HB flaps the inferior incision comes right upto the mucocutaneous junction of the septum. MT, middle turbinate; IT, inferior turbinate.

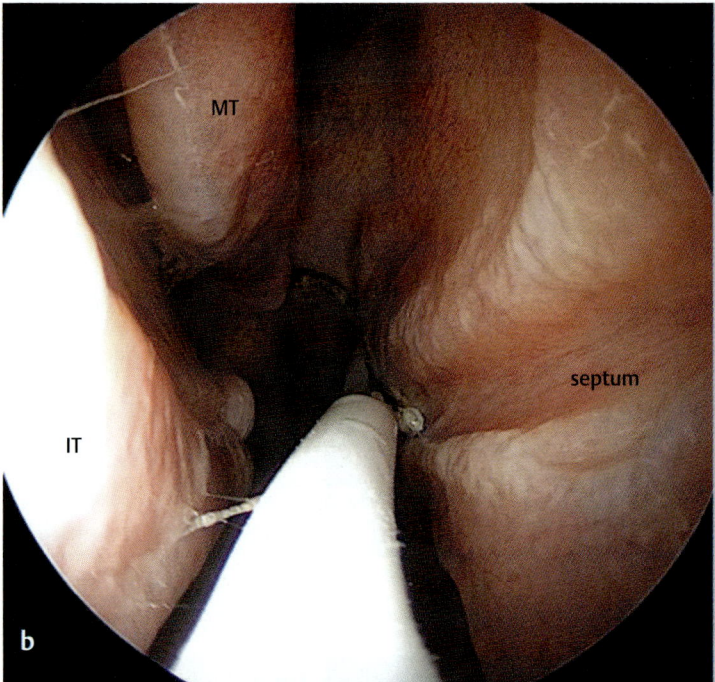

Fig. 5.7 (a-c) Image showing the beginning of inferior incision for rescue flaps and reverse flaps (on the right side). The inferior incision starts just above the eustachian tube (ET) along the arch of choana and along the inferior septum approximately till the bony cartilaginous junction. For HB flaps the inferior incision comes right upto the mucocutaneous junction of the septum. MT, middle turbinate; IT, inferior turbinate.

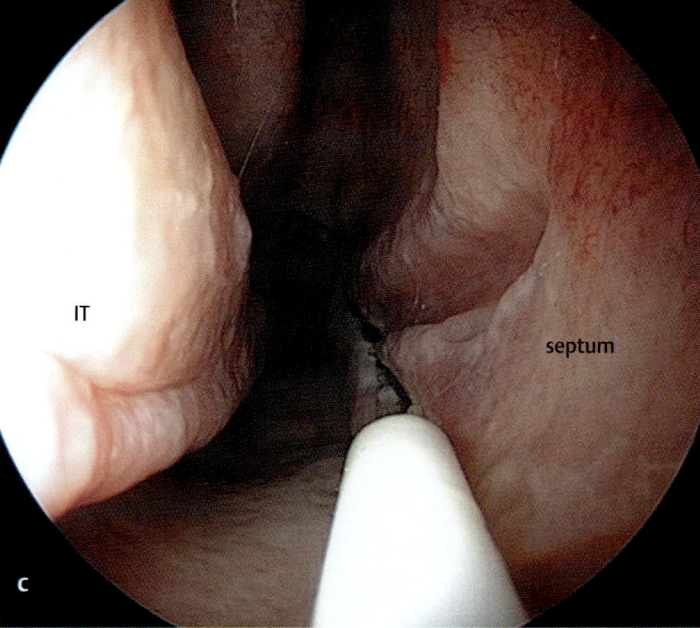

This is done bilaterally. The mucoperiosteum is elevated off the perpendicular plate and posterior vomer using an elevator and ball probe anteriorly (See **Fig. 10.2, 10.25** in chapter 10), and the bone removed using Luc's forceps (See **Fig. 10.4** in chapter 10) or straight ethmoid forceps (**Fig. 5.9**) (See **Fig. 10.5** in chapter 10), in a large piece to aid in reconstruction, should it be required. This completes the septectomy, permitting a binostril approach (**Fig. 5.10**). This means, the mucoperiosteum can droop down, allowing instrumentation and passage of the endoscope (**Fig. 5.11**). This pedicled flap maintains the septal branch of the sphenopalatine artery. Initially, this conservative approach may take a little time getting used to, but is easy after a couple of cases. It allows the mucoperiosteum to be repositioned at the end of the surgery, effectively closing the posterior septectomy and allowing for a normal-looking nasal cavity with insignificant morbidity and quick healing (**Fig. 5.12**).

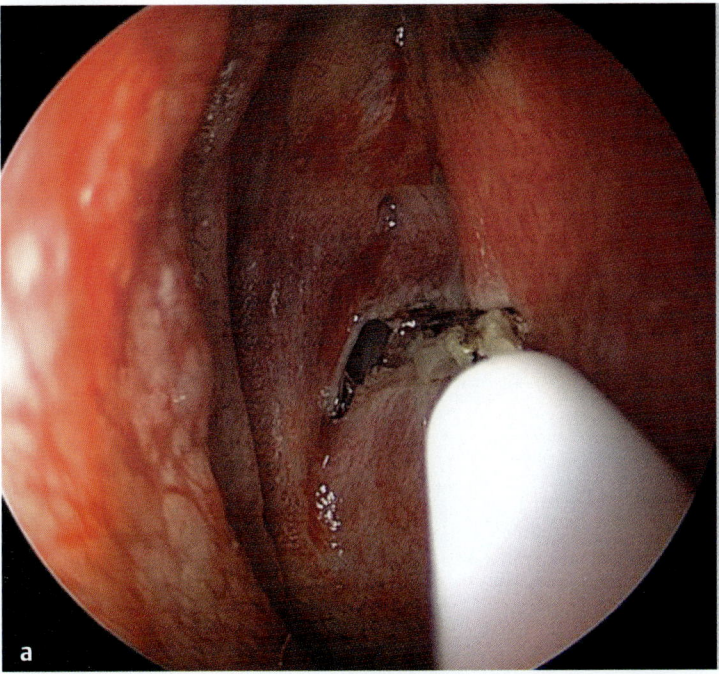

a

Fig. 5.8 **(a)** Superior incision taken from the right sphenoid ostium, for rescue flaps, HB flaps, and reverse flaps.

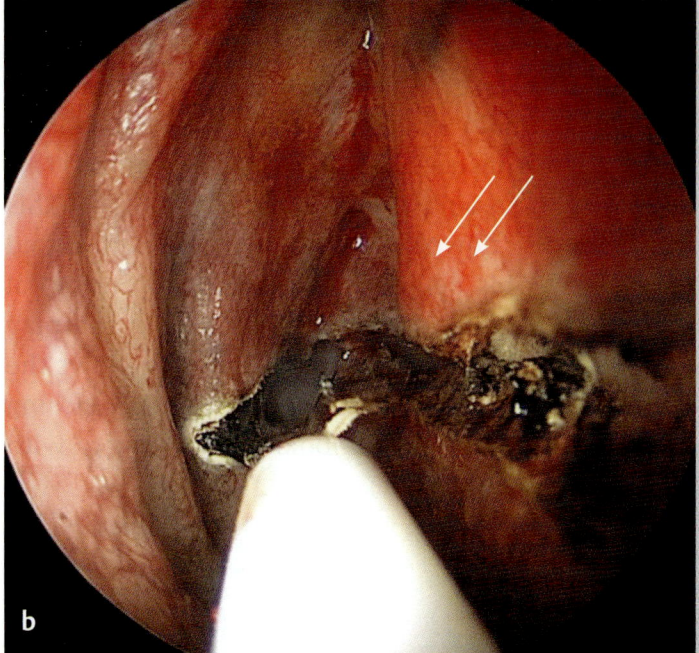

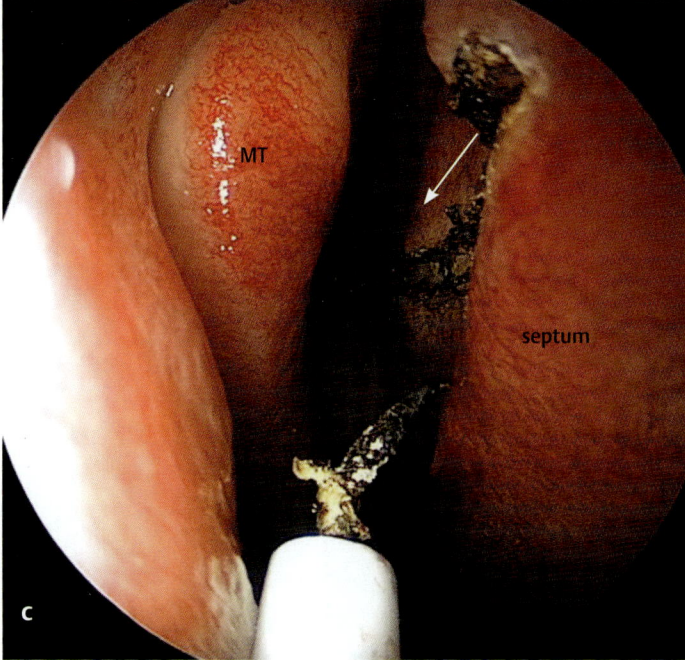

Fig. 5.8 (b, c) The incision being extended further anterior on the septum staying below the olfactory fibres (*two white arrows*). A small lateral incision is taken from the ostium to aid in downward displacement of the flap. MT, middle turbinate.

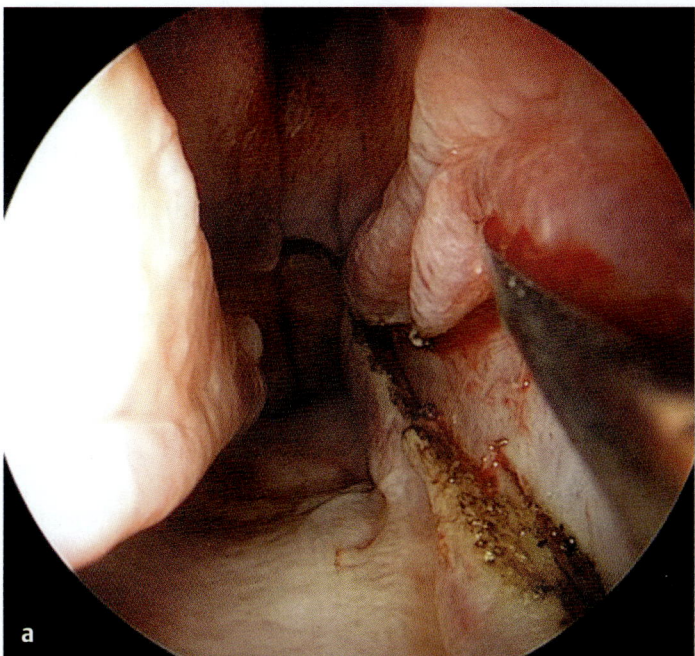

a

Fig. 5.9   Elevation of the mucoperiosteal flaps **(a)** inferiorly and **(b, c)** superiorly, using Freer's elevators (See **Fig. 10.2** in chapter 10). **(d)** Dislocation of the bony cartilaginous junction of the septum, allowing for posterior septectomy.

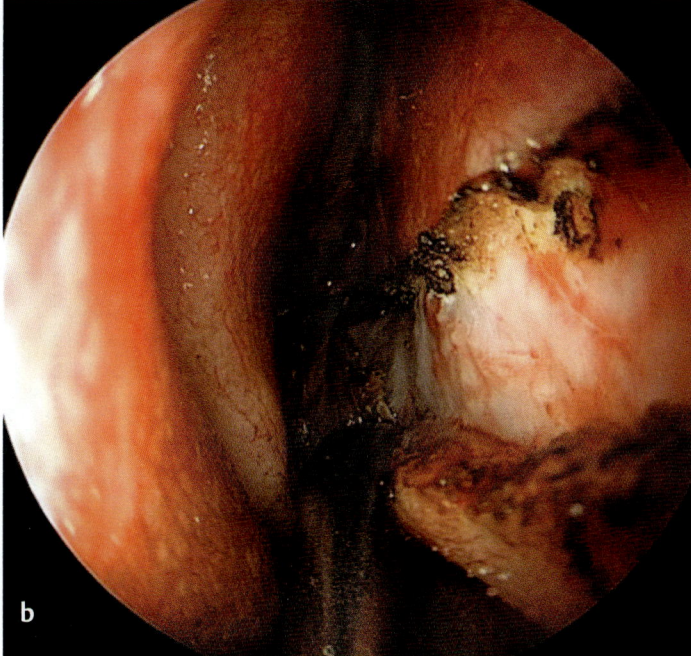

b

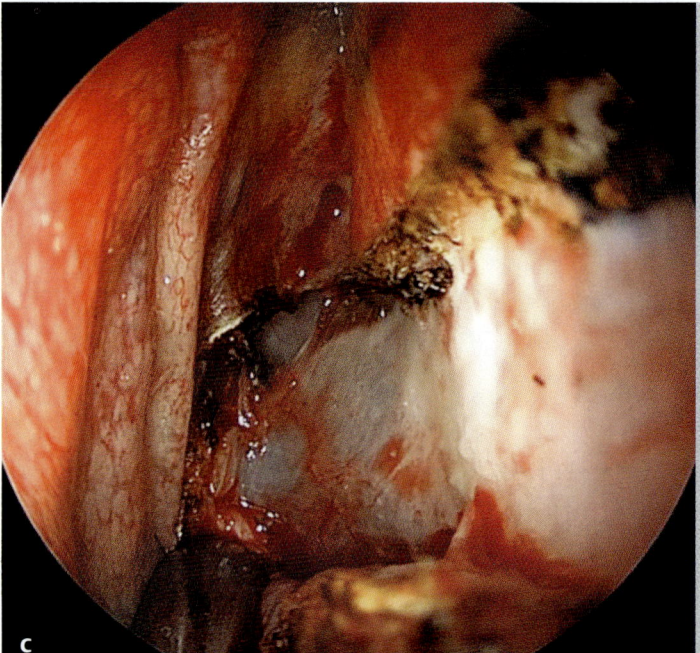

c

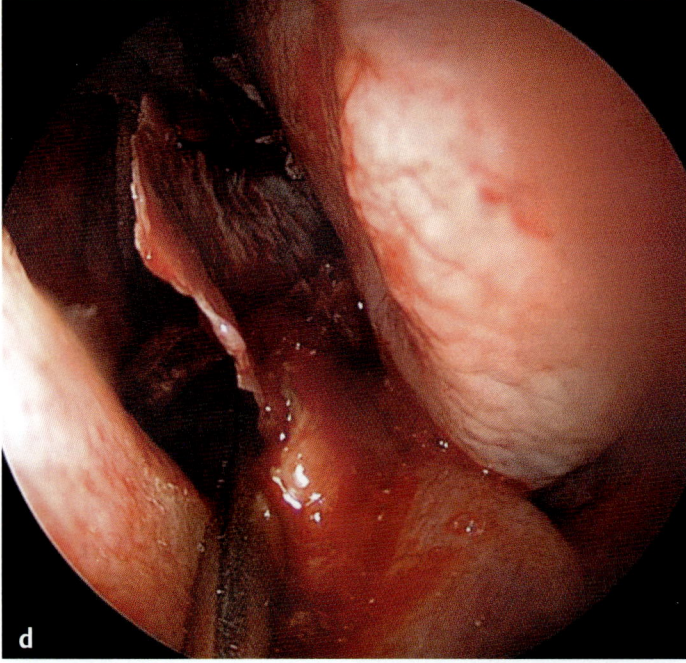

d

Fig. 5.9 Elevation of the mucoperiosteal flaps **(a)** inferiorly and **(b, c)** superiorly, using Freer's elevators (See **Fig. 10.2** in chapter 10). **(d)** Dislocation of the bony cartilaginous junction of the septum, allowing for posterior septectomy.

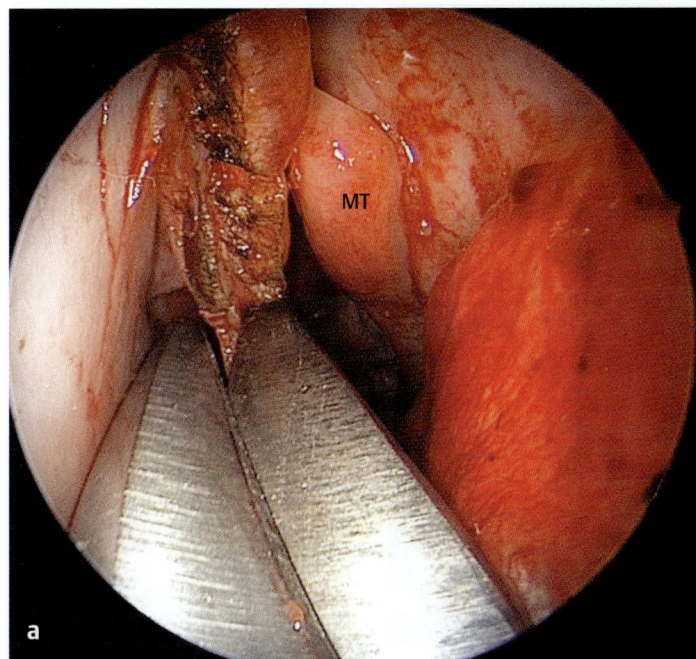

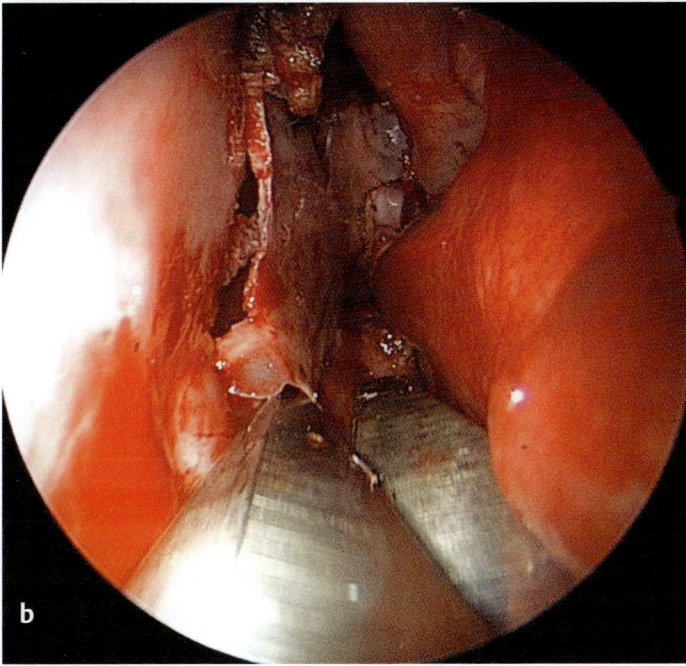

Fig. 5.10 **(a)** Controlled superior cut over the bony septum using turbinectomy scissors (See **Fig. 10.10** in chapter 10). MT, middle turbinate. **(b)** Inferior cut given by turbinectomy scissors.

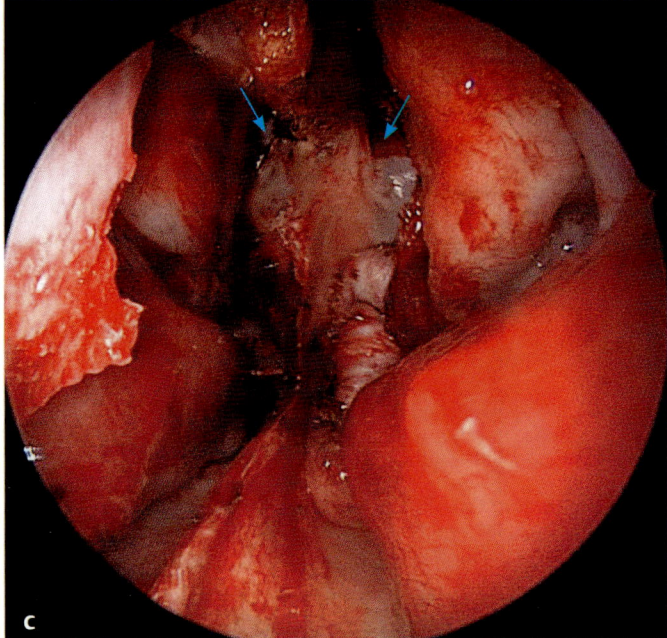

Fig. 5.10 **(c)** View after posterior septectomy, allowing for a binostril approach. Note the bilateral sphenoid ostia indicated by *blue arrows*.

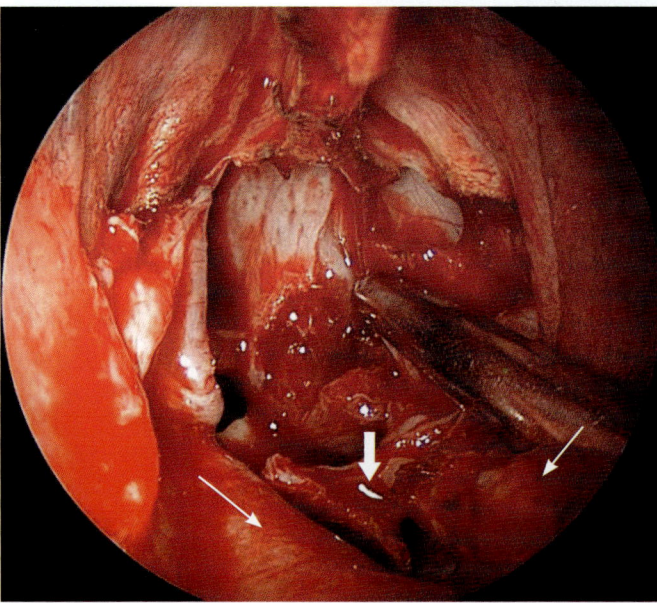

Fig. 5.11 Rescue flaps raised on both sides. The keel of the sphenoid is seen in the midline (*block white arrow*). The flaps can be pushed down and the instruments (in this picture, a suction), can be manoeuvred over the flaps (*thin white arrows*).

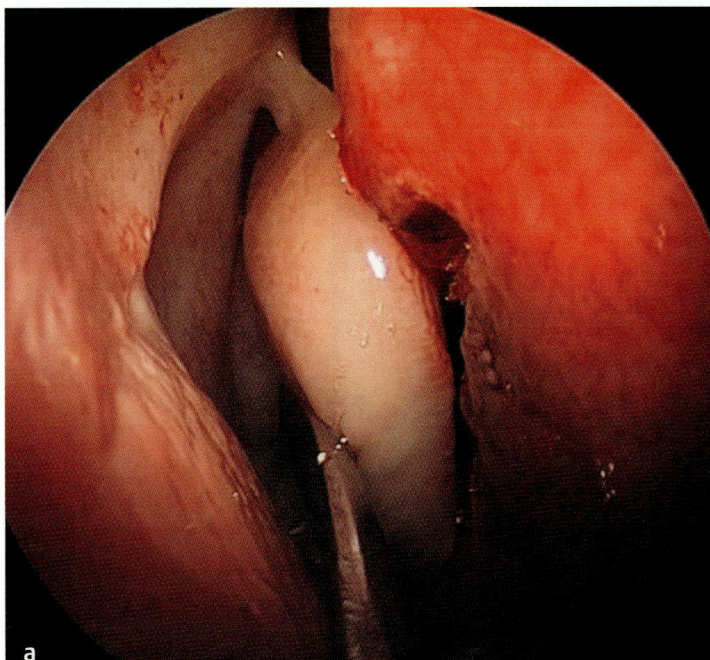

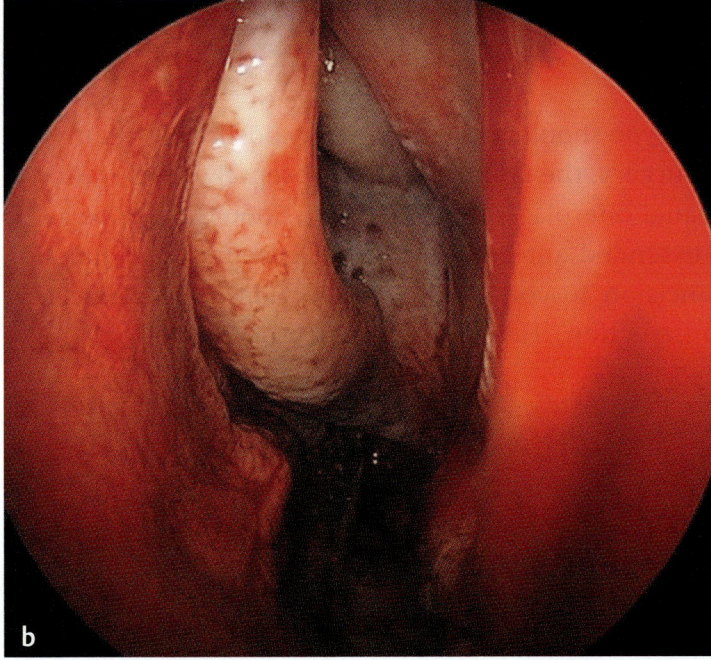

Fig. 5.12 (a, b) The rescue flaps and the middle turbinates being reposited on both sides at the end of the surgery. Note that there is very little exposed bone or raw area.

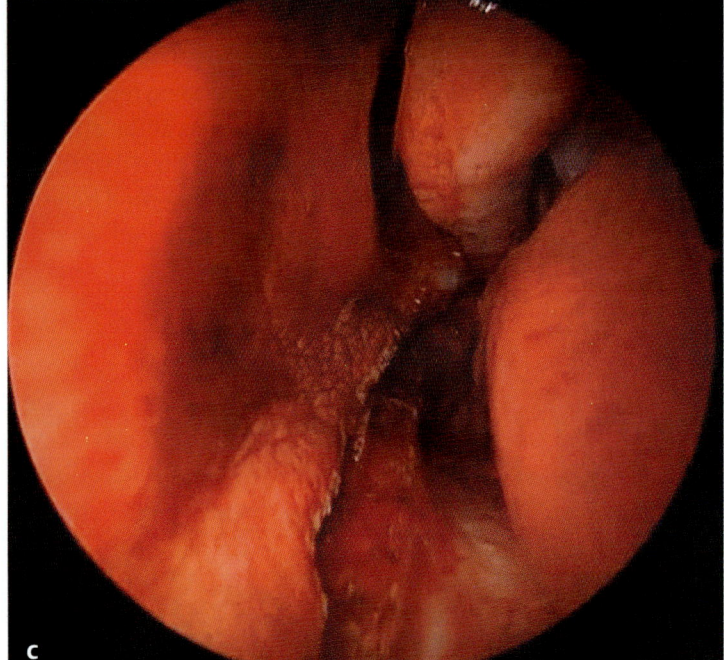

Fig. 5.12 (c) Posterior septum looks intact at the end of the surgery.

Once the flaps are raised, you should have complete exposure of the anterior sphenoid wall. In pituitary surgery, the landmark for nasoseptal flap elevation is usually the palatovaginal canal inferolaterally (**Fig. 5.13**). Should there be a CSF leak, the incisions can be extended anteriorly till the mucocutaneous junction and joined by a vertical incision to complete a Hadad flap on any one side (described in detail in reconstruction). Hence the name, rescue flap.

Sphenoidal Stage

Shoulder osteotomies are then made from the ostium downwards and then extended towards the sphenoid keel. This can be done using a drill (See **Fig. 10.8** in chapter 10) or osteotomes, (See **Fig 10.9** in chapter 10) (**Fig. 5.14**) and allows you to remove the rostrum with anterior wall in a large piece, which may be used for reconstruction. Once the sphenoid is opened, one will then have vision

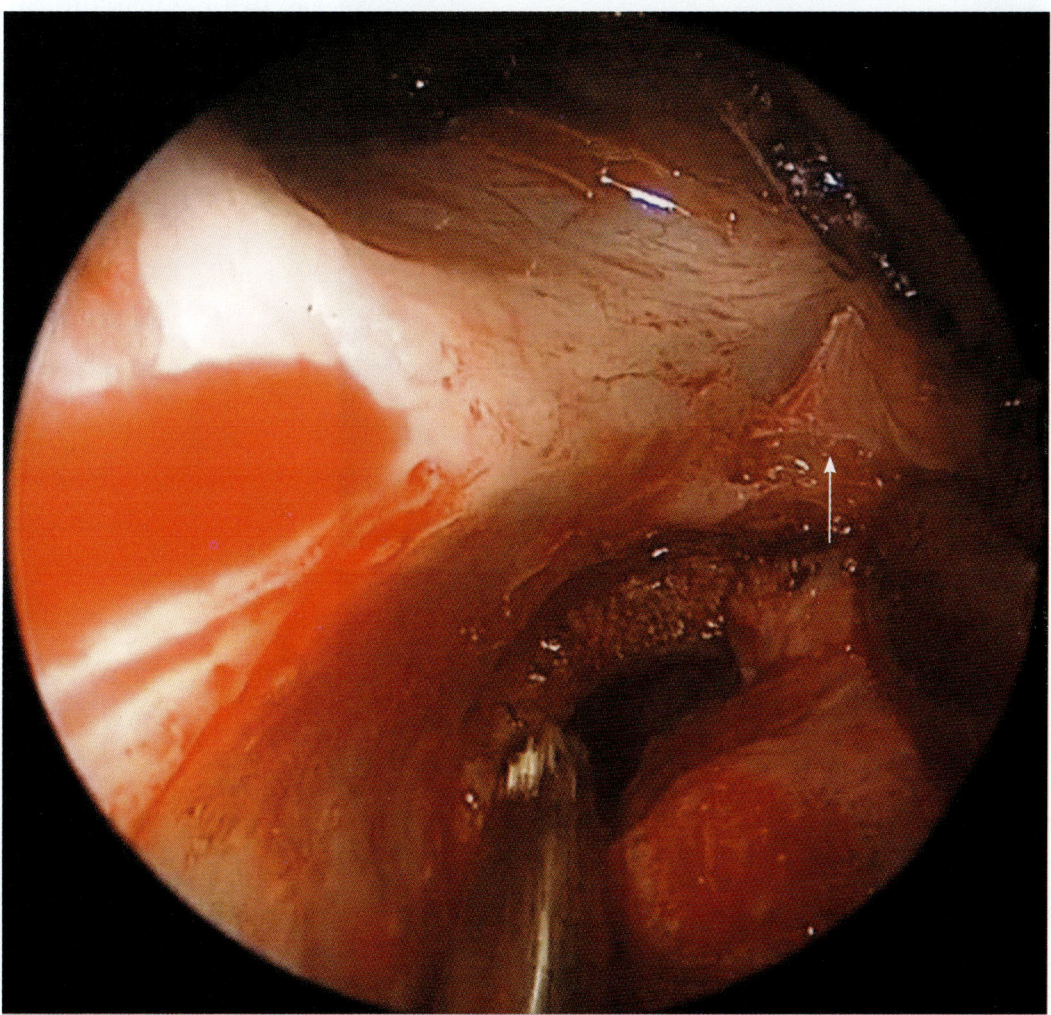

Fig. 5.13 The rescue flap/Hadad flap being raised up to the visualisation of the palatovaginal canal *(white arrow)* on the left side.

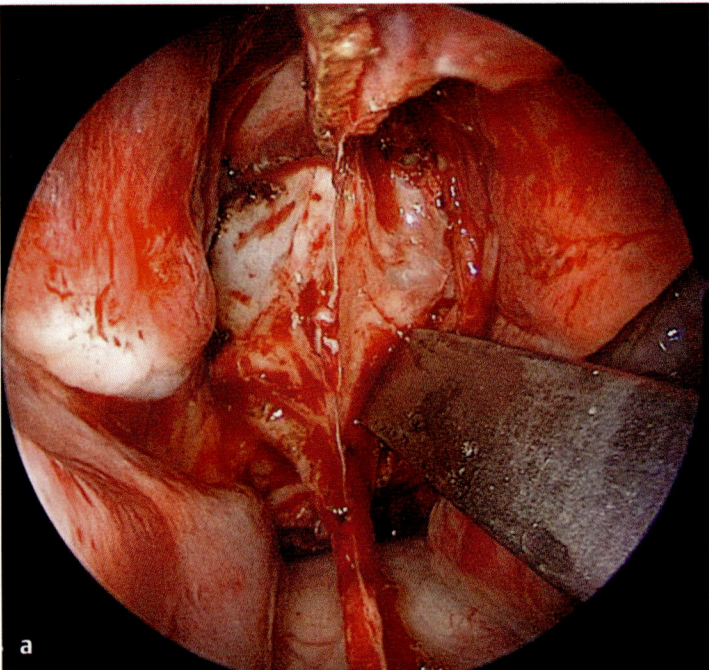

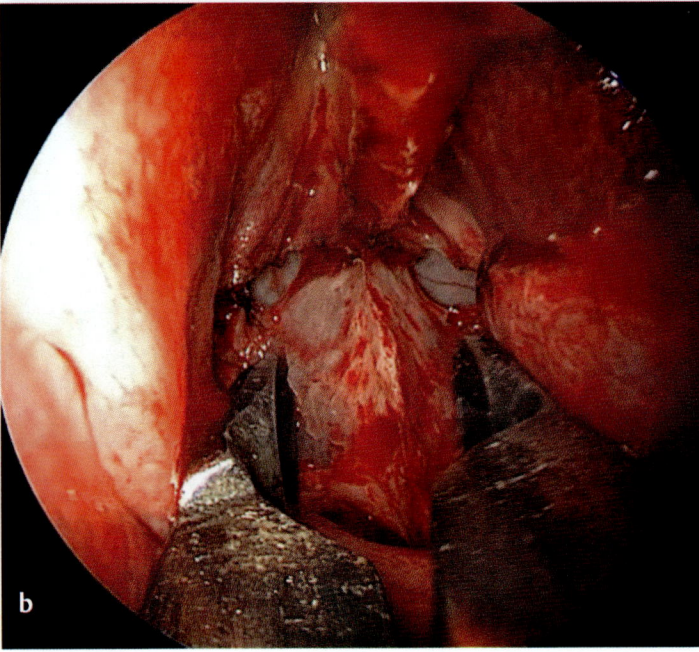

Fig.5.14 Removal of anterior wall of sphenoid using an osteotome (See **Fig. 10.9** in chapter 10) **(a)** and Luc's forceps (See **Fig. 10.4** in chapter 10) **(b)**.

of both sphenoid sinuses, and be able to appreciate the deviation of the inters-phenoid septum, presence of incomplete septations, and identify impressions of the optic canal, carotid artery, and lateral opticocarotid recess (OCR) (**Fig. 5.15**). These may be more apparent after removal of the sphenoid mucosa. It's impor-tant to remove mucosa from and around the sella to have a clear picture of the extent of sella and for safe bone removal in relation to the surrounding struc-tures (**Fig. 5.15**) (See **Figs. 10.5, 10.6, 10.7, 10.12** in chapter 10). If a Hadad flap is being used, we need to remove all the sphenoid mucosa, to allow placement of the flap on bare bone. One may often experience brisk bleeding on mucosa removal, but this is short lived, and stops after a few minutes. It also ceases with packing with cottonoids, and/or irrigation with warm saline.

If there are Onodi cells (sphenoethmoidal cells) present, then they must be opened to identify the optic canal and lateral OCR (**Fig. 5.16**). To do this, we insert an elevator (See **Fig. 10.2** in chapter 10) through the superior meatus and allow it to enter the posterior cell. One can then cut the inferior half of the superior turbinate, (See **Fig. 10.10** in chapter 10) and remove bone to communicate

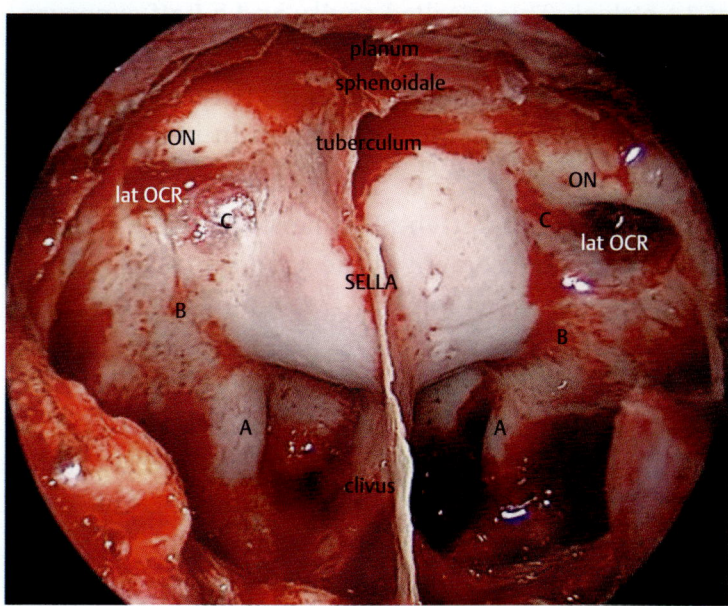

Fig. 5.15 Posterior wall of the sphenoid sinus after removal of the mucosa. After removal of the mucosa, the structures on its wall become more prominent. A, paraclival carotid; B, cavernous carotid; C, paraclinoid carotid; ON: optic nerve; lat OCR, lateral opticocarotid recess.

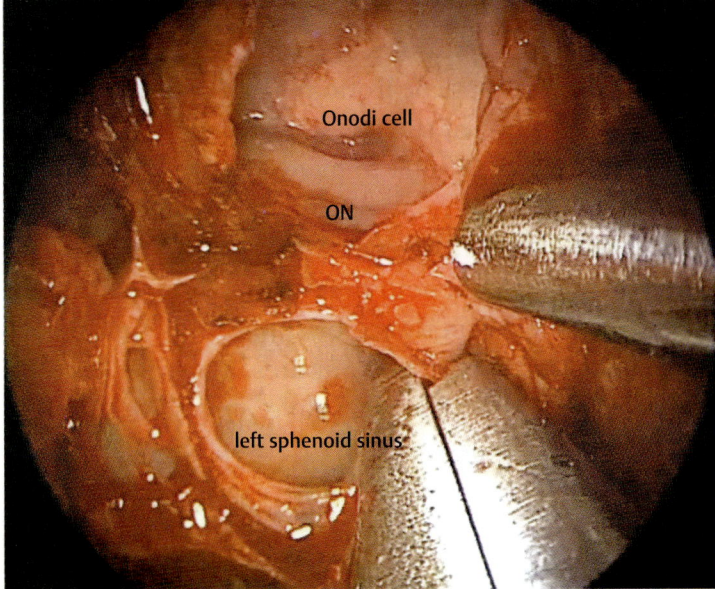

Onodi cell

ON

left sphenoid sinus

Fig. 5.16 The anterior wall of the left sphenoid sinus being opened by Kerrison's punch (See **Fig. 10.13** in chapter 10). The Onodi cell is seen on the top left corner just above the straight suction. ON, optic nerve.

the Onodi cell/posterior ethmoids with the sphenoid. This is also done when planum exposure is required, or space is at a premium, as it provides parking space for the endoscope at 11 o'clock. This is called **cavity and a half** exposure.[1] Exposure of the Onodi cells and the posterior ethmoid cells is important when the sphenoid is filled with pathology and orientation and identification of the landmarks become difficult. Posterior ethmoidectomy helps in identifying the orbital apex and trace the optic nerve until the sphenoid.

Once the exposure seems adequate, flatten all sphenoidal septa to allow ease of movement of instruments and placement of the naso-septal flap should it be required. This can be done using either a 3- or 4-mm diamond drill (See **Fig. 10.8** in chapter 10) or thru-cut forceps (**Fig. 5.17**) (See **Fig. 10.11** in chapter 10). Exposure is complete when one can visualise easily both the lateral OCRs, tuberculum, and planum (**Fig. 5.15**). Laterally, a straight suction (See **Fig. 10.12** in chapter 10) should be able to get lateral to the ipsilateral carotid. One also needs at least two suction widths under the sella bulge, and some amount of clivus may occasionally require drilling to achieve this. This will allow free movement of instruments and make surgery safer and easier.

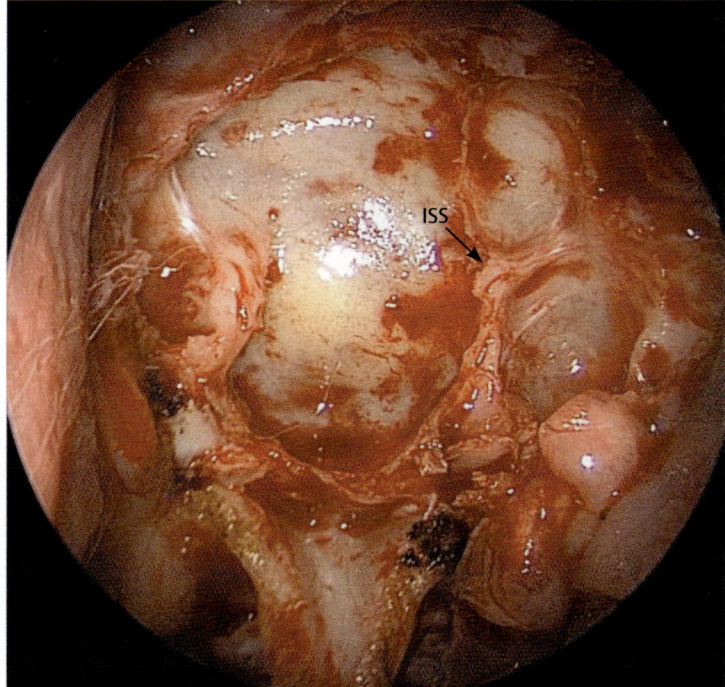

Fig. 5.17 Exposure of the sella after removing the anterior sphenoid wall and drilling of the intersphenoid septae (ISS) (*thin black arrow*).

Sellar Stage

The next step is to remove bone over the sella bulge. The bone over the sella bulge may be deficient or thinned out owing to the pressure of the tumour. In such cases, we use Kerrison's Rounger punch (See **Fig. 10.13** in chapter 10) to remove the sella bone. If the sellar floor is intact, we prefer circumferential opening with drill using a 3-mm diamond burr (**Fig. 5.18**) (See **Fig. 10.8** in chapter 10), as it is safer and avoids injury to the venous lakes and sinuses, and good exposure of medial wall of both the cavernous sinuses can be obtained. One may also use Kerrison's punches (**Fig. 5.19**) to remove bone, especially at the periphery, once it has been thinned by the burr. For extended approaches, we drill anterior to the planum sphenoidale for anterior fossa pathology and down on the clivus inferior as required depending on the extent of the tumour (described in detail in Chapter 6).

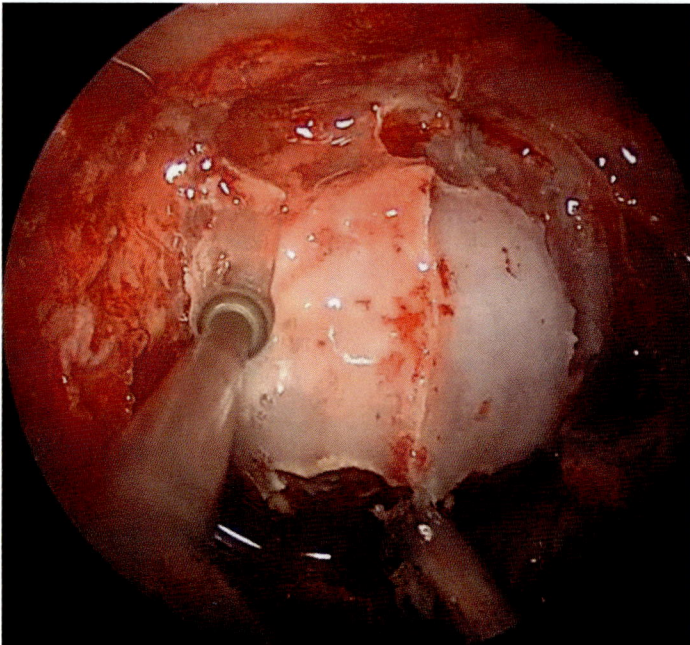

Fig. 5.18 Circumferential drilling of the sella being done using a 3-mm diamond drill (See **Fig. 10.8** in chapter 10).

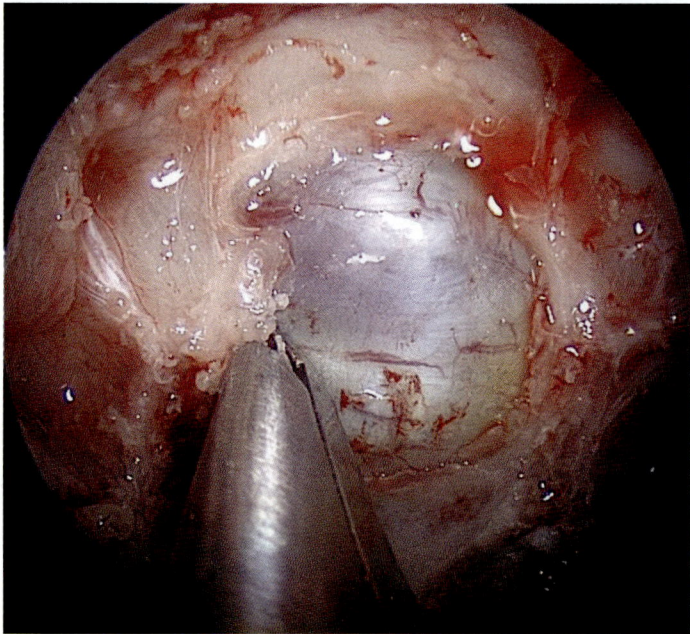

Fig. 5.19 After removal of the sellar bone, dural bulge can be seen through the bony defect. For a wider exposure, one can use a Kerrison punch (See **Fig. 10.13** in chapter 10) for removing the peripheral sellar bone.

Exposure is deemed complete when you have the **4 blue** sign. This is, cavernous edges laterally, and intercavernous sinus edge below and above the sella (**Fig. 5.20**). If bleeding from the cavernous is encountered, it will stop with cotton pledgets, use of Surgicel® or Gelfoam®. If the bleeding is persistent, or as an option, one could use Surgiflo® or Floseal®. These solutions are expensive, but the advantage is, after haemostasis, the excess material is washed away from the site, and does not cause visual obstruction of distal structures.

The process of tumour removal is always a two-surgeon, four-hand, binostril approach. The ENT surgeon now holds the endoscope and will navigate the field of view. His second hand may irrigate (if not using clear vision or Endoscrub) or assist with an instrument. The neurosurgeon can use both hands—the left with a suction and the right with the instrument of choice to aid tumour removal. This is of course for right-handed surgeons. Surgeon positioning depends on the comfort of the team. It is our practise to stand on the same (right) side of the

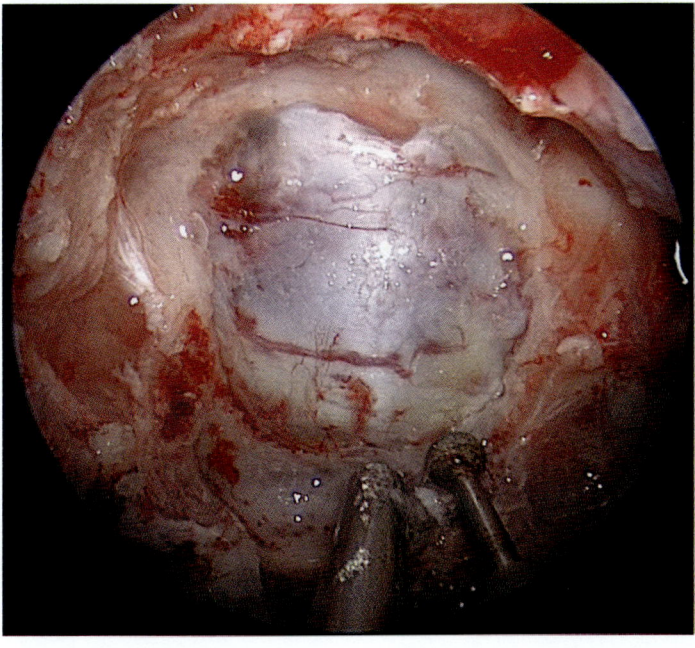

Fig. 5.20 Exposure of the sellar dura after removal of the sellar bone.

patient, with the ENT towards the head end. One may use one or two monitors on the opposite side (**Fig. 5.21**). Other teams may stand opposite each other using two monitors or one at the head end.

Dural Stage

In the early days, we started with crisscross dural incision in the form of (X) (**Fig. 5.22**) using a No. 15 surgical blade or a retractable dural knife (See **Figs. 10.15, 10.22** in chapter 10). Such an incision avoids injury to the four blues. But the crisscross incisions made it difficult to retract the dura comfortably for tumour removal. This also resulted in some of the tumour being hidden behind the dural flap. Therefore, we shifted to Y-shaped incision. This shape of incision avoids injury to the superior intercavernous sinus. It also avoids CSF leak at the junction of the anterior attachment of the sella dura and the diaphragm.

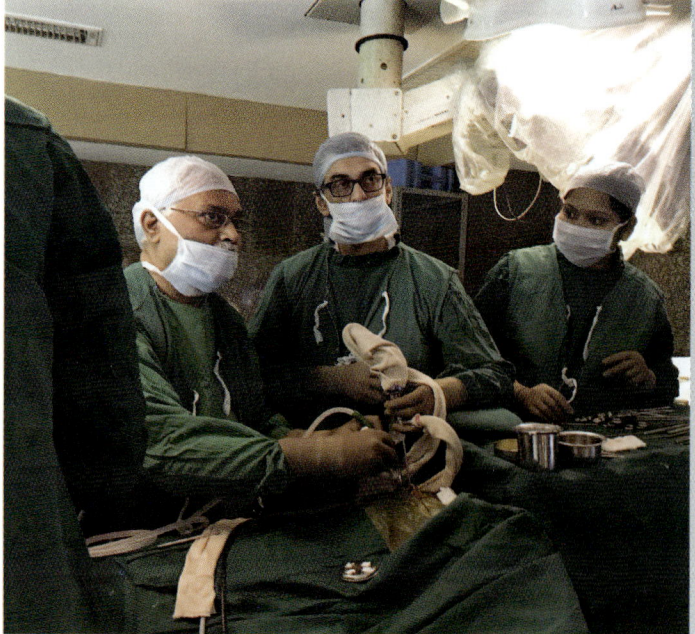

Fig. 5.21 Position of the surgeons. The otolaryngologist stands close to the head end, holding the endoscope, while the neurosurgeon works with both hands via binostril approach.

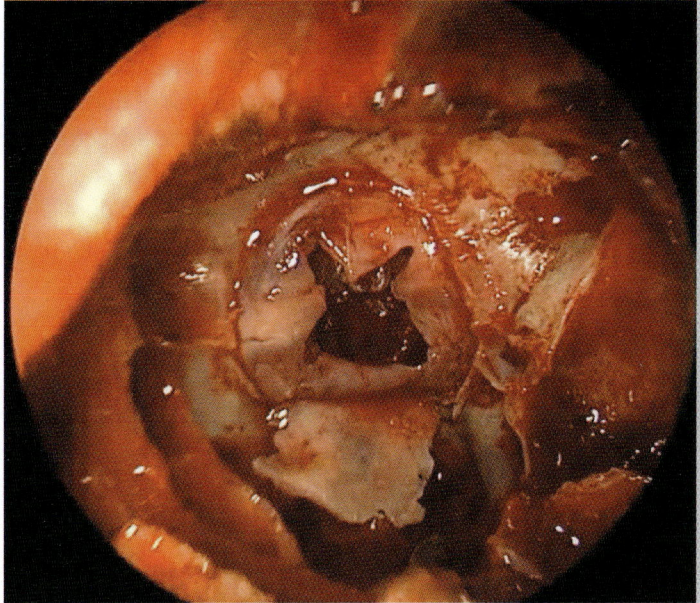

Fig. 5.22 Image showing cruciate dural incision.

Over a period of time, we moved onto deep U incision with no inferior limb. The superior flap can then be safely retracted, using a disc dissector (See **Fig. 10.16** in chapter 10).

The dura is usually incised as a low U-shaped flap, but the neurosurgeon may use a variety of preferred incisions such as the cruciate, cross, pi (π), etc (**Fig. 5.23**). Once the dura is peeled away from the tumour, a biopsy may be taken to send for histopathology (See **Fig. 10.19** in chapter 10).

Tumour removal may then be extracapsular or intracapsular. Usually, pituitary tumours, which are pulpy, can be debulked with suction alone (See **Figs. 10.12, 10.17, 10.19** in chapter 10). An extracapsular removal is desired as it ensures complete tumour removal. However this may be difficult if the tumour is very soft or very firm. In soft tumours, suction alone is sufficient. In very firm tumours, an extracapsular dissection can slightly increase the risk of getting a CSF leak as decompression of the tumour prior to removal may be difficult. With increasing experience, the extracapsular technique becomes easier and usually the favoured approach (**Fig. 5.24**).

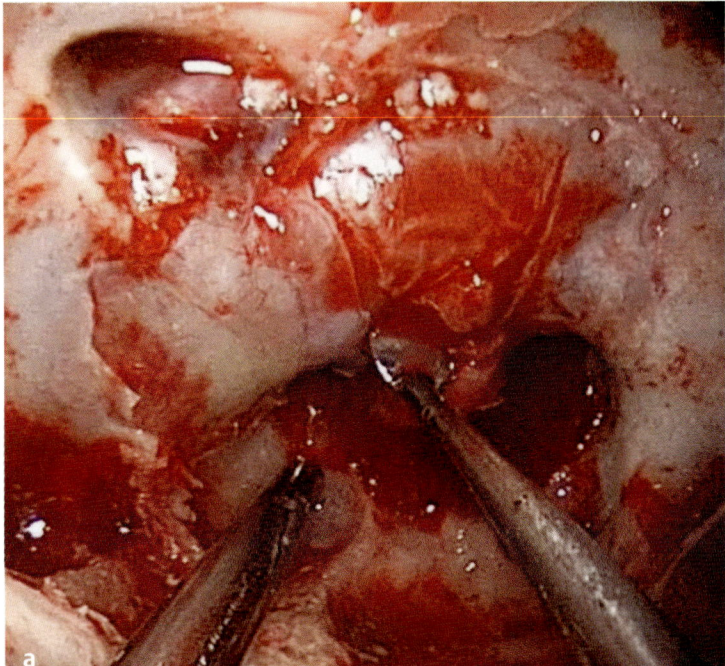

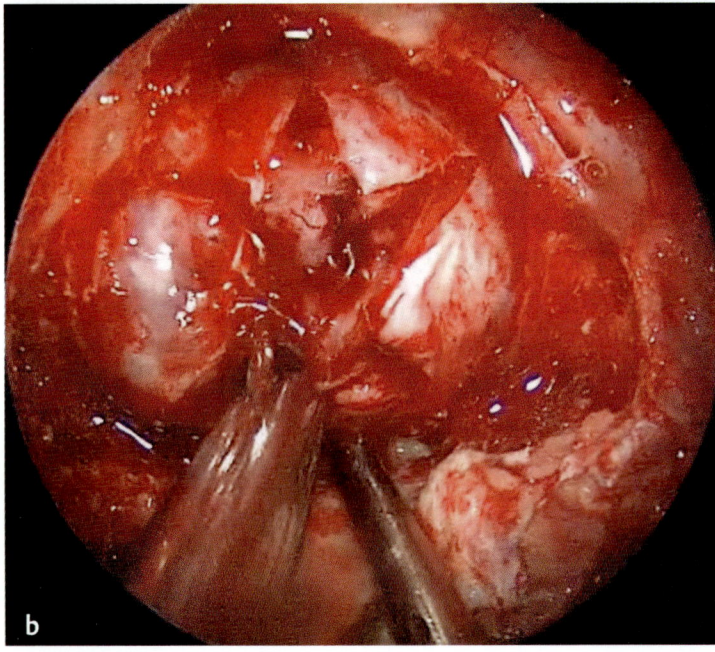

Fig. 5.23 **(a–c)** Various types of dural incision, and elevation of dural flap using disc dissectors (See **Fig. 10.16** in chapter 10). **(a)** U-shaped dural incision. **(b)** Star-shaped/stellar dural incision.

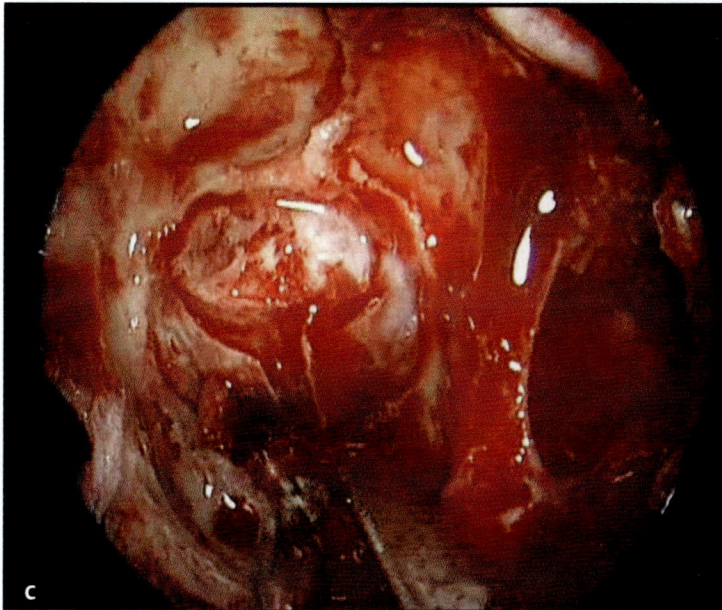

Fig. 5.23 (c) Y-shaped dural incision.

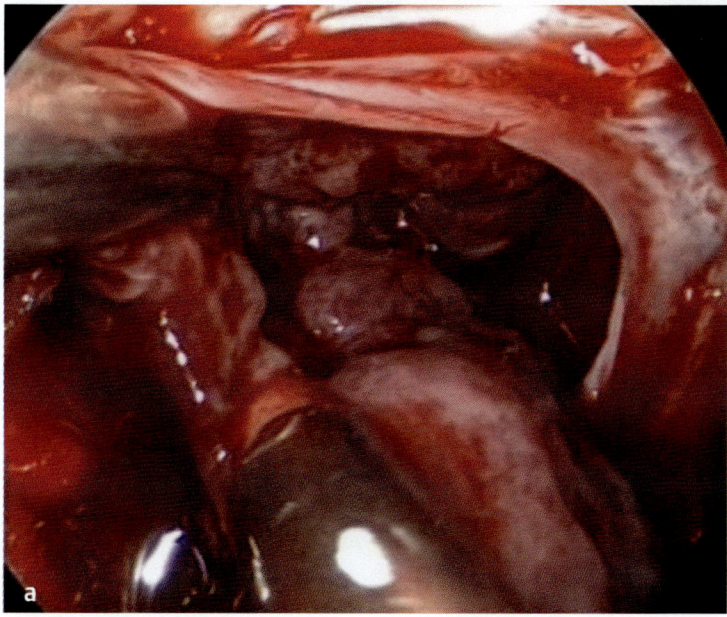

Fig. 5.24 (a–c) Picture showing extracapsular tumour dissection in case of pituitary tumour.

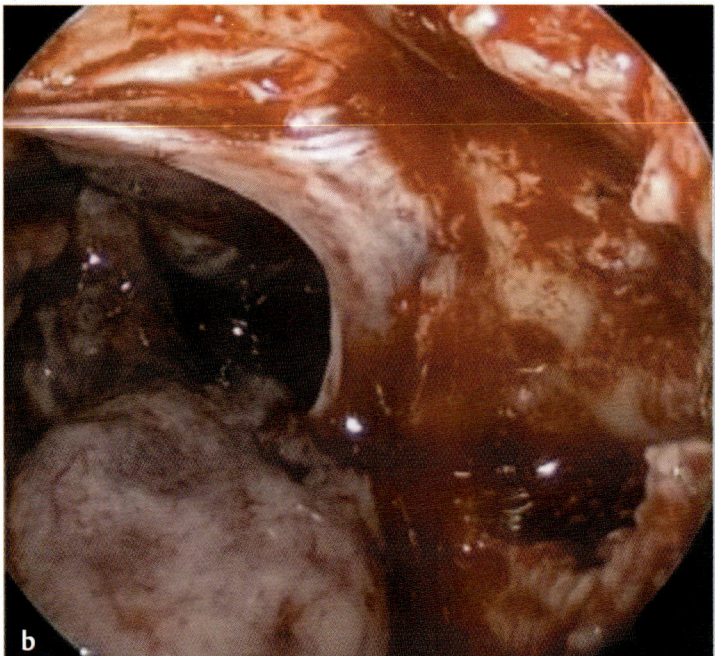

Fig. 5.24 **(a–c)** Picture showing extracapsular tumour dissection in case of pituitary tumour.

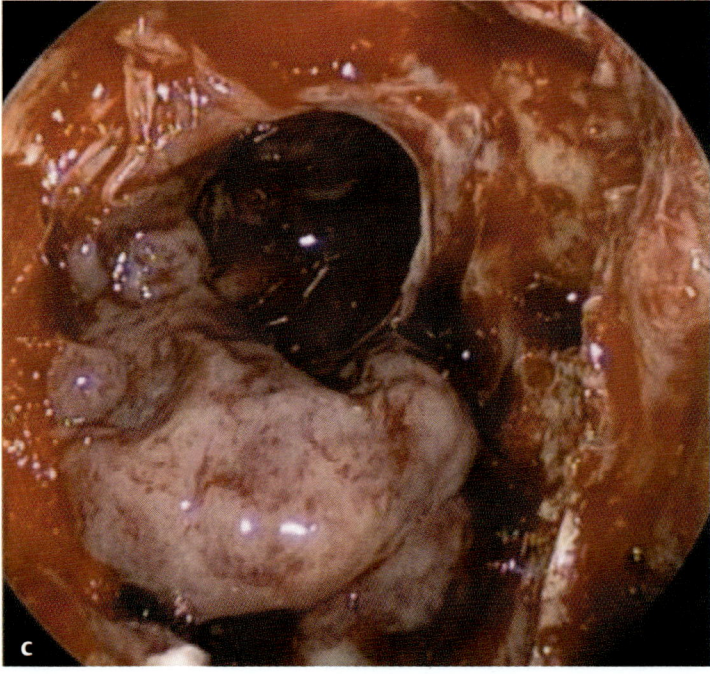

The advantage of an extracapsular excision is that one is more certain of complete tumour removal; however, there is also an increased risk of bleeding from the cavernous sinus. In an intracapsular excision, one is safer in terms of bleeding and CSF; however, there is an increased possibility of leaving behind residual tumour. In both situations, after incision of the dura, some amount of tumour is taken for biopsy and to decompress the lesion.

When doing an extracapsular excision, we have to find the plane between the dura and the pseudocapsule of the tumour (**Fig. 5.24**). One can then proceed to go around the tumour, decompressing as necessary, until the entire tumour has been delivered. The surgeons must be gentle and patient whilst dissecting to avoid the above complications, as well as to maintain the plane of dissection.

With an intracapsular dissection, one continues with tumour decompression within the tumour capsule using suction, curettes, or forceps (See **Figs. 10.12, 10.17, 10.18, 10.19, 10.20** in chapter 10) (**Fig. 5.25**).

Tumour decompression follows a sequence. Removal always starts inferiorly, then continues laterally towards the cavernous walls, and finally superiorly, but from a posterior to anterior direction, to prevent premature descent of the diaphragm sella. Early supero-anterior dissection results in the diaphragm coming down early and restricting vision and hampering proper dissection and removal of posterior and lateral tumour (**Fig. 5.26**). During dissection from the lateral and the superior walls, one can usually start seeing the normal pituitary gland (**Fig. 5.27**). A good idea of the position of the normal pituitary gland can be obtained pre-operatively from the MRI scans (T1W images, post-contrast) (**Fig. 5.28**). The walls of the cavernous sinus dura can be well identified with pulsations of the internal carotid artery. Extension of the tumor in the cavernous sinus is best removed by curved suction introduced from the opposite side.

Dissection from the diaphragm should also be carefully done so that the pituitary stalk is not disturbed. In a large tumour, one may have to retract the diaphragm upwards to make sure that tumour from posteriormost part of the cavity, in the recess just above the dorsum sella can be removed.

Conventionally, surgeons used angled curettes for tumour removal (See **Fig. 10.18** in chapter 10); this is now changing to the increased use of suctions (See **Figs. 10.12, 10.17, 10.20** in chapter 10). Part of the reason is better exposure

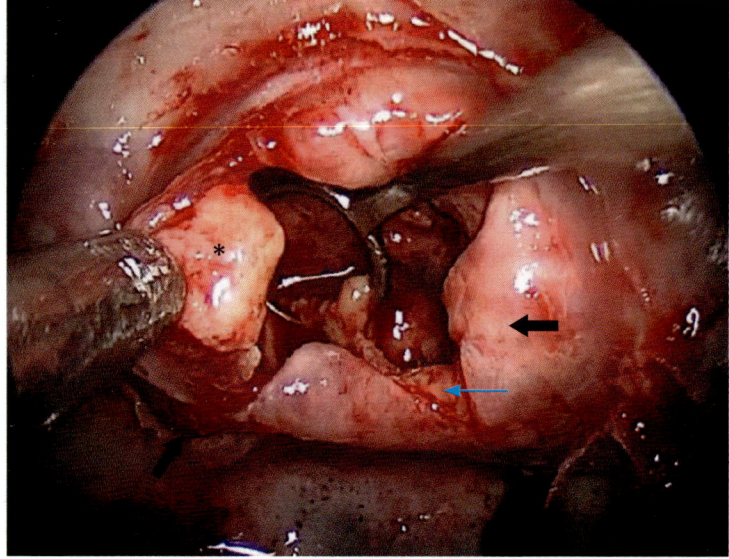

Fig. 5.25 Intra-operative picture of intracapsular dissection of tumour (*), using ring curette and keyhole suction (See **Figs. 10.12, 10.18** in chapter 10). The capsule of the tumour is marked by *blue arrow. Black arrow* is on the dura.

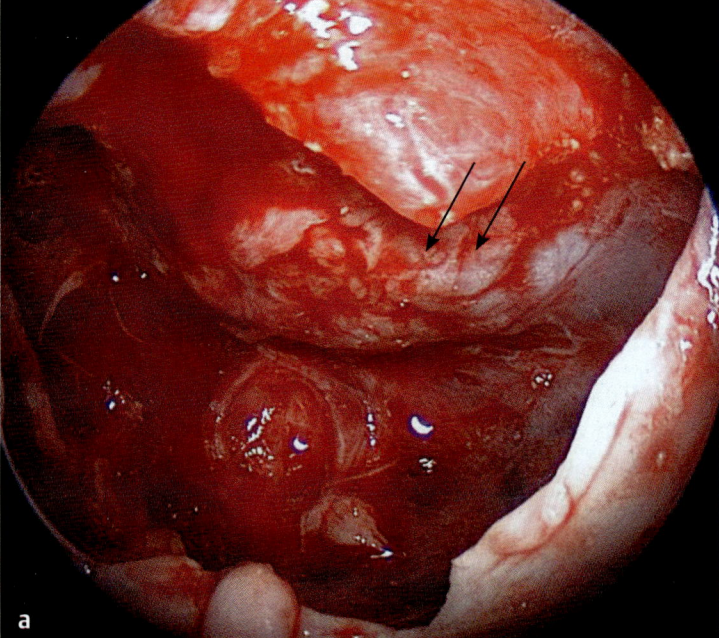

Fig. 5.26 **(a)** The diaphragm marked by two *thin black arrows* is seen prolapsing through the sella after tumour removal.

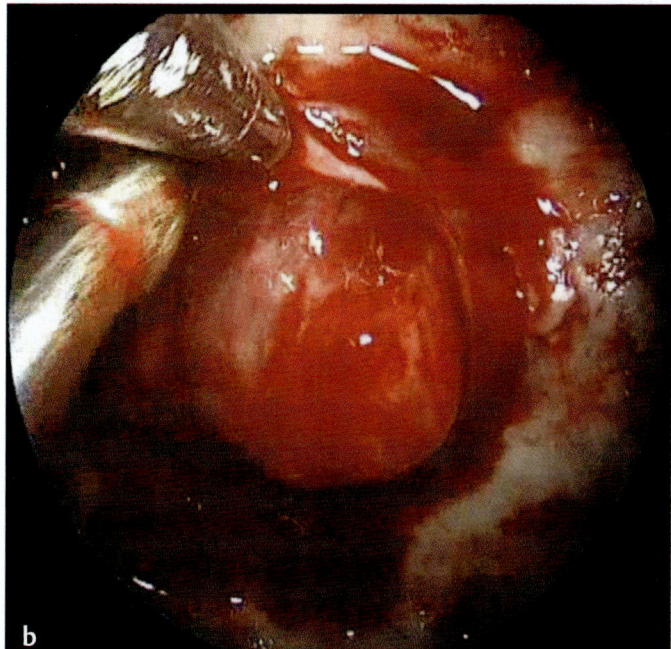

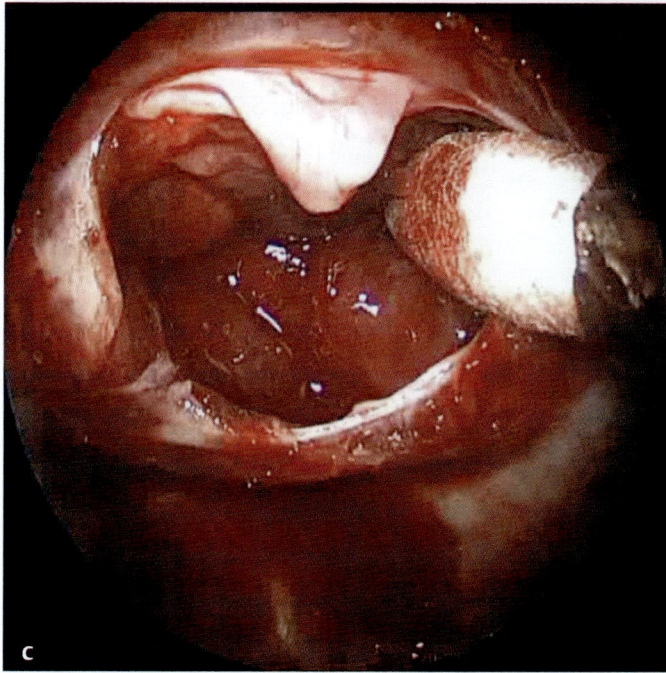

Fig. 5.26 **(b)** Such untimely descent obscures further view of the sella and the suprasellar region. **(c)** The descended diaphragm is being retracted with the help of a cotton swab loaded on a straight suction. The posterior wall of the sella now comes into view.

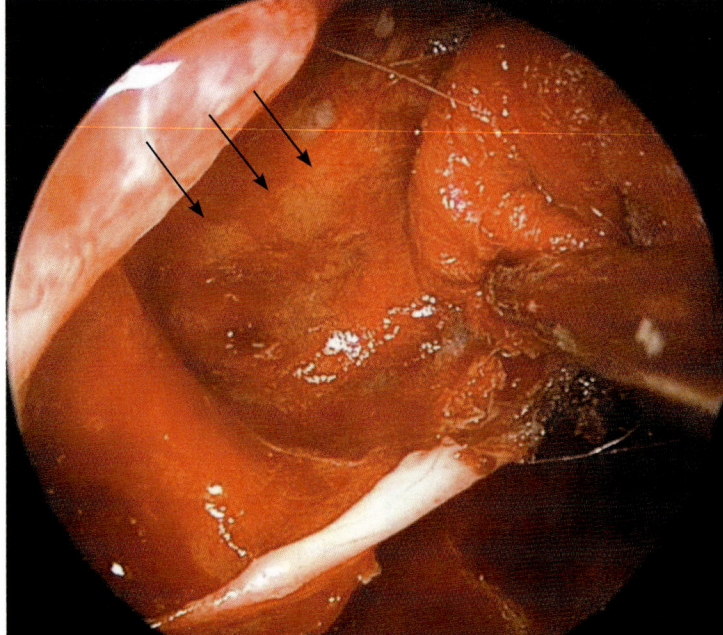

Fig. 5.27 The sellar cavity is seen after tumour removal. The normal pituitary gland with a slightly yellow hue is seen at the postero-superior wall on the right (*thin black arrows*). The cavernous carotid prominence is seen in this picture from 7 to 9 o'clock position.

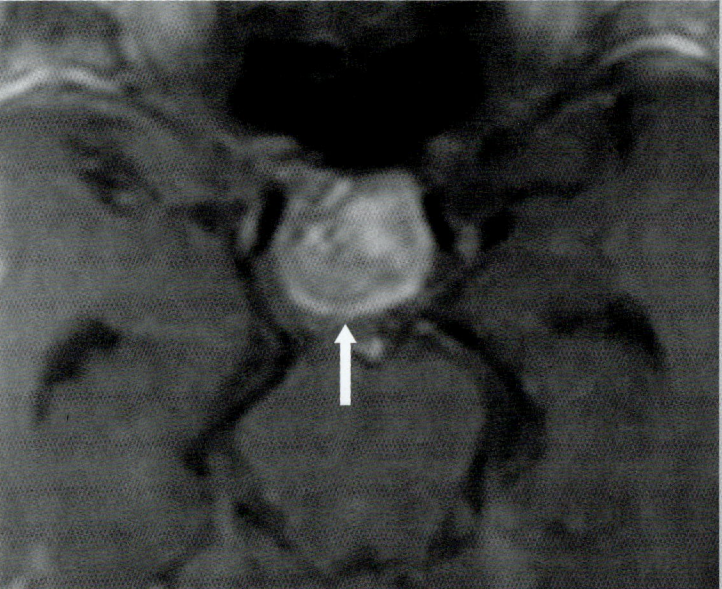

Fig. 5.28 MR T1-weighted post-contrast image of the same patient as shown in **Fig. 5.27**. The normal pituitary gland is seen as a bright curvilinear line seen on the right (*white block arrow*), posterior to the tumour.

from bone removal and also better vision from the endoscope. This allows for tumour removal under vision as against the blind curettage of earlier days. The magnification and ability to look around corners with the endoscope also ensures more complete tumour removal with fewer complications.

<u>Dissection of microadenomas:</u> For microadenomas, a different approach has to be taken. Precise location of the adenomas is pre-operatively indicated by magnetic resonance imaging (MRI) scans, which is explored and the normal gland is left untouched (**Fig. 5.29**). Rarely, a portion of the normal gland close to the adenoma may be removed, especially for Cushing's disease.

Once tumour removal is complete, it is vital to achieve good haemostasis prior to closure. It is not a good idea to overpack a cavity with Gelfoam® or Surgicel® as this may result in pressure on the cavernous sinus or optic nerves. On the other hand, neither it is advisable to leave the cavity without any haemostatic agent as a haematoma formation can also result in a similar complication. Haemostasis can be achieved with minimal packing, bipolar cautery, or irrigation with warm saline. One may also use Floseal® or Surgiflo® (**Fig. 5.30**).

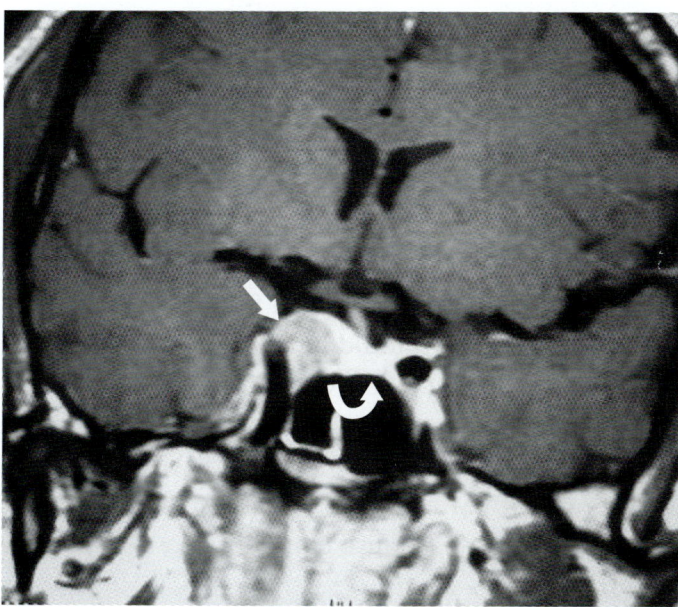

Fig. 5.29 Post-contrast T1-weighted MR scan in a secretory microadenoma (Cushing's disease) showing the tumour on the right side of the normal pituitary gland is marked by (*straight white block arrow*) marked by increased uptake of the contrast (*curved white arrow*). The pituitary stalk is seen clearly. It is necessary to delineate the tumour from the normal pituitary on pre-operative scans so that the dural incision can be pre-planned.

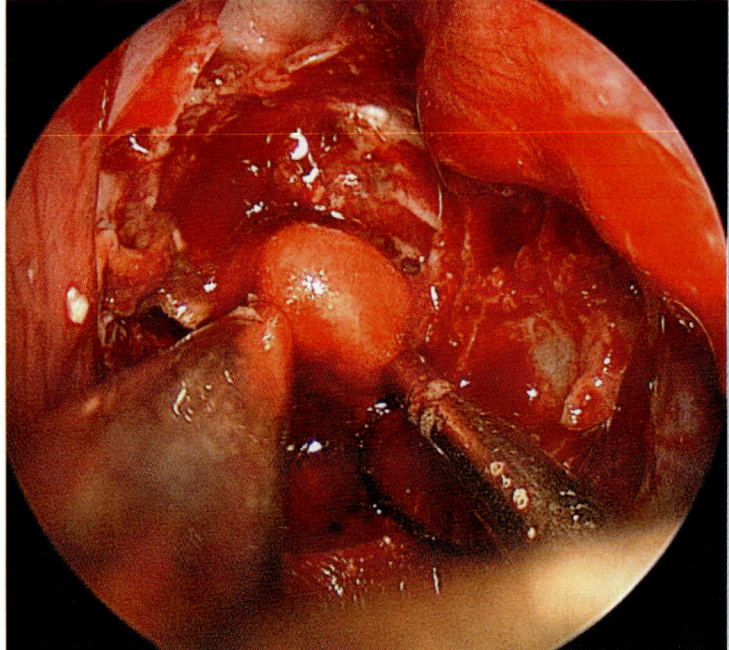

Fig. 5.30 Floseal® is being used as a haemostatic agent for left cavernous sinus bleed.

Reconstruction

If there has been no CSF leak and requisite haemostasis achieved, it is not essential to close the sella cavity. If desired, one may put a single layer of Gelfoam® or Surgicel® (**Fig. 5.31**). Alternatively, one could also use a bone flap or mucosa or mucoperiosteum to close the cavity (**Fig. 5.32**). This is of course crucial if there has been a CSF leak. Level 1 leaks can be easily closed with fat and glue or periosteum/fascia and glue (**Fig. 5.33**). Larger leaks should be closed with a pedicled vascular flap such as the HB flap. In the absence of a vascularised septal flap, a multilayer repair is done (**Fig. 5.34**). Useful materials include fat, fascia, mucoperiosteum, bone, cartilage, and tissue glue. The HB flap or vascularised pedicled septal flap has become the workhorse of CSF repair and reconstruction due to its robustness and ability to take up within 72 hours compared to 5 days for a free flap.

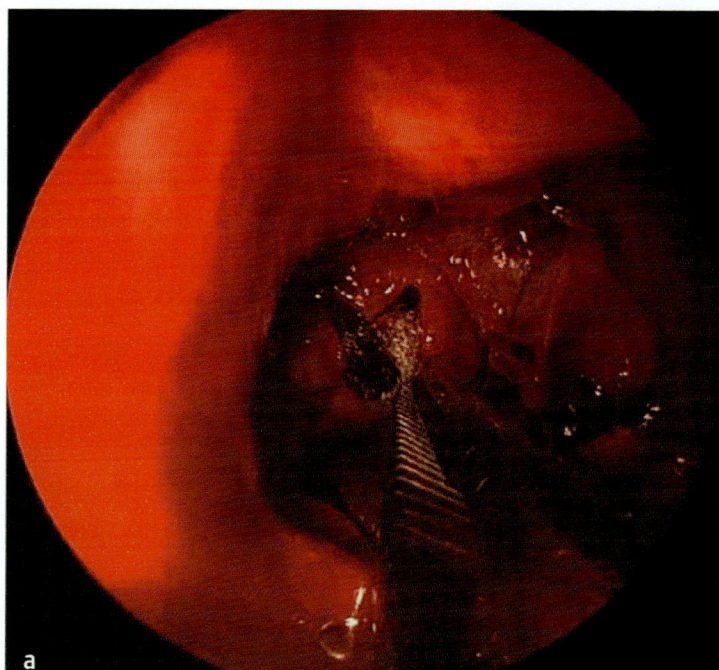

Fig. 5.31 (a, b) After complete removal of tumour and with no CSF leak, the sella is packed with a single layer of Surgicel®.

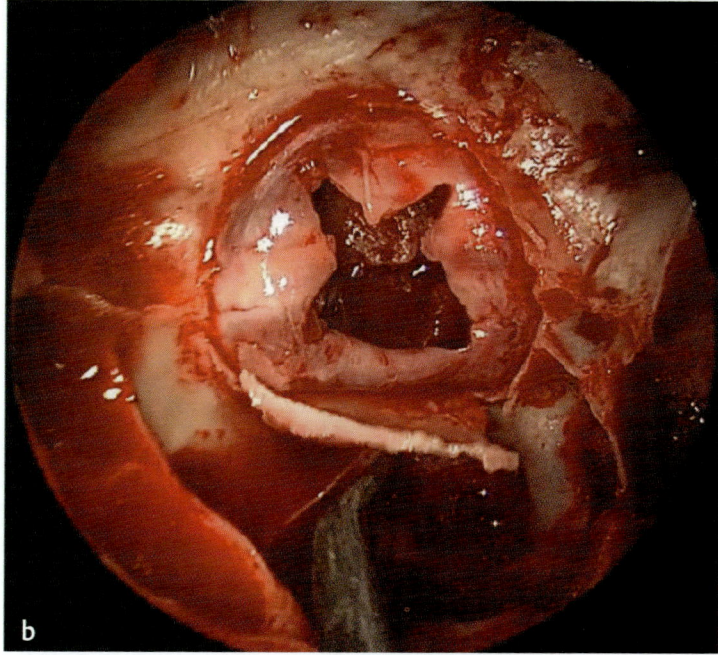

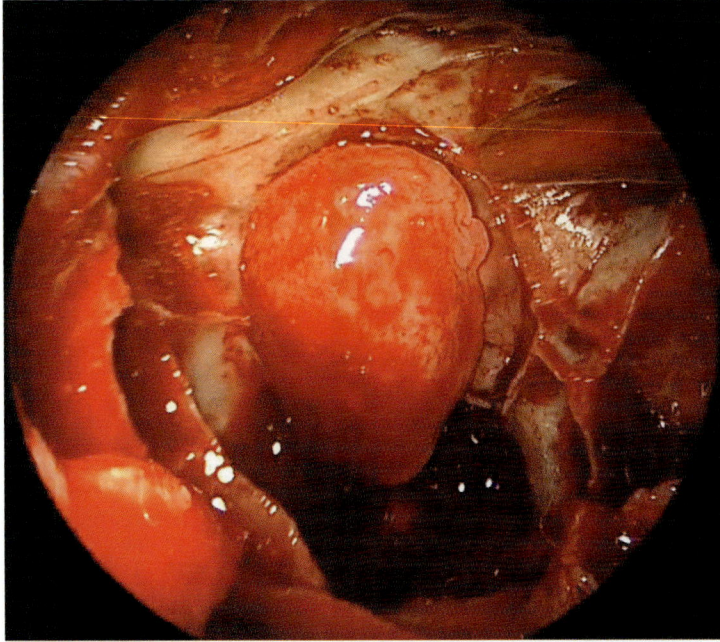

Fig. 5.32 In this case, bone with periosteum from a middle turbinate conchoplasty, is being used to close the sella. The conchal bone graft is being used from earlier conchoplasty.

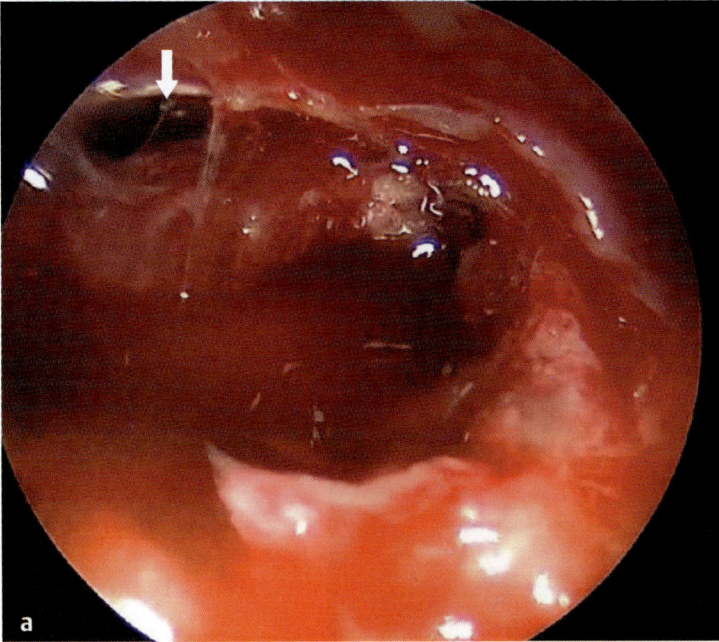

Fig. 5.33 **(a)** Dural defect seen in diaphragm sellae at the end of pituitary tumour dissection (*white block arrow*).

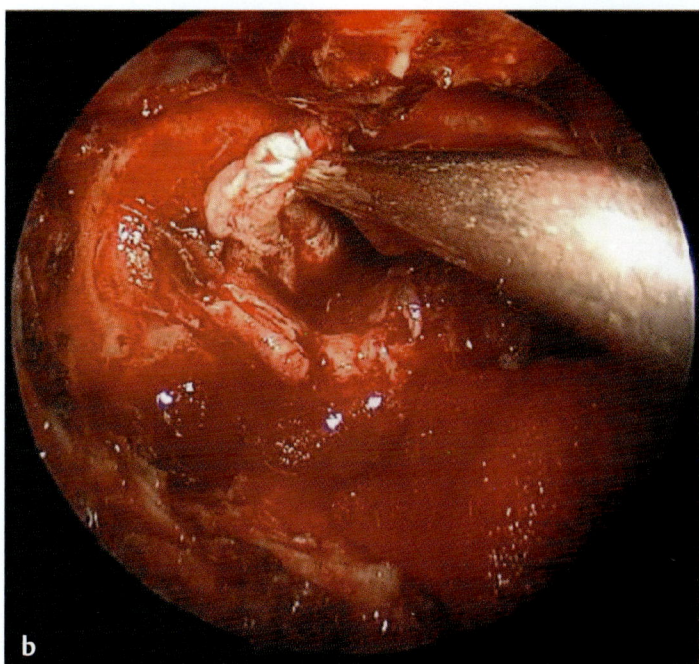

Fig. 5.33 (b, c) The same defect is being closed by fascia lata **(b)** and fat **(c)**.

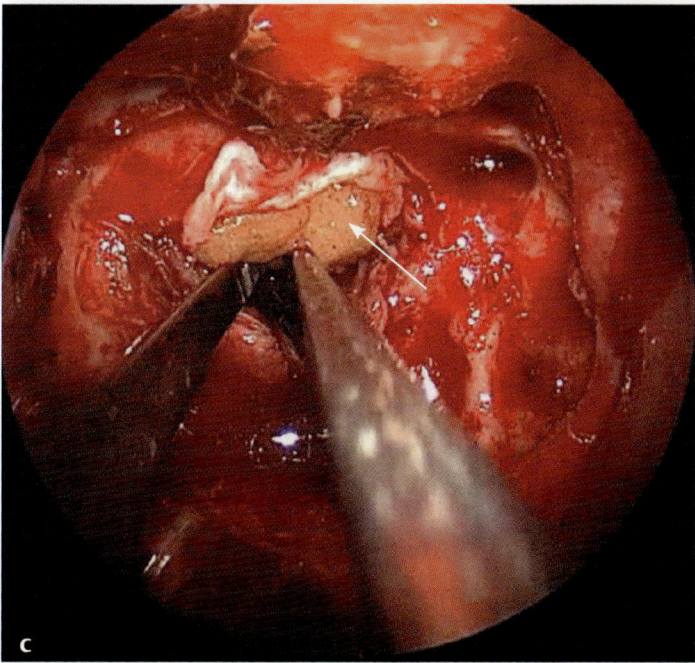

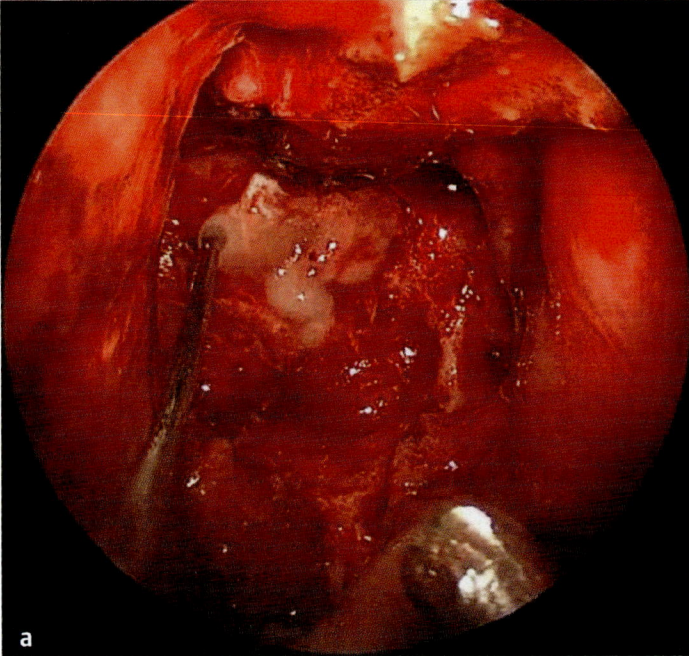

Fig. 5.34 **(a, b)** After the dural defect is plugged with fascia and fat as shown in **Fig. 5.33**, the reconstruction is sealed with glue **(a)** and reinforced with mini Hadad flap **(b)**.

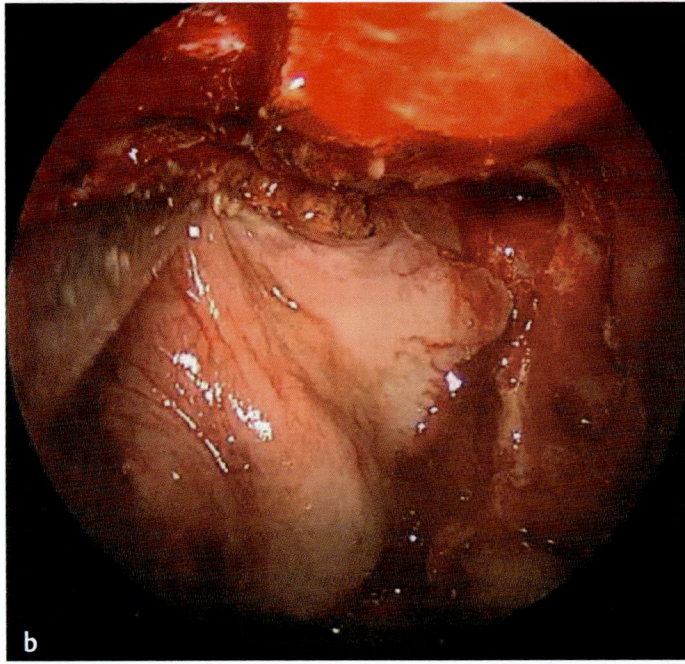

Nasoseptal flap (HB flap): The initial incisions are exactly as described in the rescue flap section. From there, we proceed anteriorly towards the mucocutaneous junction. As one comes anterior to the cartilage–bone junction of the septum, the incision arches superiorly and continues near the septal angle before becoming vertical at the mucocutaneous junction (**Fig. 5.35**). This part of the incision may occasionally be difficult as it is difficult to maintain vision at its highest point. Care must also be taken not to go through the cartilage with the incision and damage the opposite mucoperichondrium. Inferiorly, the incision comes anterior along the nasal floor, before curving upwards at the mucocutaneous junction to join the superior incision. The inferior incision may be at the base of the septum, floor of the nose, or even under the inferior turbinate, depending on the width of the flap required (**Fig. 5.36**) (See **Fig. 10.3** in chapter 10). Widely expanded sellas and large bony defects will require wider flaps and this assessment must be made at the start of surgery, as the flap is usually harvested prior to the bone work. If uncertain, take a flap significantly wider than anticipated. The length of the flap depends on pneumatisation of the

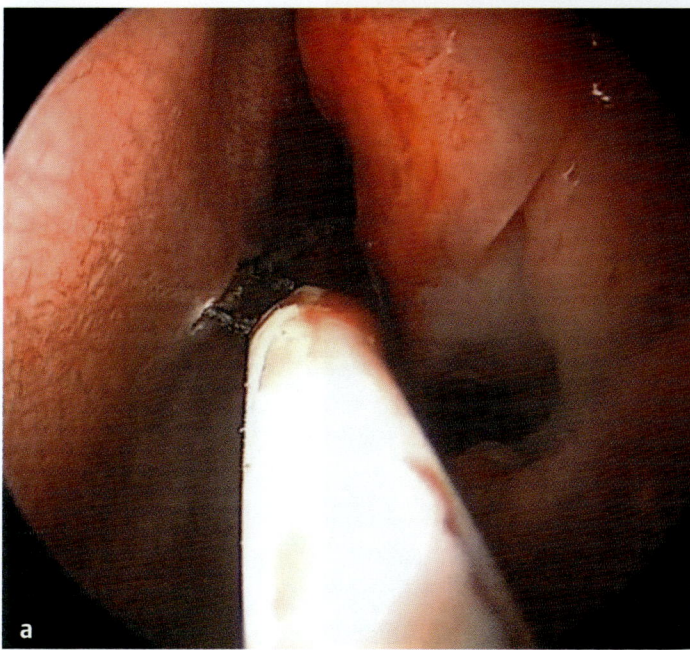

Fig. 5.35 (a–c) Intra-operative images showing incision being taken for HB flap on the left side. The superior HB incision is seen swinging up at the level of the septal bony–cartilaginous junction marked roughly by the anterior face of the middle turbinate. Anteriorly, the limit of the HB flap is up to the mucocutaneous junction of the septum. The instrument in use is a monopolar needle cautery (See **Fig. 10.3** in chapter 10).

103

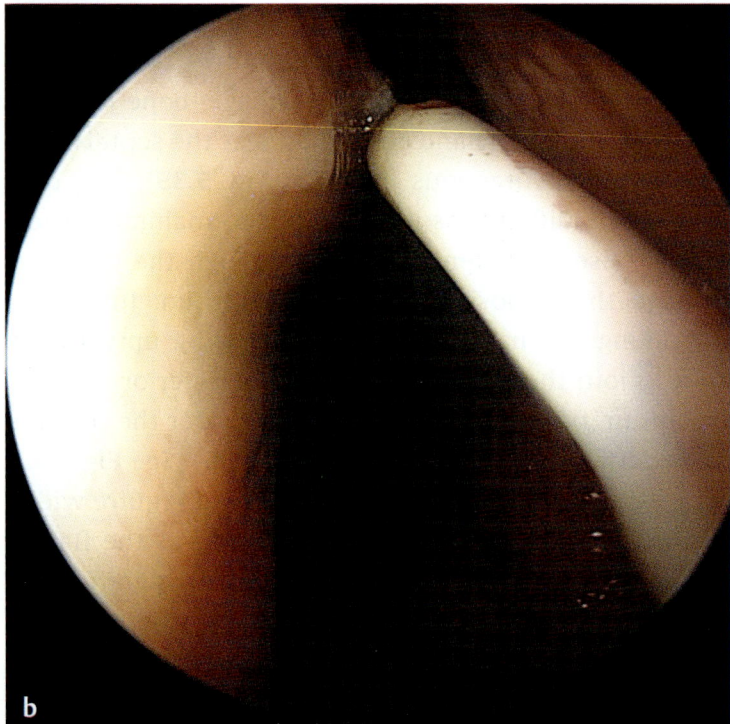

b

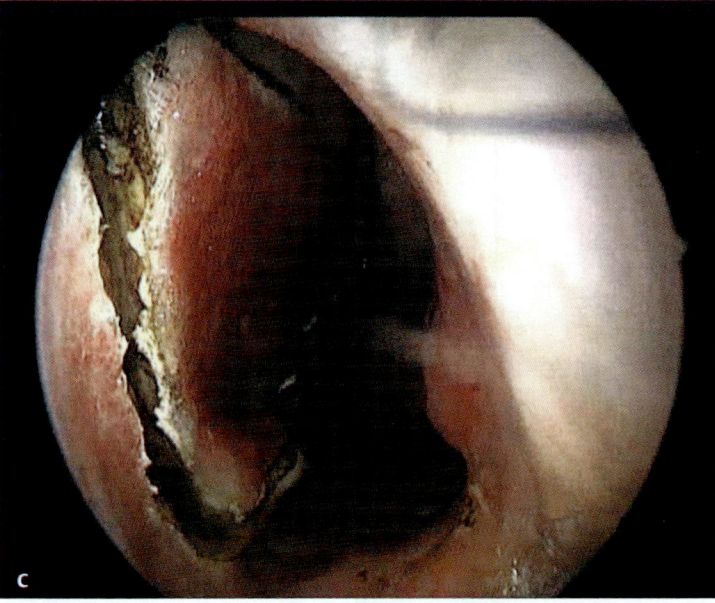

c

Fig. 5.35 (a–c) Intraoperative images showing incision being taken for HB flap on the left side. The superior HB incision is seen swinging up at the level of the septal bony–cartilaginous junction marked roughly by the anterior face of the middle turbinate. Anteriorly, the limit of the HB flap is up to the mucocutaneous junction of the septum. The instrument in use is a monopolar needle cautery (See **Fig. 10.3** in chapter 10).

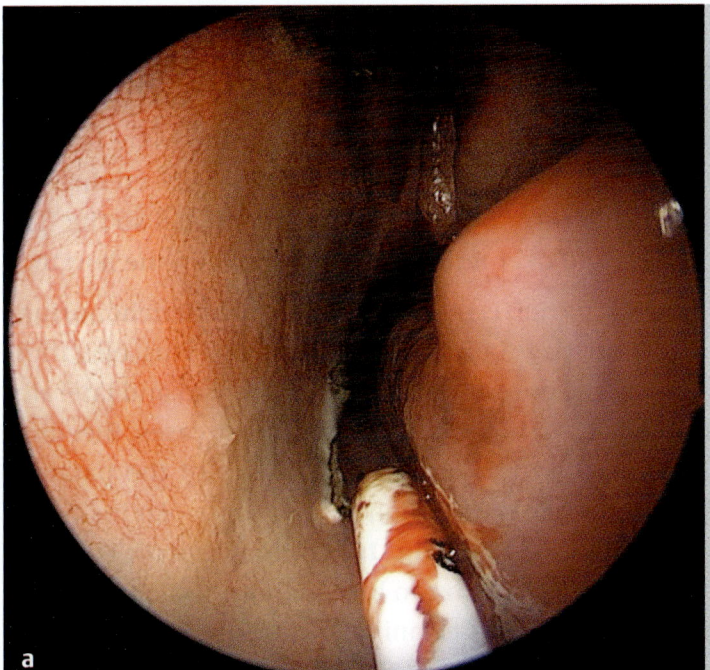

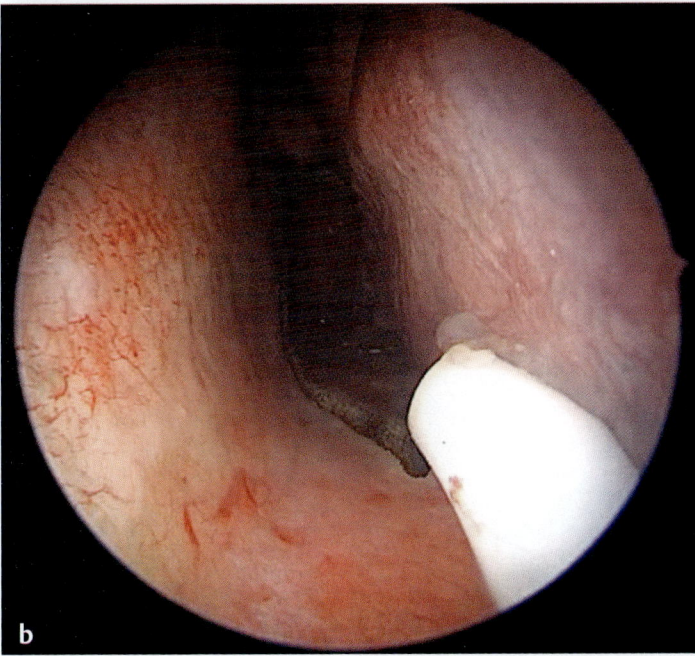

Fig. 5.36 **(a, b)** Image showing inferior incision being taken for HB flaps. The inferior HB incision over the hard palate is variable depending on the expected size of the sellar defect. The inferior incision can come down to the floor of the nasal cavity or even under the inferior meatus.

sphenoid sinus as well as the defect site. For example, a planum defect requires a longer flap than a clival defect. Also, a sinus well pneumatised under the sella will need a longer flap as compared to a pre-sellar pneumatisation. The flap must always run along the floor and clivus in contact with bone en route its final placement. This is to ensure there is no contraction of the flap if placed directly (in air). For this purpose, it is mandatory to lower the sphenoid keel so the flap can 'walk' in easily and not have to go over a ridge that will shorten the length.

Once the incision is complete, the flap is raised with the mucoperichondrium and mucoperiosteum from the cartilage and bone (**Fig. 5.37**). This elevation moves along posteriorly, exposing the anterior wall of the sphenoid and laterally till the palatovaginal canal (**Fig. 5.13**). This is sufficient in most cases. Bleeding may be encountered anteriorly and posteriorly from branches of the palatine arteries, and so it is our preference to take the incision with a monopolar insulated needle cautery, the tip bent by 60 degrees (See **Fig. 10.3** in chapter 10). This also prevents oozing from the superior edge, which can be annoying as it comes onto the endoscope, which then requires frequent cleaning. Whilst elevating the flap,

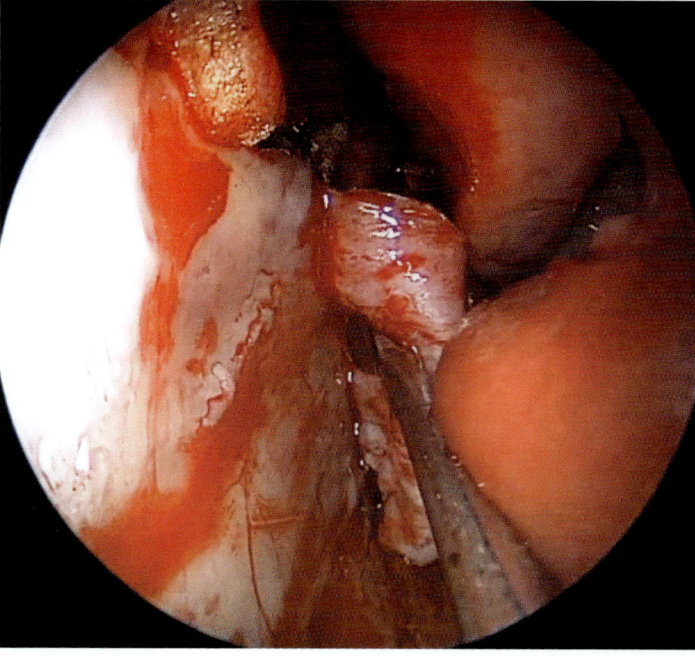

Fig. 5.37 Image showing elevation of the mucoperichondrium of a Hadad flap on the left side. The anterior incision is given at the mucocutaneous junction.

it is vital not to perforate it for reasons of closure and vasculature. The flap must reach the target area easily without stretch (**Fig. 5.38**) (See **Figs. 10.12, 10.21** in chapter 10). One can increase the reach of the flap by placing a little fat on the sphenoid posterior floor to help 'elongate' the flap (**Fig. 5.39**). The flap must be in contact with bone surrounding the defect site for best uptake. Hence, no fat, fascia, intervening mucosa, or tissue glue should be interposed between bone and flap at the site of repair. Glue may be put on top of the flap to maintain position and provide extra security for the repair. A layer of Gelfoam®, Surgicel®, or even fat is kept on top of the flap to provide a buffer, before placing the nasal pack (**Fig. 5.40**). This is to make certain that the flap is not pulled when removing the nasal pack. We prefer to use Merocel® nasal packs as against Foley's catheters, as we feel it provides a more even pressure on the repair(**Fig. 5.41**). These packs are usually kept for 4 to 5 days and the patient is advised bed rest. Lumbar drains are kept with larger defects or if the CSF pressure is high for 2 to 4 days. The patient will receive an antibiotic for 4 to 7 days.

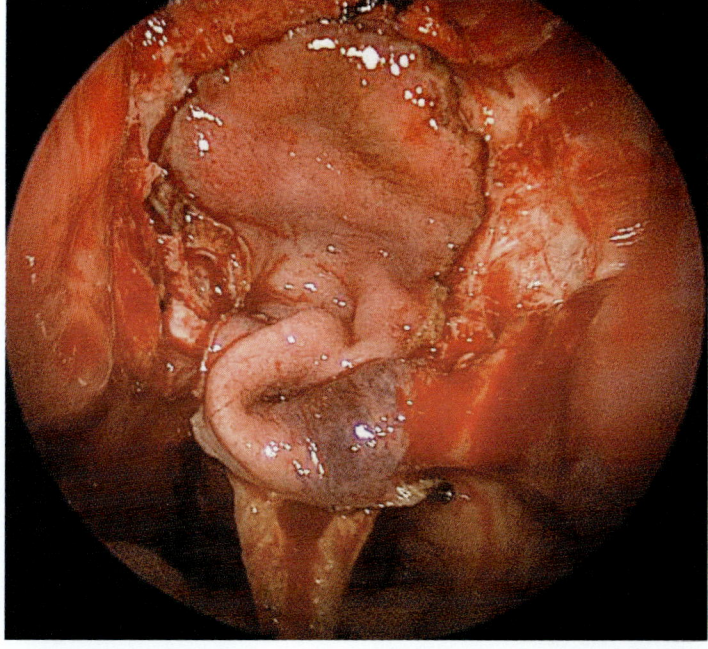

Fig. 5.38 The HB flap in its final position. It is placed over the sella without any stretch or twisting of the flap.

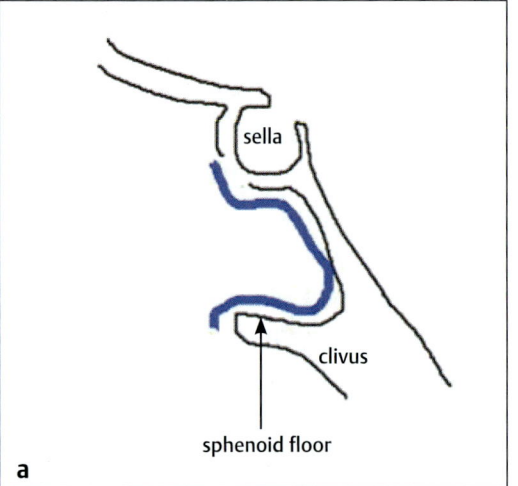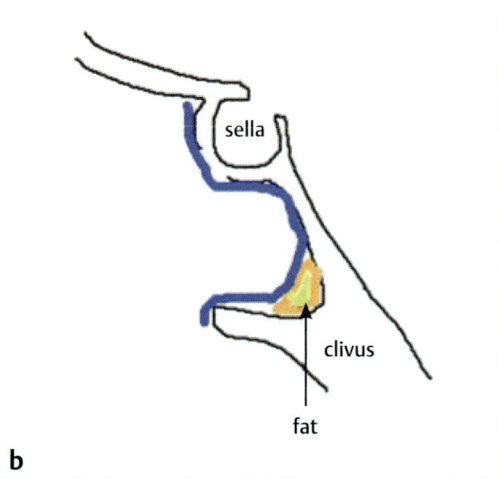

Fig. 5.39 **(a)** HB flap (blue) climbing over the floor of the sphenoid floor. **(b)** A fat blob placed in the sphenoid sinus helps in apparent lengthening of the HB flap, so that it reaches up to the superior wall of the sella.

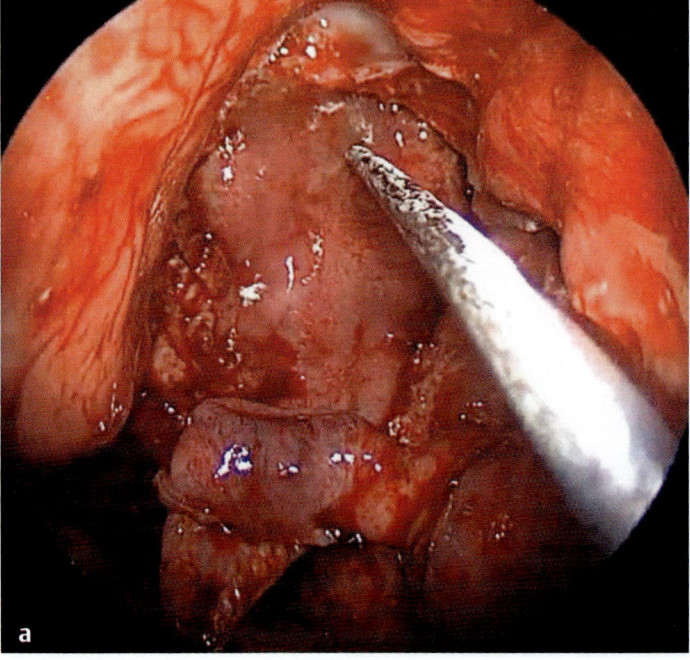

Fig. 5.40 **(a, b)** The Hadad flap is secured with glue in its final position.

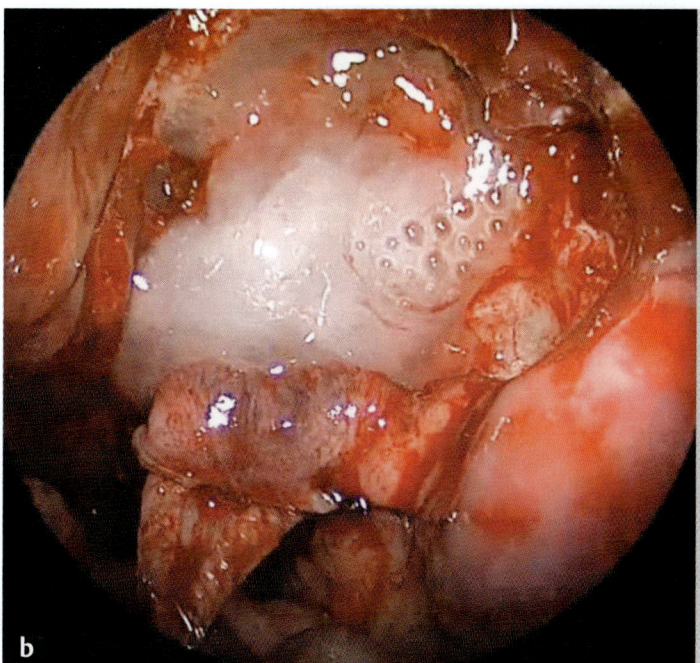

Fig. 5.40 **(a, b)** The Hadad flap is secured with glue in its final position. **(c, d)** A layer of glue, fat, and adequate Gelfoam is placed over the HB flap for extra support and cushioning, so that the flap is not pulled off with pack removal (**Figs.5.40c, 5.40d**)

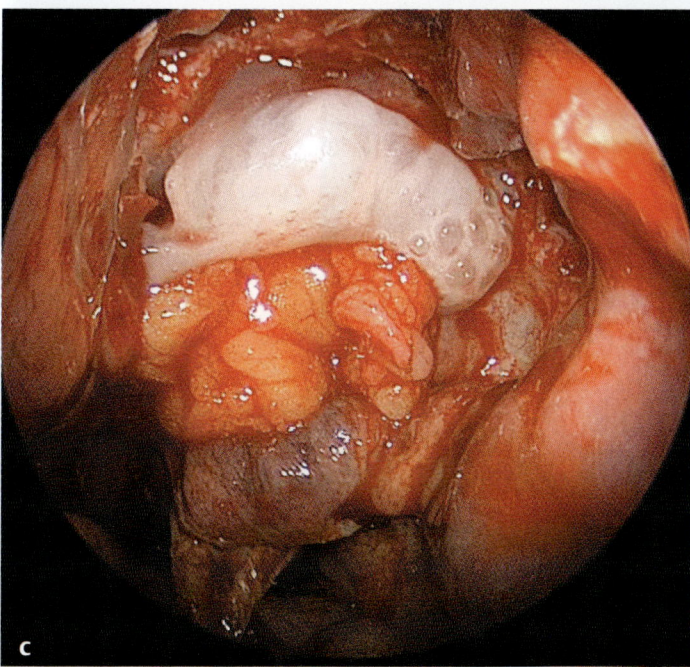

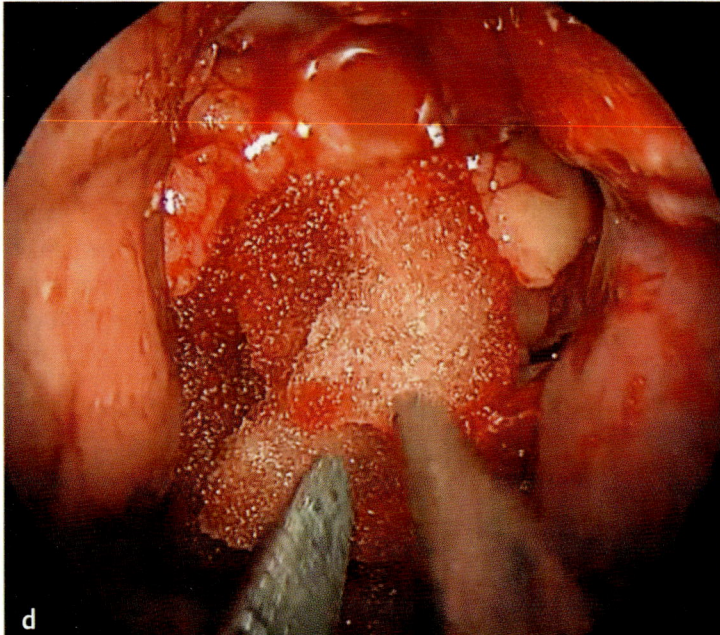

d

Fig. 5.40 (c, d) A layer of glue, fat, and adequate Gelfoam is placed over the HB flap for extra support and cushioning, so that the flap is not pulled off with pack removal (**Figs. 5.40c, 5.40d**)

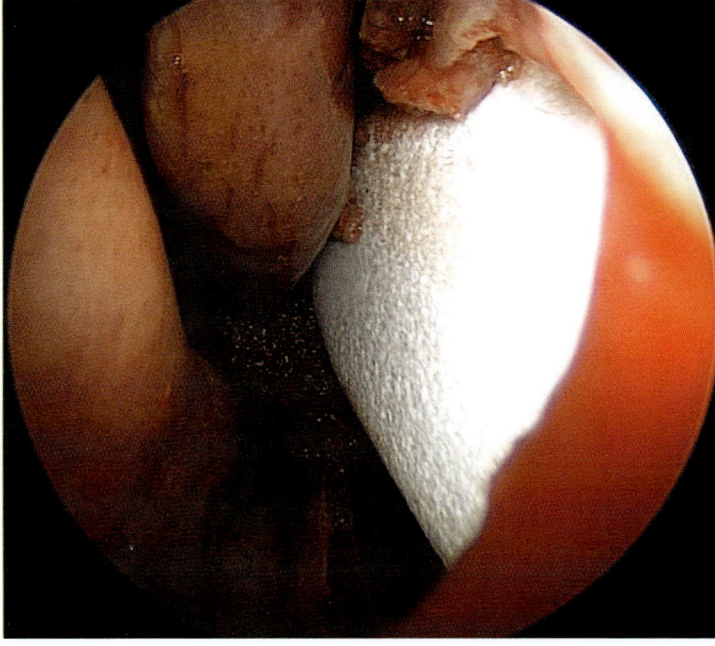

Fig. 5.41 A Merocel pack on the side of elevation of the HB flap. This pack is kept in situ for 3 to 5 days till the flap is taken up.

In case of multilayered repairs, there are no rules. We could use fat or fascia as an underlay graft, and bone or cartilage at defect level and then fascia or periosteum as an overlay graft. Dura substitutes may also prove to be useful. Tissue glue is used at different levels provided it does not occupy space between layers.

Reverse flap: With the elevation of HB flap and posterior septectomy, the anterior portion of the septal cartilage remains bare and devoid of any mucosa. If left alone, this bare cartilage may form the nidus for excessive crust formation in the anterior nasal cavity. Hence, to hasten the process of mucosalisation and healing, the septal flap from the opposite side can be reversed and utilised to cover the bare anterior cartilage. Reverse flap is essentially like a rescue flap, only based anteriorly. The horizontal parallel incisions are similar to a rescue flap. The anterior incisions end at the level of the bony cartilaginous junction of the septum (**Fig. 5.42**). The two incisions are joined posteriorly over the sphenoid, thus sacrificing the septal branch of the sphenopalatine artery (**Fig. 5.43**). This flap is reversed onto the opposite side through the posterior septectomy and sutured anteriorly to the caudal cutaneous strip of the septum (**Fig. 5.44**).

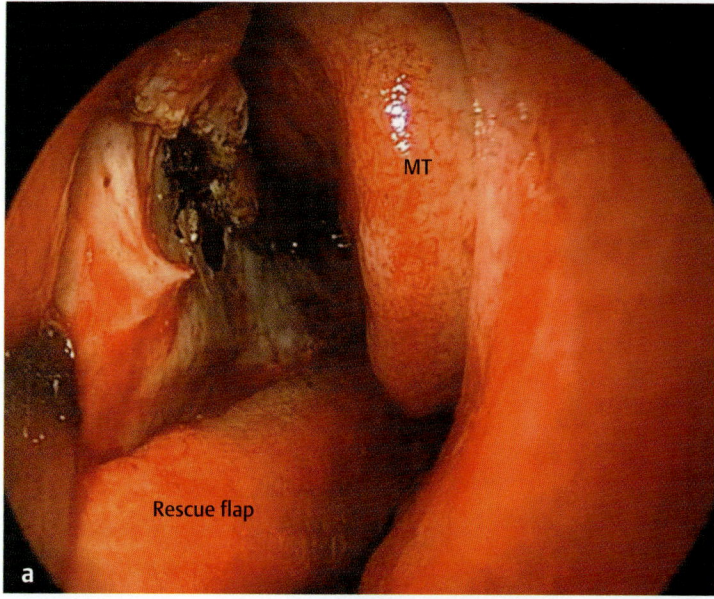

Fig. 5.42 (a) The horizontal incisions of rescue flaps come up to the level of bony–cartilaginous junction of the septum. MT, middle turbinate.

111

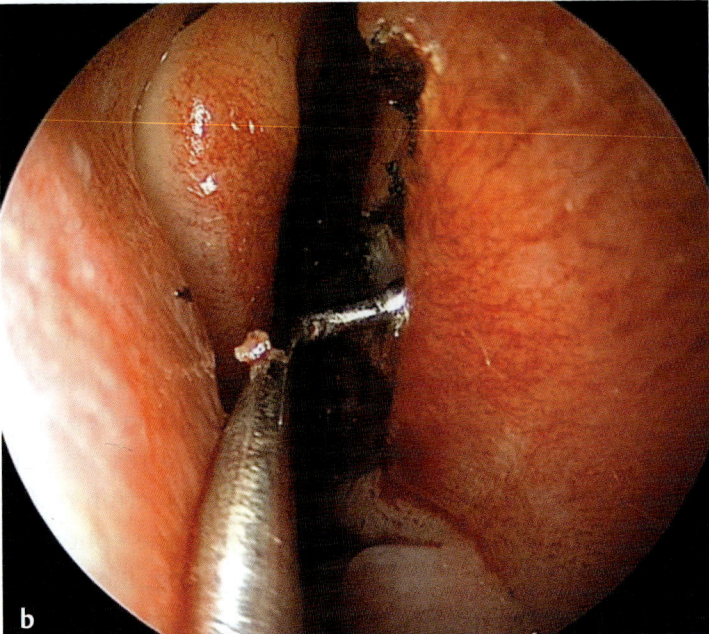

Fig. 5.42 **(b)** Anterior elevation of the rescue flaps using ball probe (See **Fig. 10.25** in chapter 10).

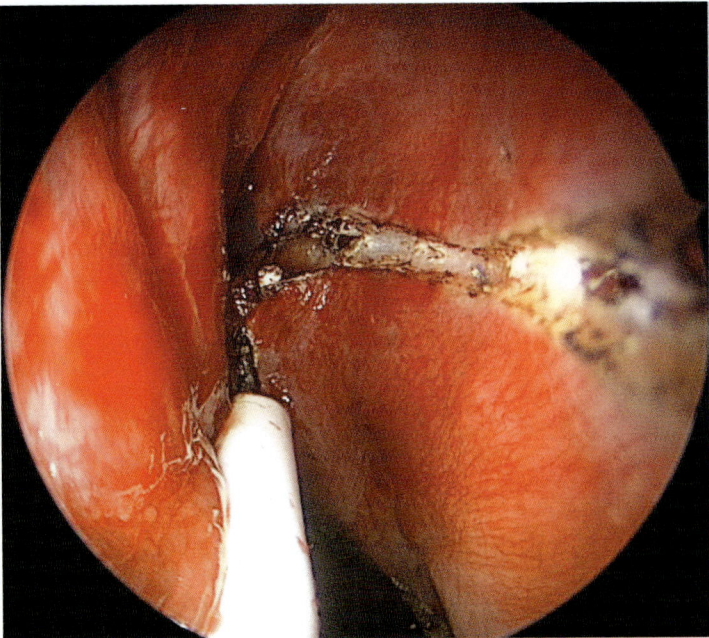

Fig. 5.43 The posterior incision in a reverse flap given over the sphenoid anterior face from the sphenoid ostium to the choana. This incision sacrifices the septal branch of the sphenopalatine artery. The superior incision is like that of a rescue flap.

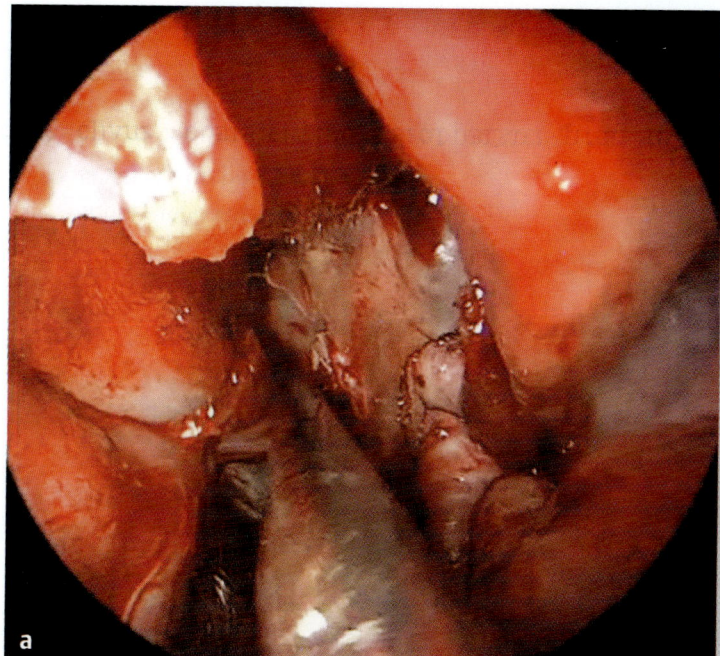

Fig. 5.44 **(a–e)** The reverse flap is swung from the right side through the posterior septectomy and is sutured on the left side to the mucocutaneous junction.

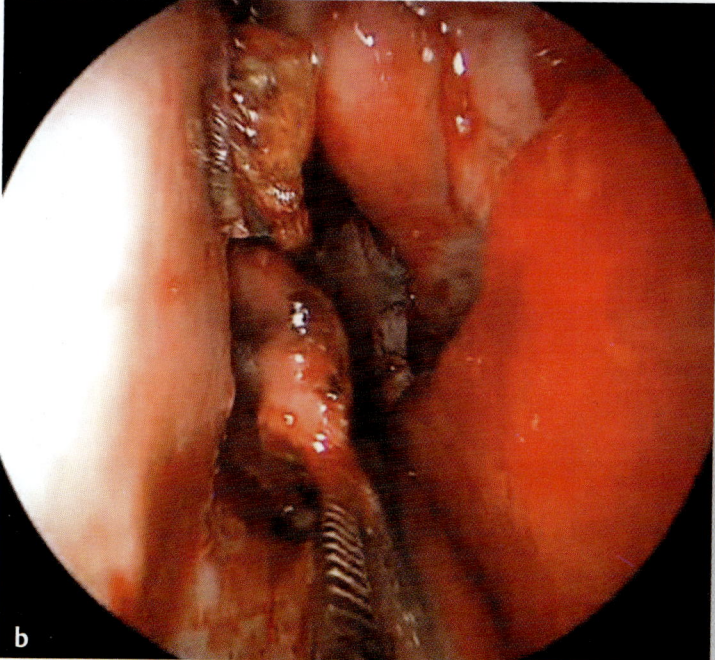

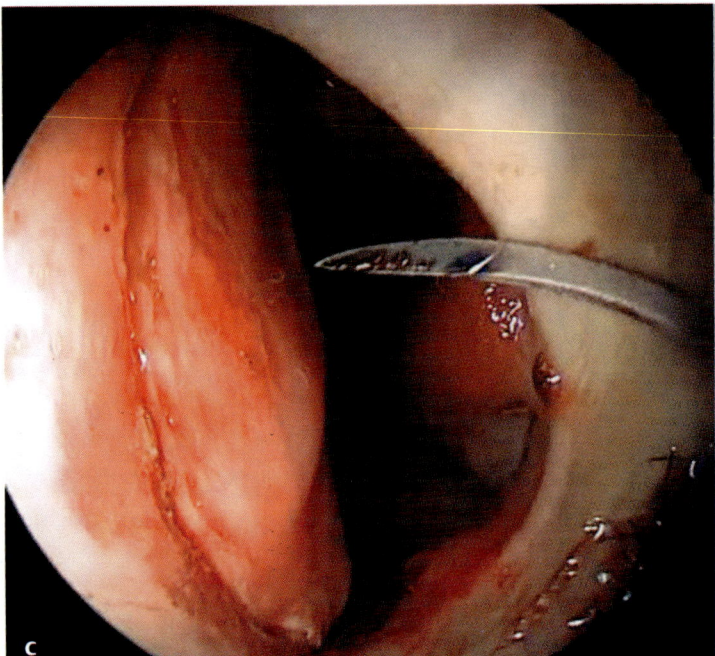

Fig. 5.44 (a–e) The reverse flap is swung from the right side through the posterior septectomy and is sutured on the left side to the mucocutaneous junction.

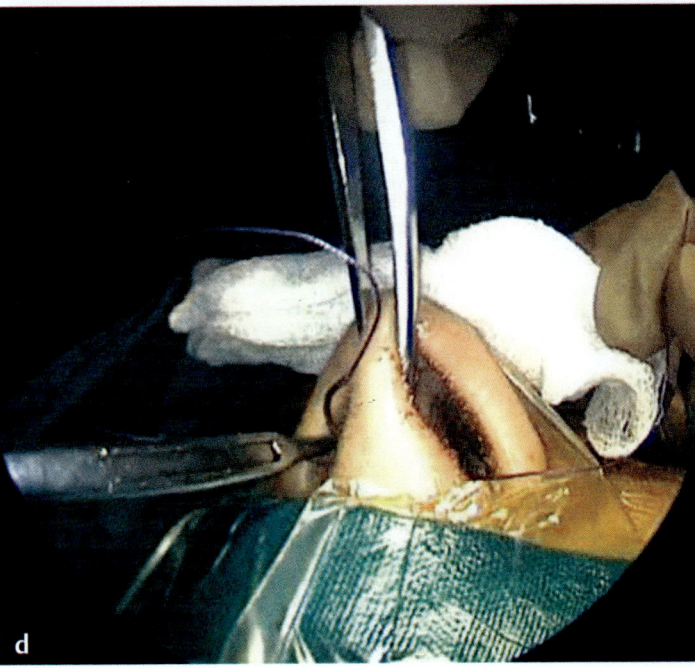

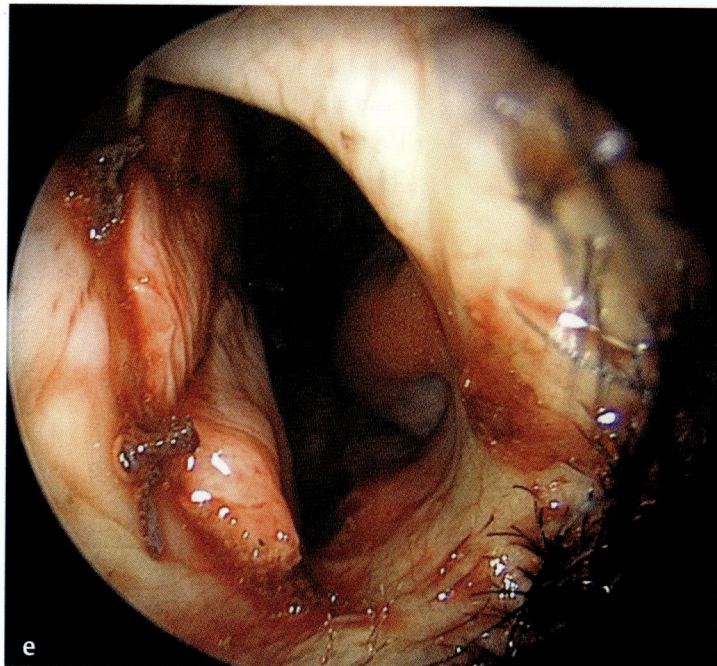

Fig. 5.44 (a–e) The reverse flap is swung from the right side through the posterior septectomy and is sutured on the left side to the mucocutaneous junction.

Reserve flaps: These are based on sphenopalatine artery. These flaps are lateral nasal wall, middle turbinate, or inferior turbinate flaps. Lateral nasal wall flaps are extremely useful large flaps elevated over the lateral nasal wall using the mucoperiosteum anterior to the uncinate process, inferior turbinate, and floor of the nose. They are reserved for those cases in which a HB flap cannot be harvested, for example, in revision cases. Flaps elevated from the middle turbinate are smaller and can be used for smaller defects or to augment a primary flap. Inferior turbinate flaps are longer and larger and can extend to the floor of the nose extending till an incision is taken on the anterior part of the inferior turbinate (**Fig. 5.45**).

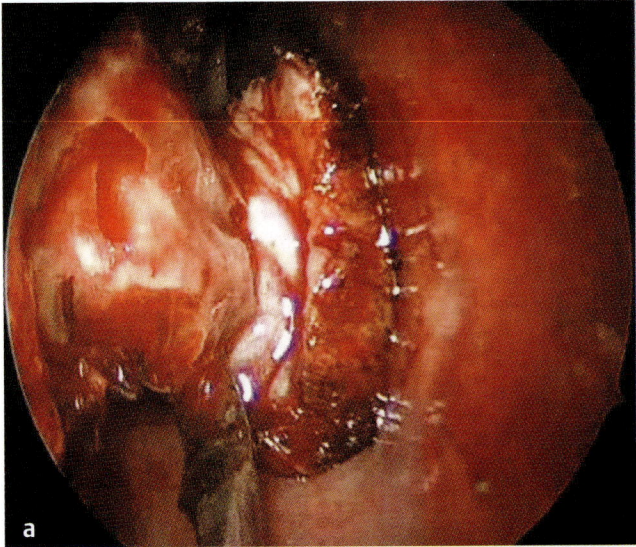

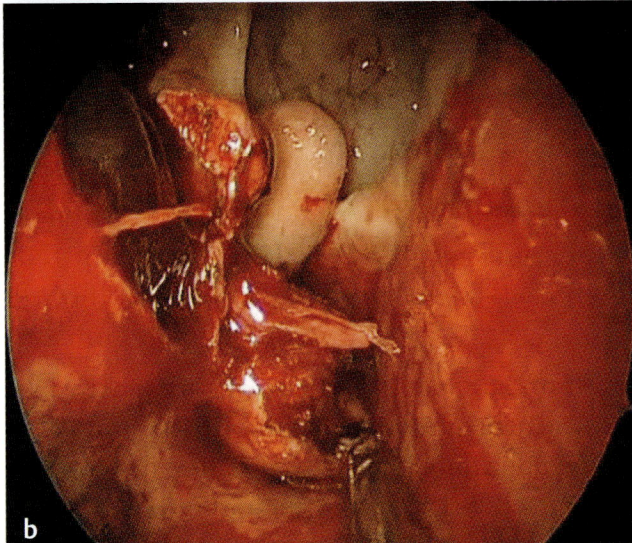

Fig. 5.45 Reserve flap (inferior turbinate) is being elevated on the right side from the **(a)** anterior and **(b)** posterior end of the inferior turbinate bone.

Reference

1. Kassam AB, Gardner PA, eds. Endoscopic Approaches to Skull Base. Prog Neurol Surg. Basel, Karger; 2012;26:21–26

Extended Endonasal Transsphenoid Surgeries

Nishit Shah and C. E. Deopujari

Extended endoscopic skull base surgery, like any other surgery, is based on the principle of optimum bone removal to achieve maximal exposure. Barring complex intra-axial tumours, majority of skull base midline and paramedian tumours can be tackled by extended skull base surgery. The surgical exposure has to be done beyond the tumour edges as judged by navigation in its horizontal and vertical axes.

Indications for sagittal midline plane lesions are as follows:

- Giant pituitary adenomas.
- Macroadenomas with anterior extension.
- Craniopharyngiomas.
- Planum/tubercular/clival meningiomas.
- Chordomas.
- Odontoidectomy.
- Other/ miscellaneous tumours or lesions.

Neuro-navigation is considered indispensable for extended skull base approaches as it helps in defining bony and soft tissue landmarks intra-operatively. Intra-operative use of Doppler helps in localising major vessels, preventing inadvertent injury. The surgical team must familiarise themselves with the usage of angled endoscopes, angled instruments, and curved suctions, for the precision of extended endonasal dissection.

The transsphenoidal corridor is the first step in most extended approaches such as transplanar, transtubercular, transclival, and transcavernous.

Transplanar / Transtubercular Approach

The boundaries for a transplanar / transtubercular exposure are as follows:

- *Anteriorly*: The cribriform plate–planum sphenoidale junction (posterior ethmoid artery).

- *Posteriorly*: The sella.

- *Laterally*: Medial aspect of opticocarotid recesses (OCRs).

For this approach, it is imperative to do bilateral posterior ethmoidectomies in order to gain complete exposure of the planum sphenoidale, and orbital apex. The planum is drilled using a 3-mm diamond drill (See **Fig. 10.8** in chapter 10) until it is egg-shelled (**Fig. 6.1**) and then removed using fine dissectors or Kerrison's punch (See **Fig. 10.13, 10.26** in chapter 10). The punch is used more like a hook, and only the tip of the Kerrison's punch is used to remove the bone (**Fig. 6.2**). The superior intercavernous sinus is cauterised using vertical bipolar pistol grip forceps (See **Fig. 10.27** in chapter 10) and sacrificed (**Fig. 6.3**). Cauterisation of this sinus is done strictly in the midline to avoid any injury to the inferior hypophyseal arteries as these arteries also supply the visual pathways. The tuberculum sellae is freed from the planum sphenoidale anteriorly and the medial OCR laterally. The tuberculum is then gently dissected and removed. The bone resection continues across the tuberculum to the planum, thus affording access to the suprasellar cistern. Bone removal may be continued anteriorly upto the posterior ethmoid arteries should it be required. The bone removal is completed to reach the falciform ligament and the posterior ethmoid arteries.

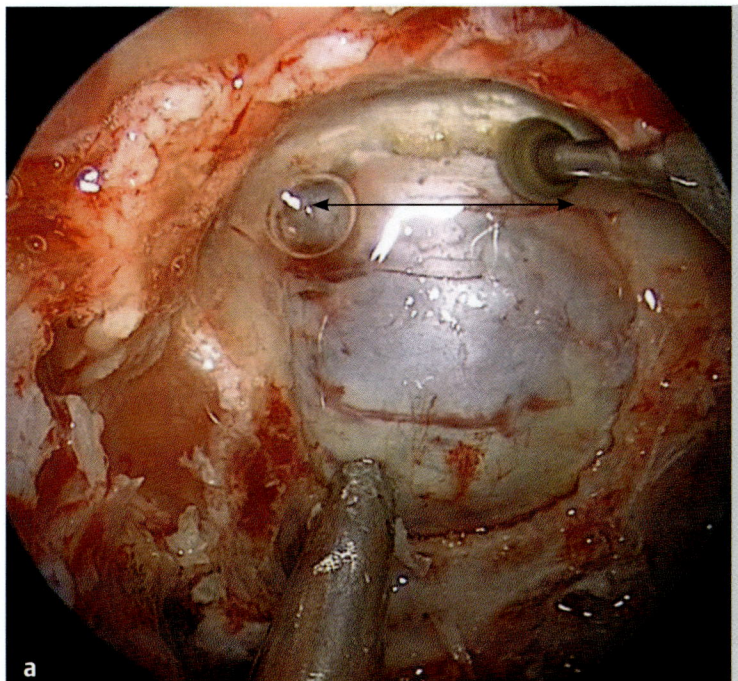

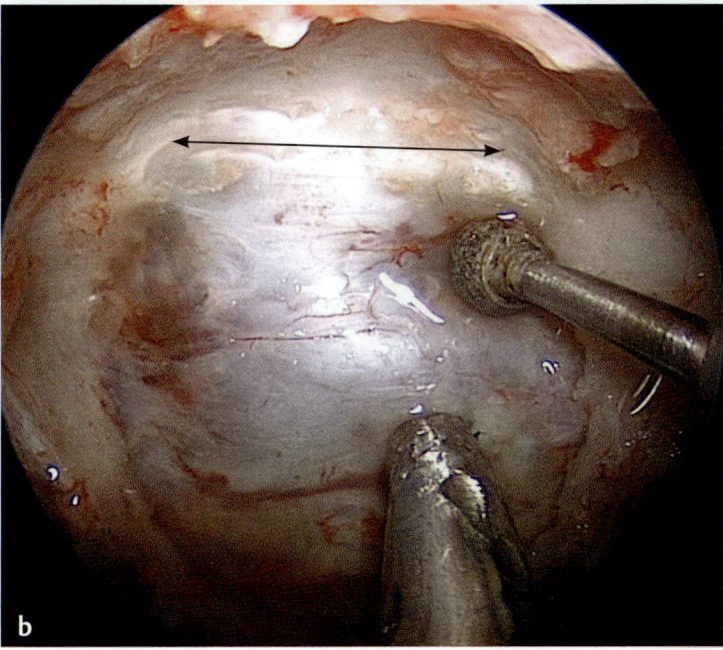

Fig. 6.1 (a, b) Transtubercular approach. After exposure of the sella, the tuberculum (*double-headed black arrow*) is drilled using a 3-mm diamond drill.

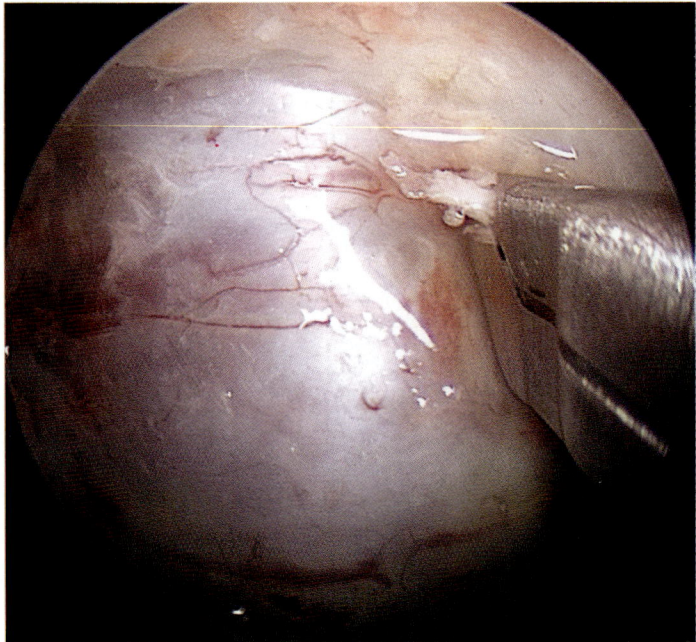

Fig. 6.2 The peripheral part of the tuberculum is removed using Kerrison's punch as a hook (See **Fig. 10.13** in chapter 10).

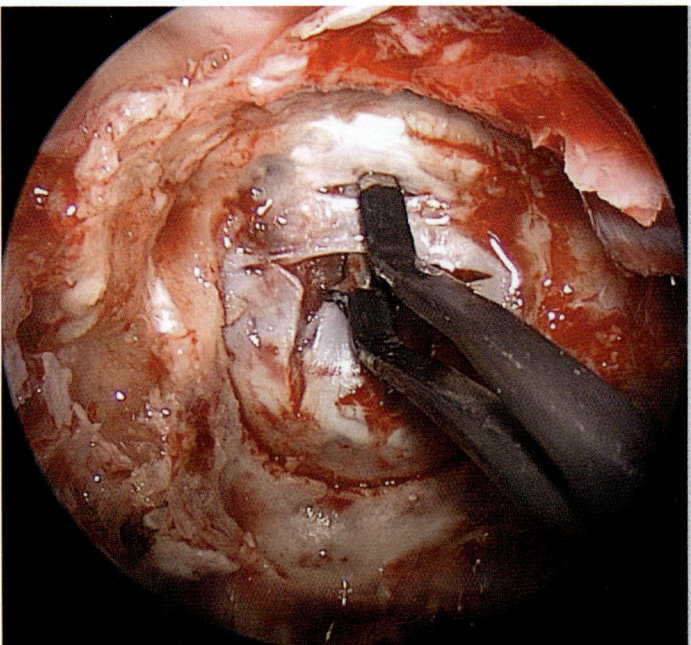

Fig. 6.3 Cauterisation of the superior intercavernous sinus (SICS), using vertical bipolar, is strictly done in the midline to avoid injury to the inferior hypophyseal artery (See **Fig. 10.27** in chapter 10).

Bone removal for the transplanum approach is said to resemble a chef's hat (**Fig. 6.4**). The inferior exposure is restricted by the median OCR but can widen considerably superior to the optic nerves.

Few examples of sellar–suprasellar lesions, planum/tubercular lesions are described in **Fig. 6.5–6.9**.

Reconstruction

One major fear deterring most surgeons for extended approaches is failure to create a watertight seal between the nasal cavity and the intracranial cavity.

The extended trans-sphenoid approaches come with an inherent risk of dural defect and cerebrospinal fluid (CSF) leak. It is almost always advisable to harvest a pedicled nasoseptal flap at the start of surgery for reconstruction in anticipation of a CSF leak. We make sure that the Hadad flap to be harvested for transtubercular/transplanar surgeries is longer than for regular trans-sellar surgeries as obviously the site of defect is way anterior. This means that the anterior vertical incision of the Hadad flap needs to come right at the

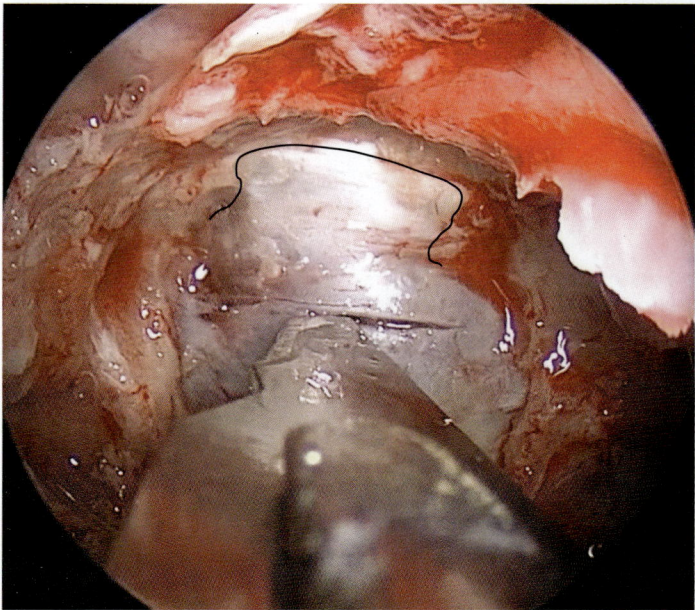

Fig. 6.4 The chef's hat appearance typically seen after drilling out of the tuberculum and the planum (outlined in black). The inferior constriction is due to the medial OCRs.

121

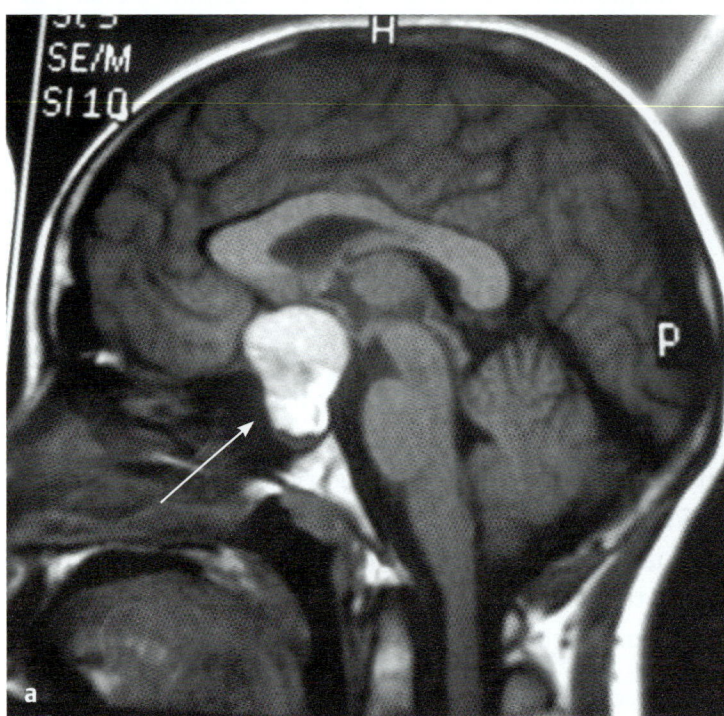

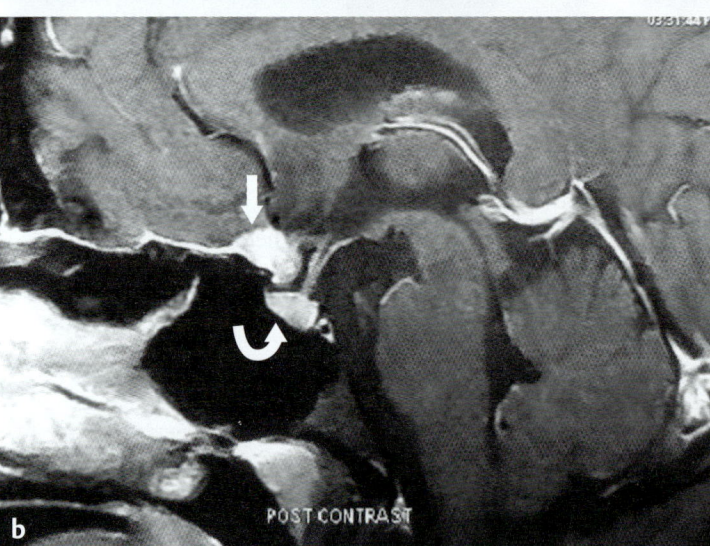

Fig. 6.5 **(a)** T2-weighted MRI sagittal view showing sellar–suprasellar heterogenous lesion (*thin white arrow*) is suggestive of craniopharyngiomas. Such a lesion warrants a transtubercular approach for complete exposure and resection of the tumour. **(b)** T1-weighted MRI sagittal view showing a planum sphenoidale meningioma (*straight white block arrow*). The normal pituitary gland is seen completely separated from the tumour (*curved arrow*). Such cases warrant a transplanar approach.

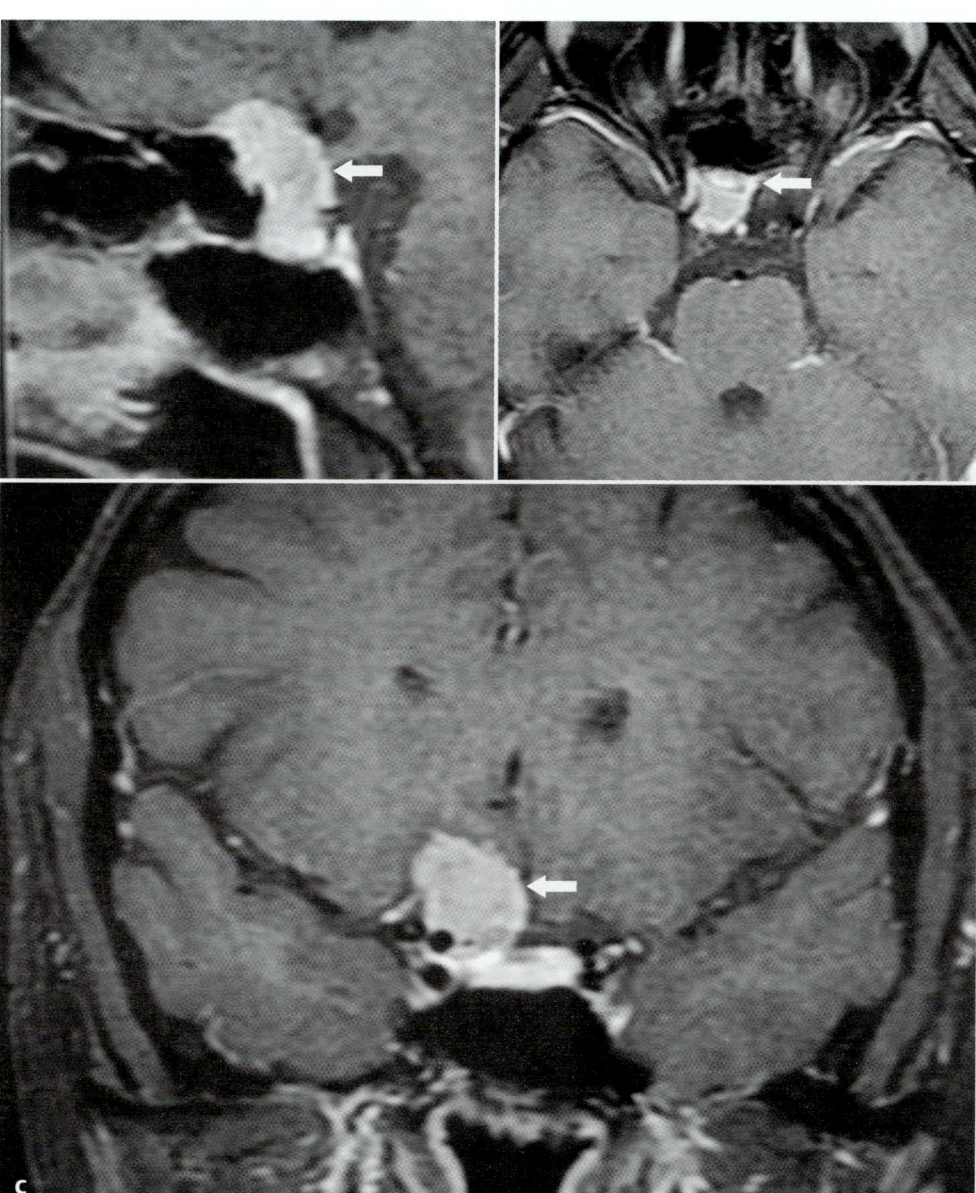

Fig. 6.5 **(c)** Planum meningioma (*short white block arrow*) is seen on sagittal, axial, and coronal axes, with little or no displacement of the carotids. Transplanum approach was taken for complete excision of the tumour.

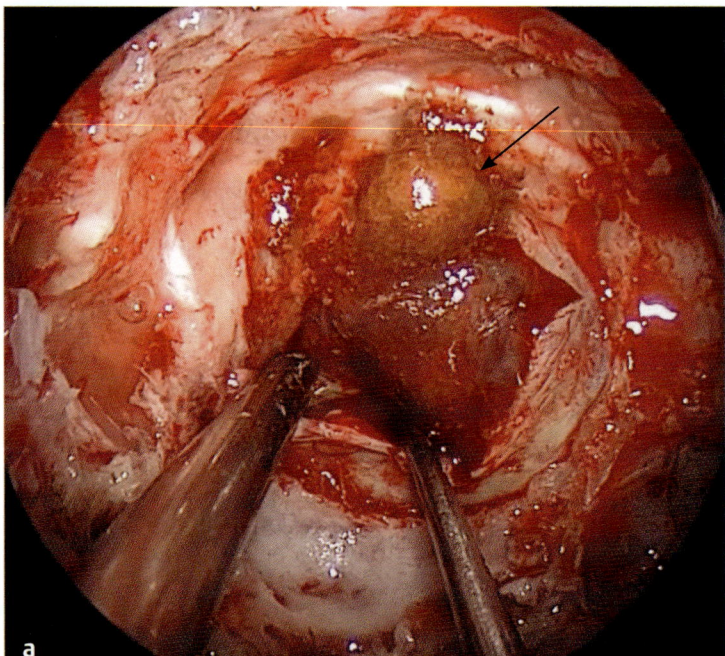

a

Fig. 6.6 (a–f)
Extracapsular excision
of craniopharyngioma.
Note the typical
xanthochromatic material
(machine oil) shown in
long black arrow **(a)** and
calcific material being
removed in **(e)**. **(f)** The
last bit of the capsule of
the craniopharyngiomas
being cut off using
sharp dural scissors (See
Fig. 10.22 in chapter 10).

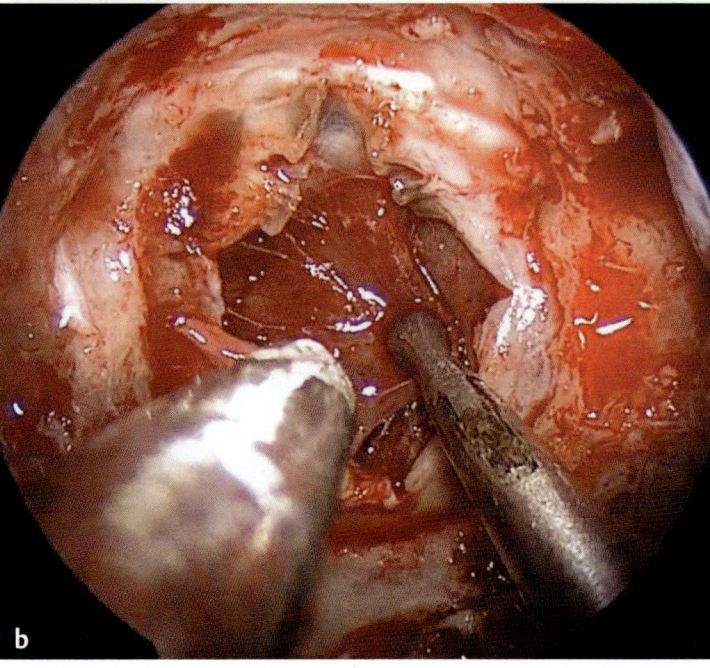

b

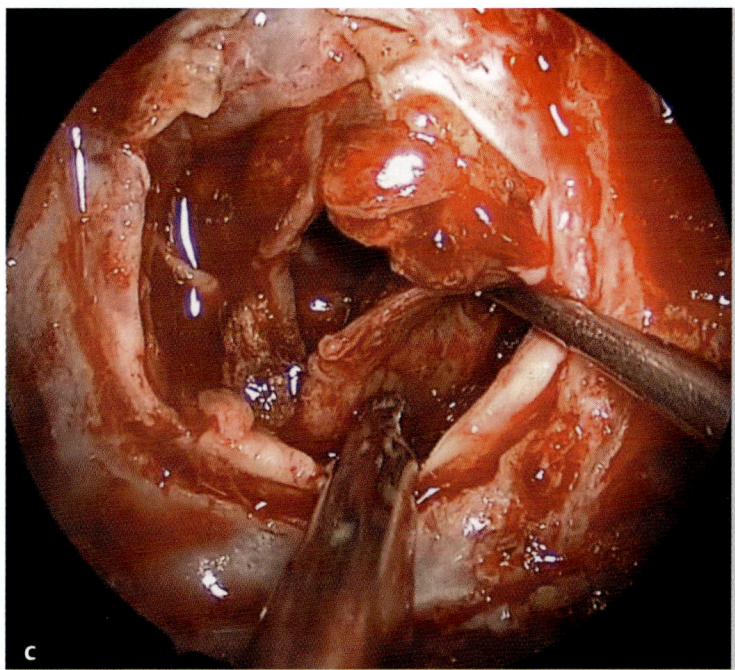

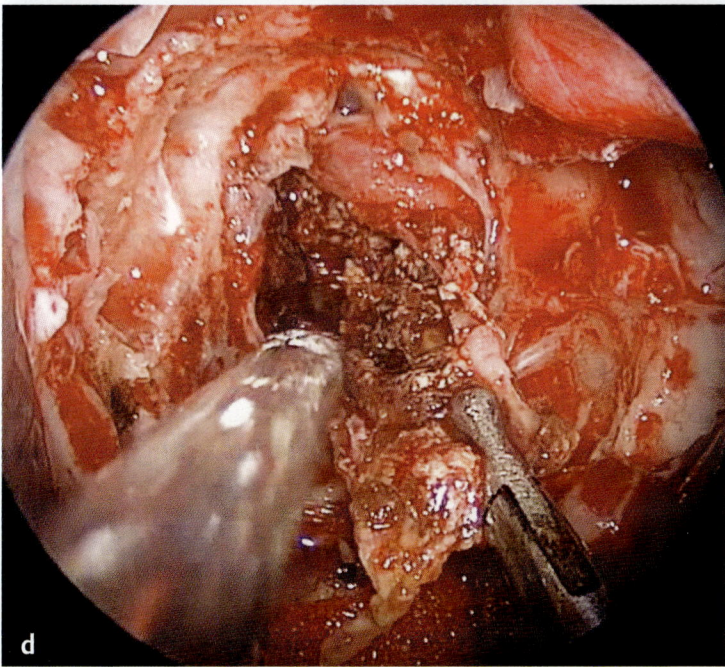

Fig. 6.6 (a–f) Extracapsular excision of craniopharyngioma. Note the typical xanthochromatic material (machine oil) shown in *long black arrow* **(a)** and calcific material being removed in **(e)**. **(f)** The last bit of the capsule of the craniopharyngiomas being cut off using sharp dural scissors (See **Fig. 10.22** in chapter 10).

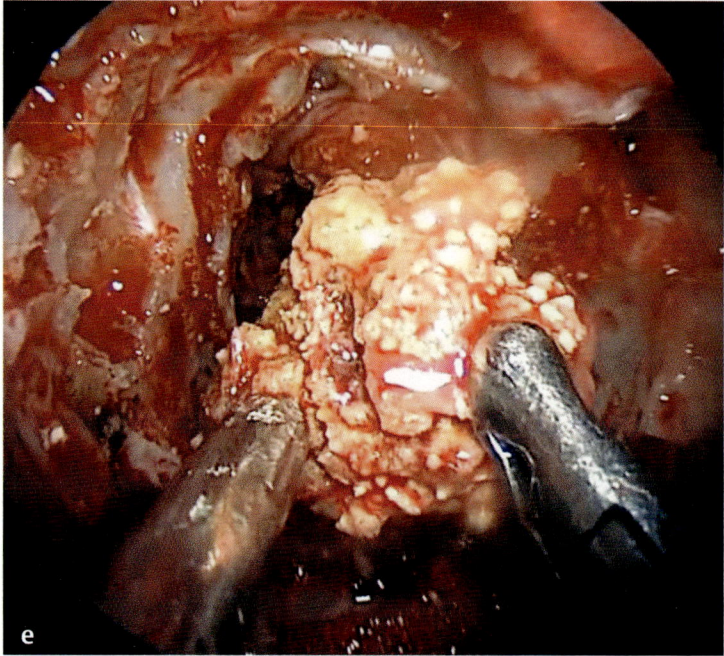

e

Fig. 6.6 (a–f) Extracapsular excision of craniopharyngioma. Note the typical xanthochromatic material (machine oil) shown in *long black arrow* **(a)** and calcific material being removed in **(e)**. **(f)** The last bit of the capsule of the craniopharyngiomas being cut off using sharp dural scissors (See **Fig. 10.22** in chapter 10).

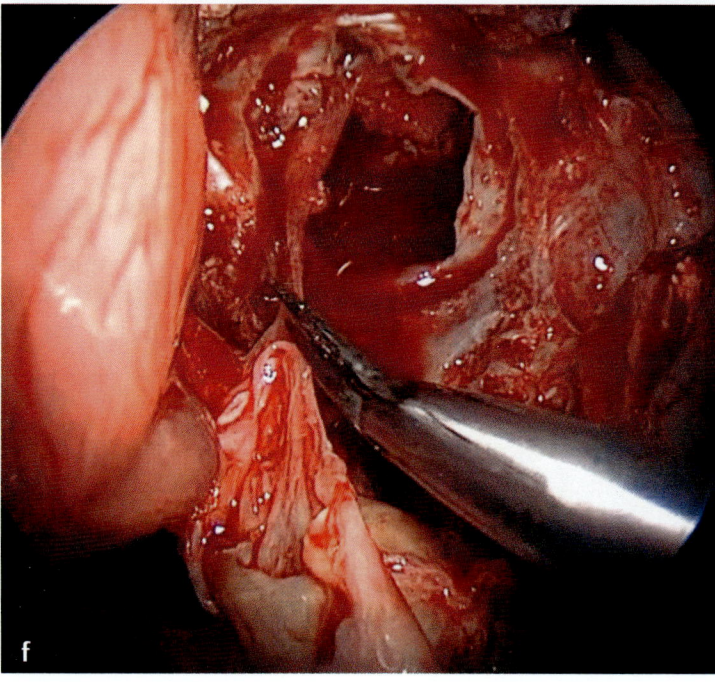

f

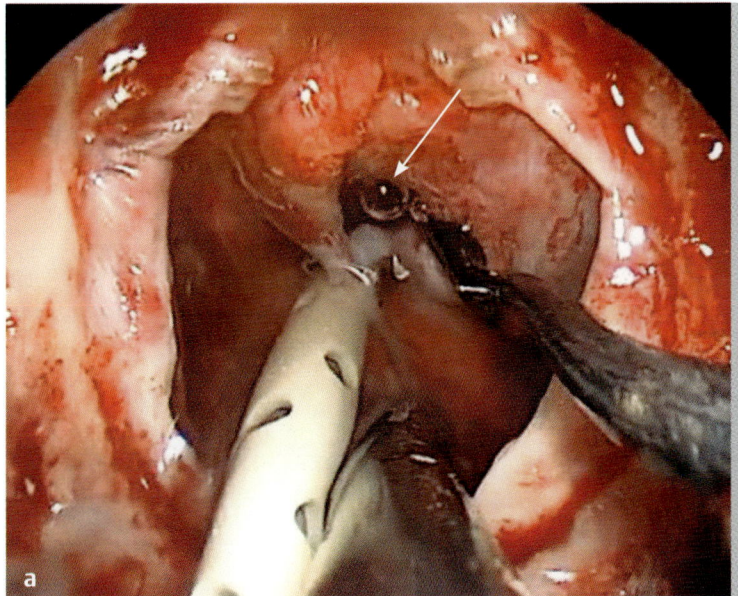

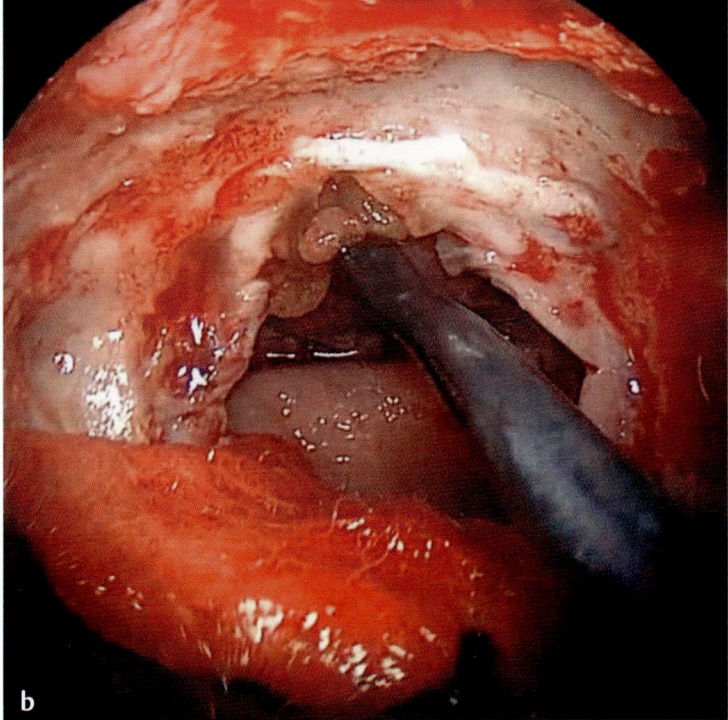

Fig. 6.7 (a–f) Reconstruction of tubercular defect created after excision of craniopharyngioma shown in **Fig. 6.6**.
Fig. 6.7 (a) Dural defect is seen (*single white arrow*).
(b) Plugged with fat with the help of silver dissector.

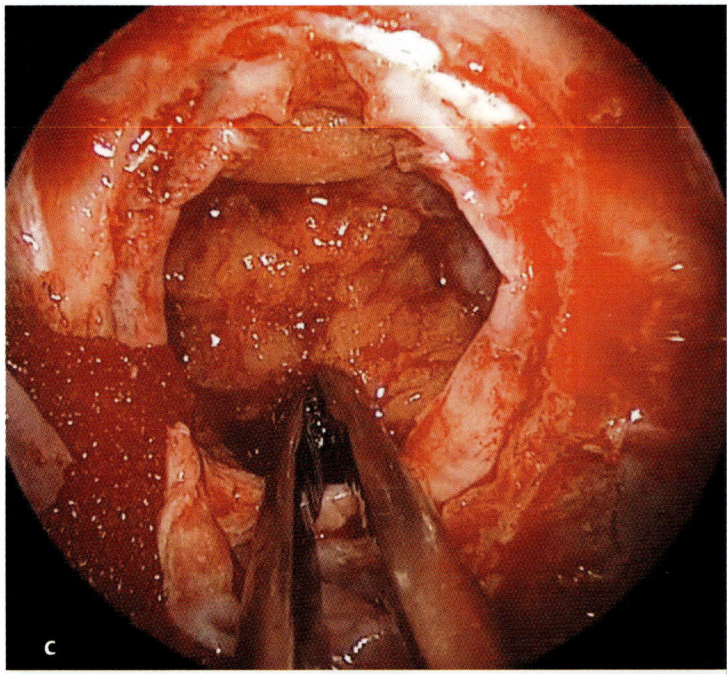

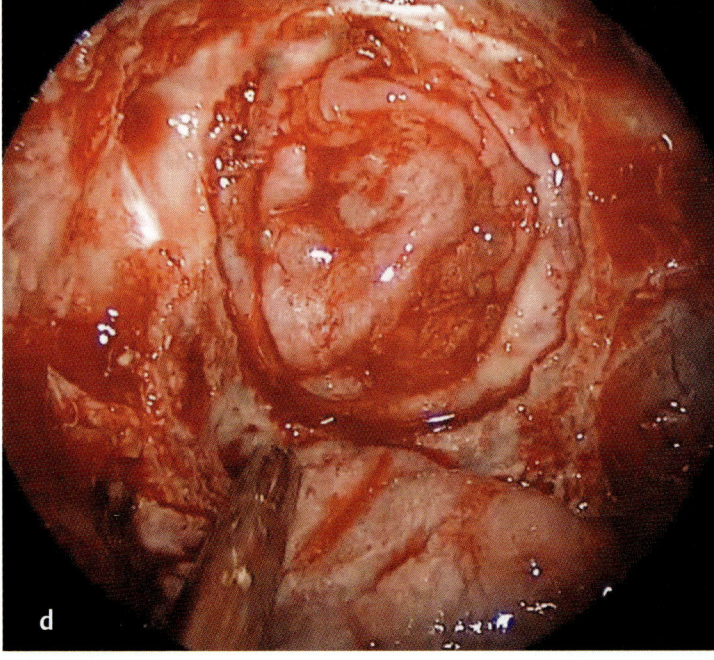

Fig. 6.7 **(c)** Sella is being packed by fat. **(d)** The sellar defect is closed by underlay free fascia graft.

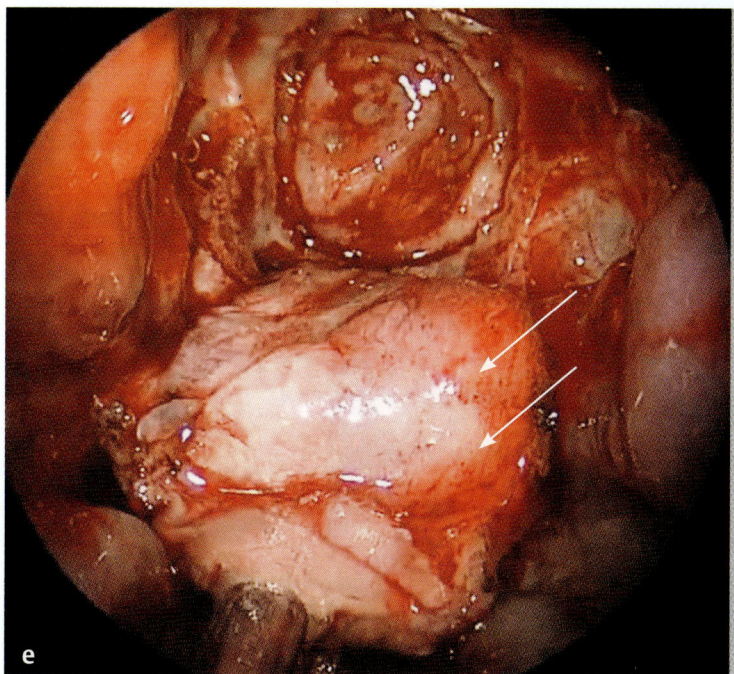

Fig. 6.7 (e, f) The free fascia graft repair is reinforced by Hadad flap (*double white arrow*).

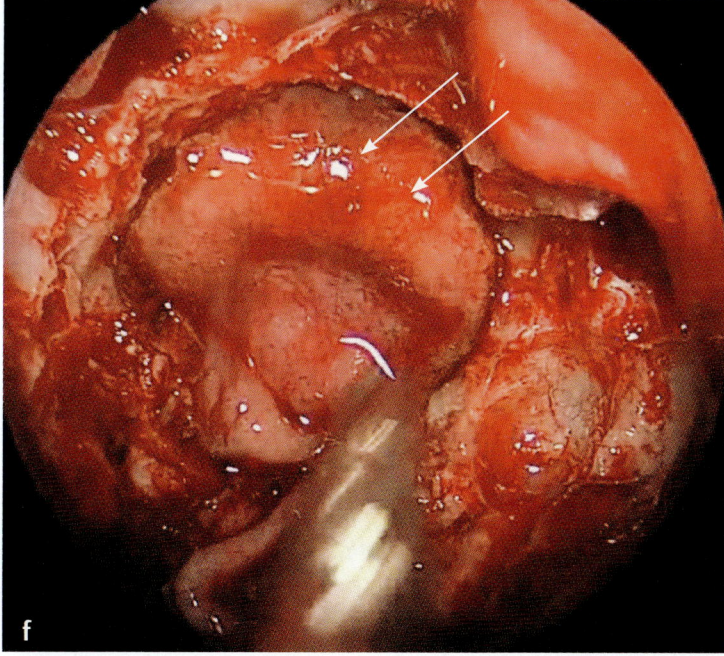

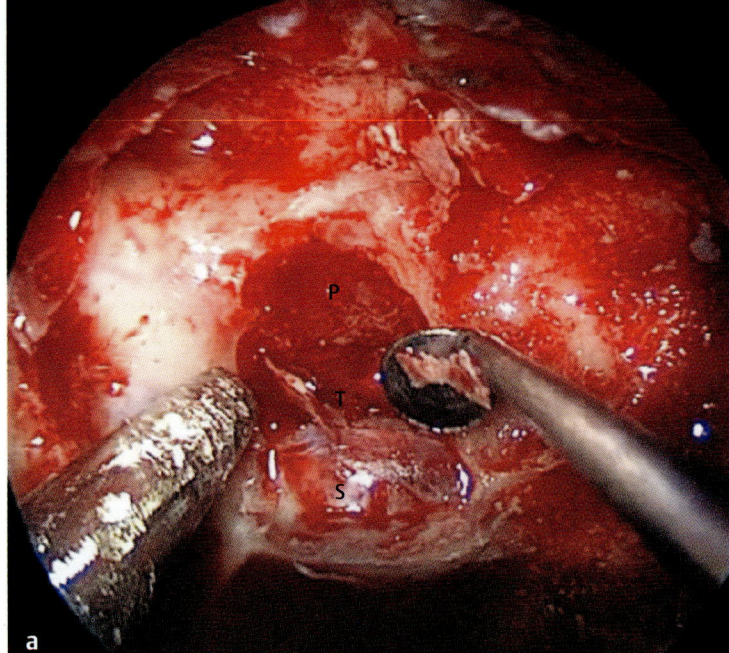

Fig. 6.8 Excision of planum meningioma shown in **Fig. 6.5c**. **(a)** Exposure of the sella (S), tuberculum (T), and planum (P). **(b)** View after cauterisation of SICS. The planum meningioma (PM) is distinctly seen above the sella.

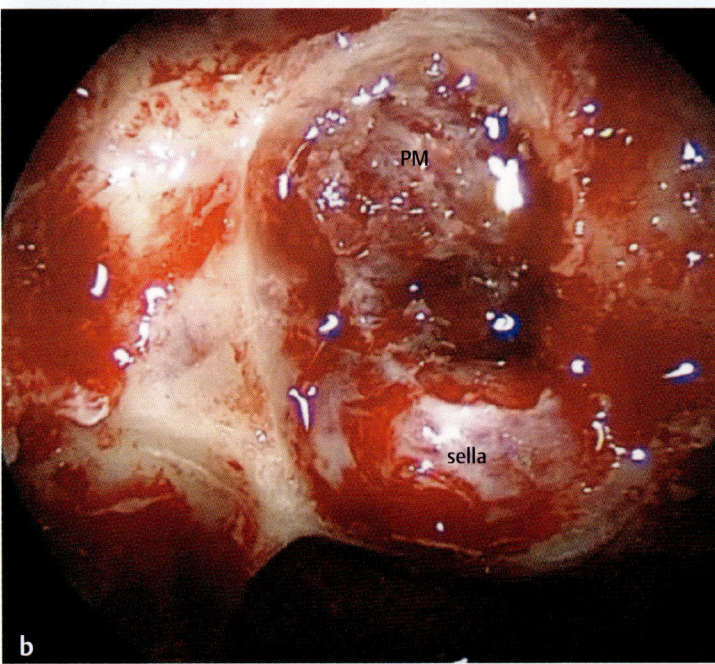

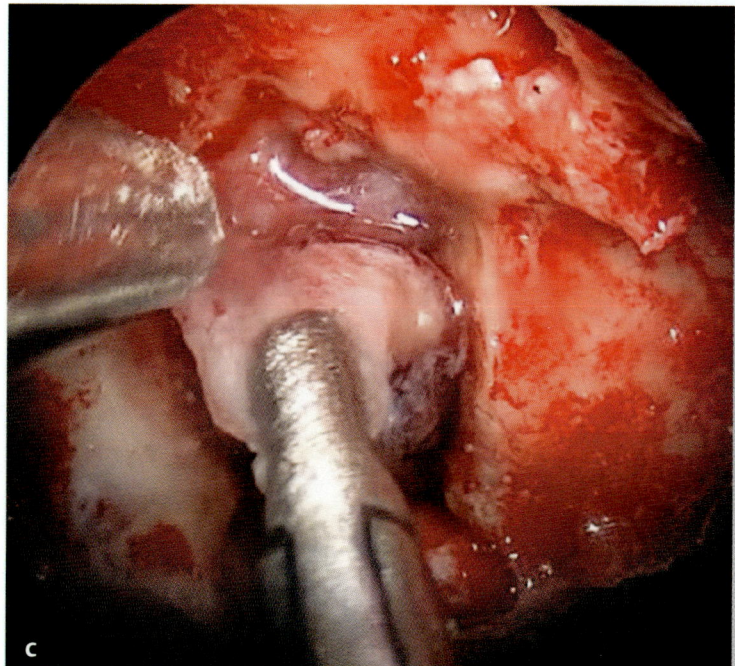

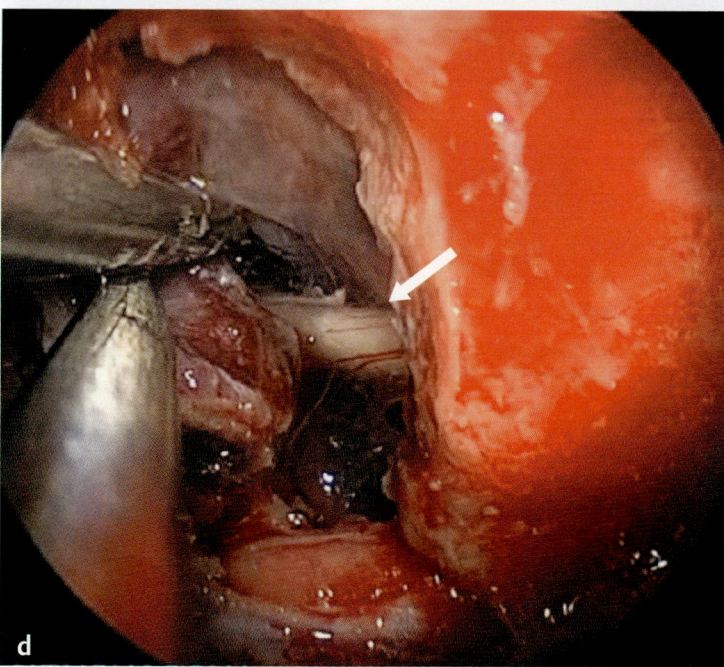

Fig. 6.8 (c, d) Piecemeal excision of the meningioma using combination of blunt and sharp instruments. Note: the left optic nerve coming into view **(d)** (*long white arrow*).

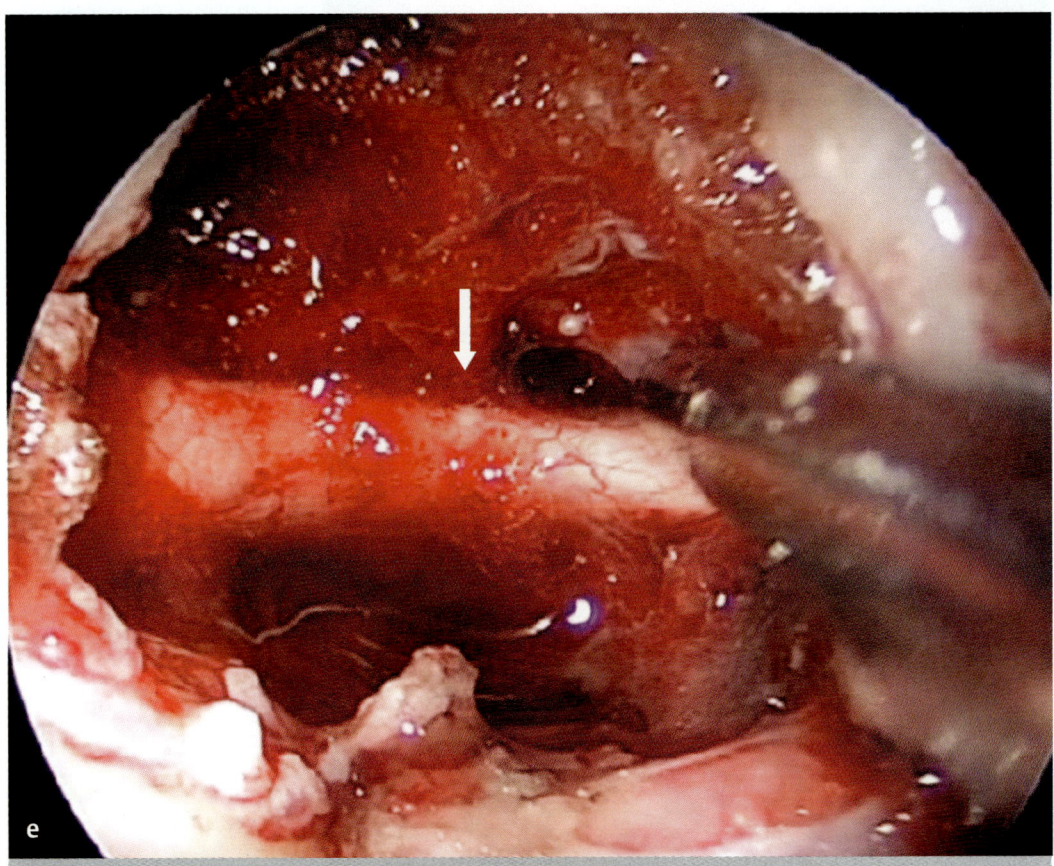

Fig. 6.8 **(e)** View after complete excision of the planum meningioma. Optic chiasm is marked by *white arrow*.

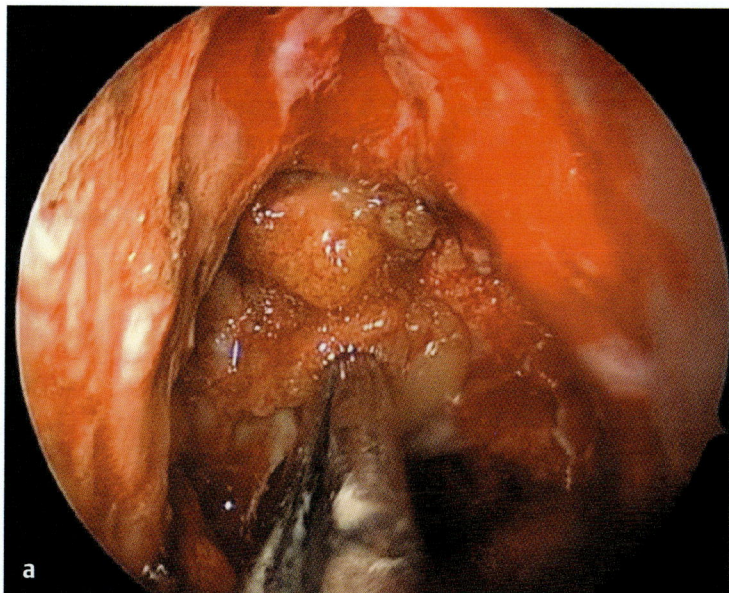

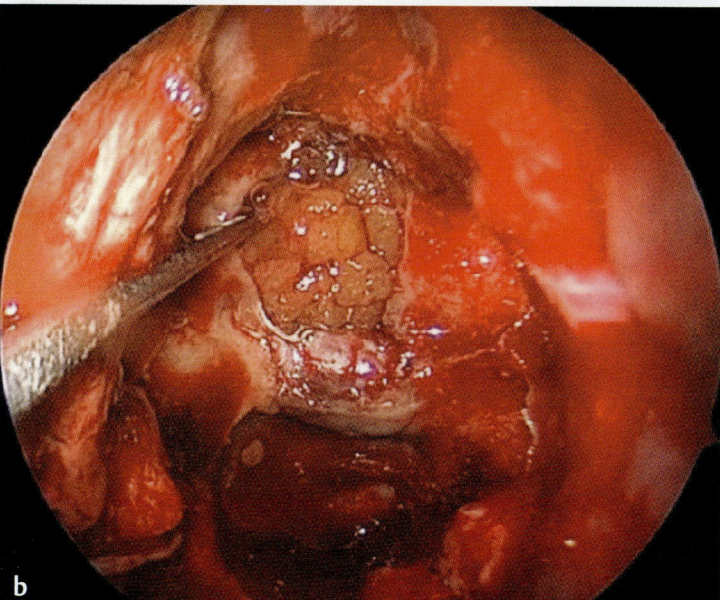

Fig. 6.9 Reconstruction of the defect shown in **Fig. 6.8e**.
Fig. 6.9 (a, b) Planum defect being closed by fat plug and being reinforced by glue.

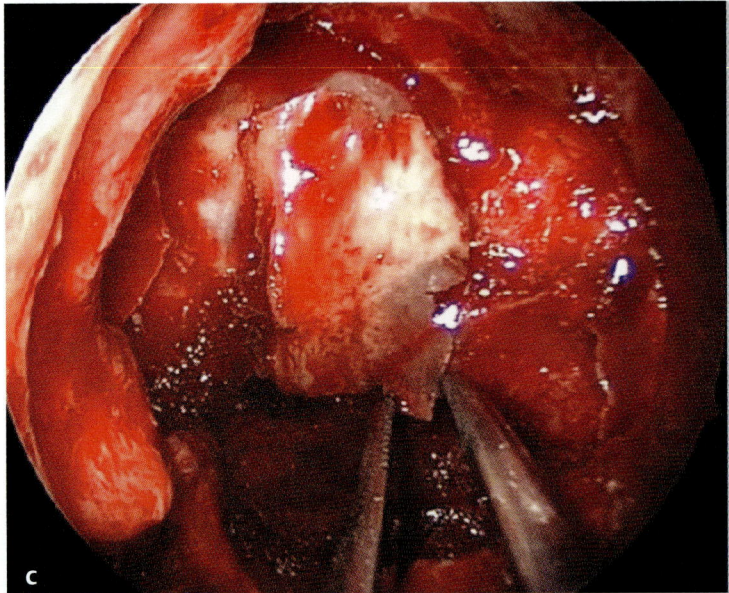

Fig. 6.9 (c) Free bone graft (sphenoid keel in this case) used to wedge in to close the bony sellar defect. (d) Final closure done with the Hadad flap.

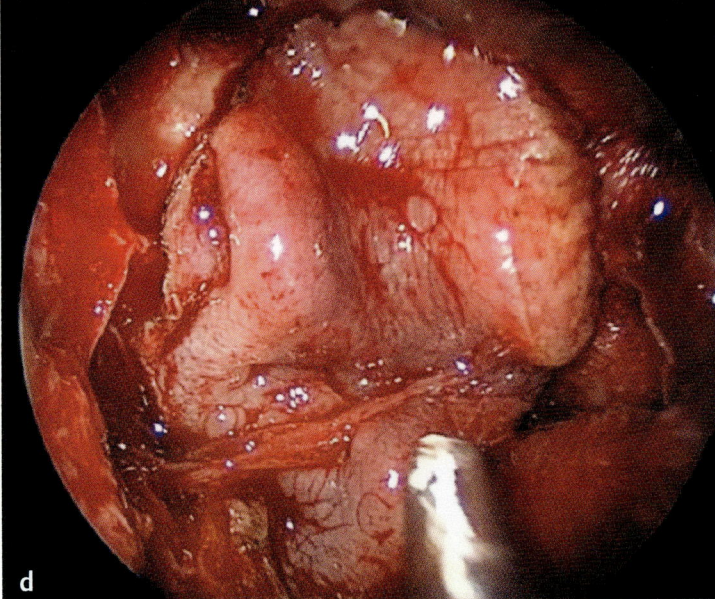

mucocutaneous junction of the septum. In cases where the Hadad flap cannot be harvested (e.g. in revision cases, or cases with septal perforation), one may opt for free repair using fat, fascia, and glue (**Figs. 6.7, 6.9**) or harvest a Reserve flap from the lateral nasal wall (refer to chapter 5 section Reconstruction).

Transclival Approach

The upper clivus is bound by the dorsum sellae and the posterior clinoids. In order to gain access to the basilar artery, which is situated posteriorly, it is essential to remove the dorsum sella and the posterior clinoids. Clival lesions generally displace the paraclival carotids and the basilar venous plexus, which aid in endoscopic resection (**Fig. 6.10**). The extent of drilling of the clivus depends on the extent of the lesion. Use of neuro-navigation system is mandatory. The floor of the sphenoid sinus is completely drilled and made flush with the lower two-thirds of the clivus. Like any other approach, it is important to keep critical landmarks in the field of vision, which are paraclival carotids, medial pterygoids, and vidian canals on either side (**Fig. 6.11**). An inverted U-shaped pharyngeal flap may be elevated in order to expose the clivus, which may later also aid in reconstruction (**Fig. 6.12**). The clival bone is drilled using a coarse 3-mm diamond burr with the aid of neuro-navigation. Clival drilling is a time-consuming process as one may encounter continuous bleeding from the bone marrow (**Fig. 6.13**). This is controlled by continuous irrigation, and/or bone wax. Once the inner cortex is reached, it may be drilled with a diamond drill, or Kerrison's punch or fine dissector (See **Figs. 10.8, 10.13, 10.26** in chapter 10). Once the inner clival cortex is removed, the dura with the basilar plexus is exposed (**Fig. 6.14**). Bleeding from the basilar plexus can be significant and is controlled by fibrillar collagen or Floseal®. Often however, the bleeding may not be significant due to the presence of pathology in that area.

The limitations of endoscopic transclival surgery are the cases with lateral tumour extension to the jugular bulb, carotid canal, or cavernous sinus or in cases with tumour present up to the foramen magnum extending to the occipital condyle or the lowermost part of the dens. In such scenarios, endoscopic approach is contraindicated or is at least combined with transcranial approach.[1]

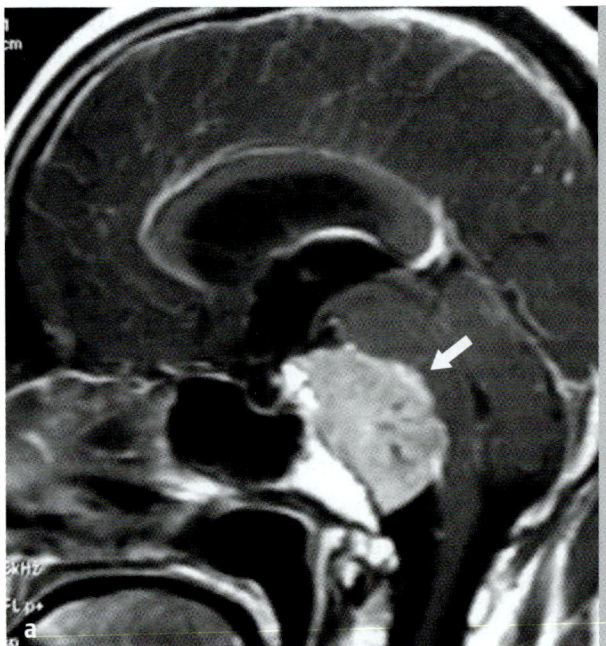

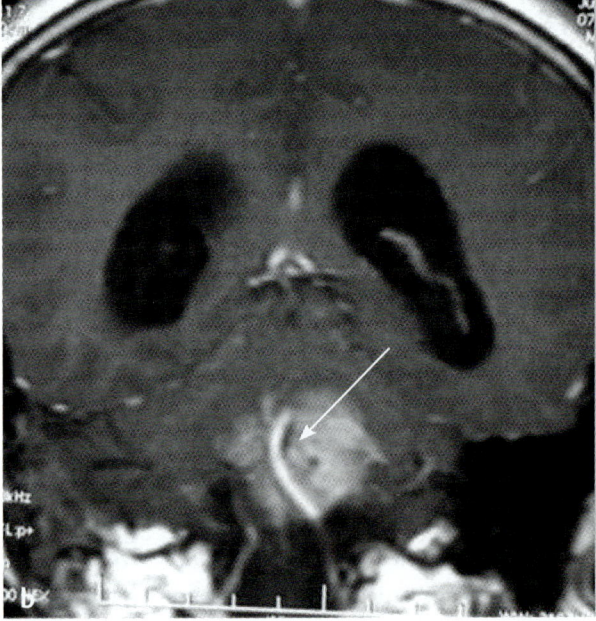

Fig. 6.10 **(a, b)** Clival meningioma (*short white block arrow*), occupying the entire clivus, seen to displace the basilar artery (*long white arrow*) posteriorly obstructing the fourth ventricle causing hydrocephalus (seen by enlargement of lateral ventricles). Lesion was excised by transclival approach.

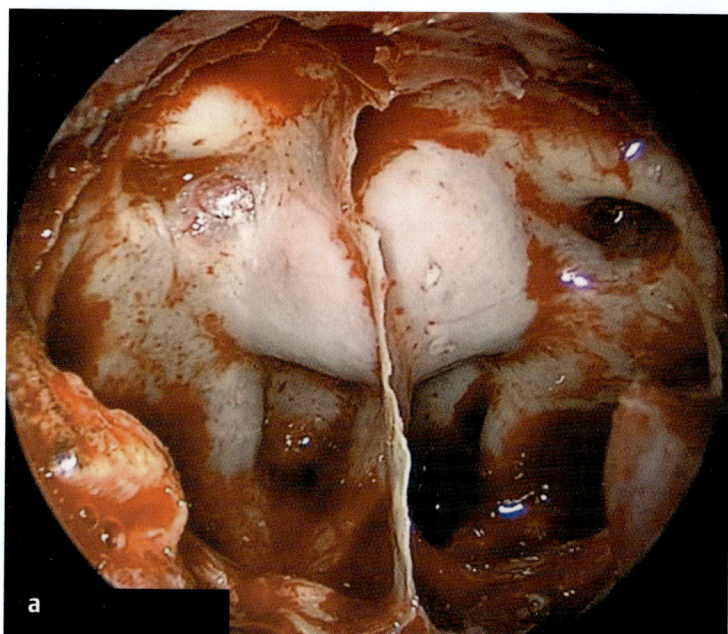

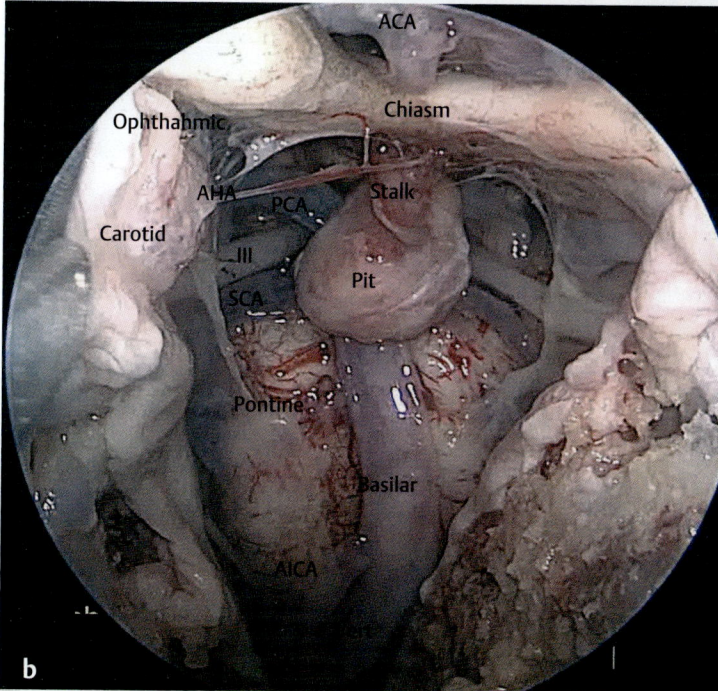

Fig. 6.11 **(a)** Critical landmarks in the field of vision for transclival surgery. **(b)** Cadaveric picture of the retroclival anatomy. AHA, anterior hypophyseal artery; Pit, pituitary gland; III, oculomotor nerve; ACA, anterior cerebral artery; PCA, posterior cerebral artery; SCA, superior cerebellar artery; AICA, antero-inferior cerebellar artery; Vert, vertebral artery.

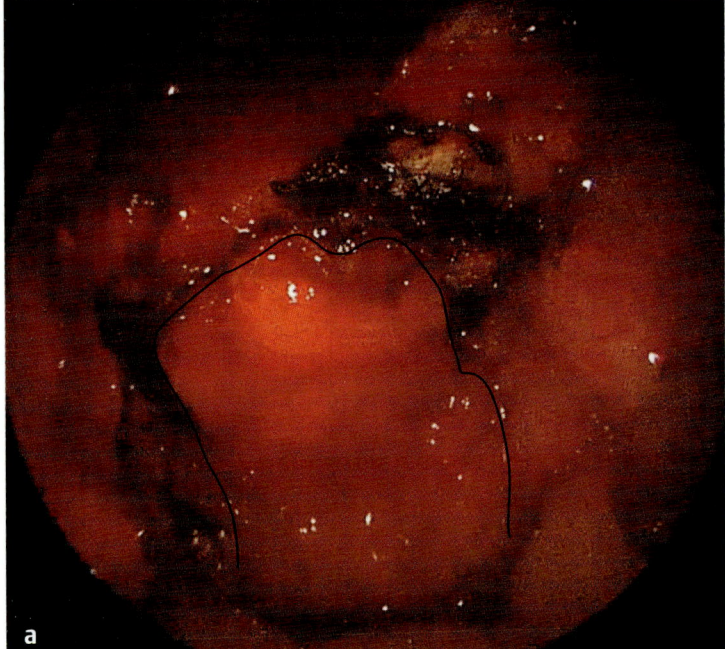

Fig. 6.12 **(a, b)** Inverted U-shaped pharyngeal flap (outlined in black) is elevated in order to expose the lower clivus. This same flap may be used for reconstruction or it may be juxtaposed with the Hadad flap to close the defect.

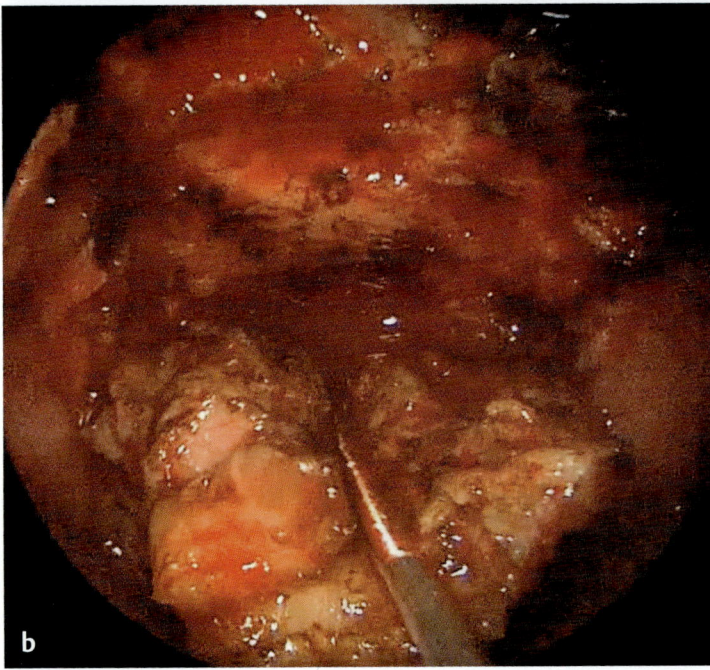

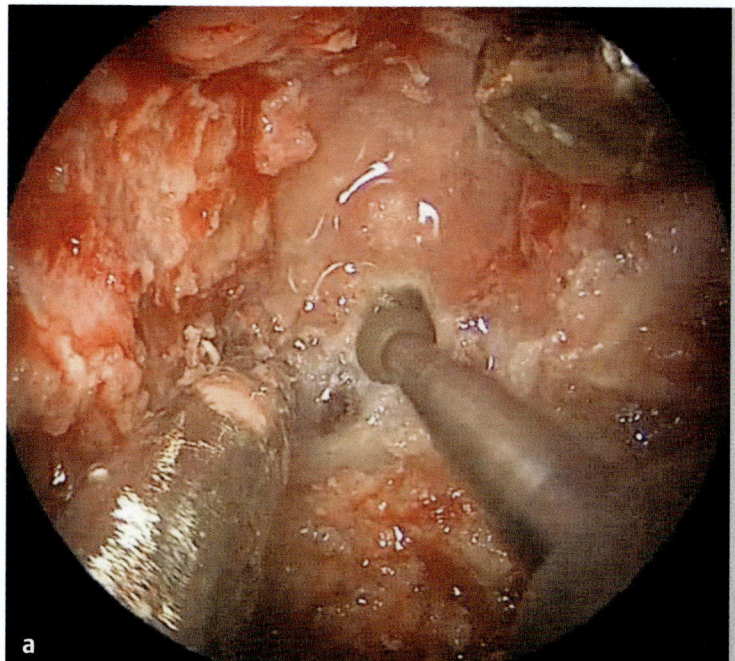

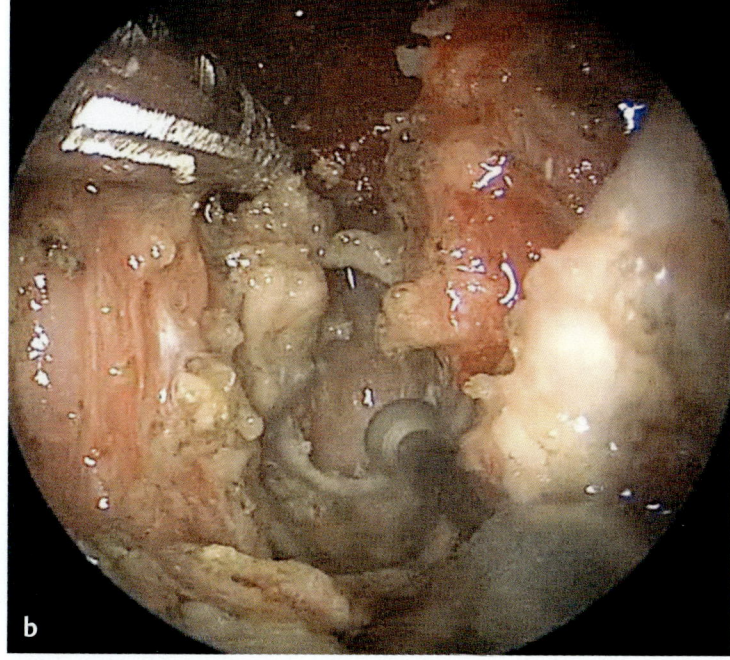

Fig. 6.13 **(a)** Drilling of the clival bone initially using cutting burr and intra-operative navigation at every step until the inner cortex is reached. **(b)** Once the inner cortex is reached, the burr is switched to diamond for further drilling.

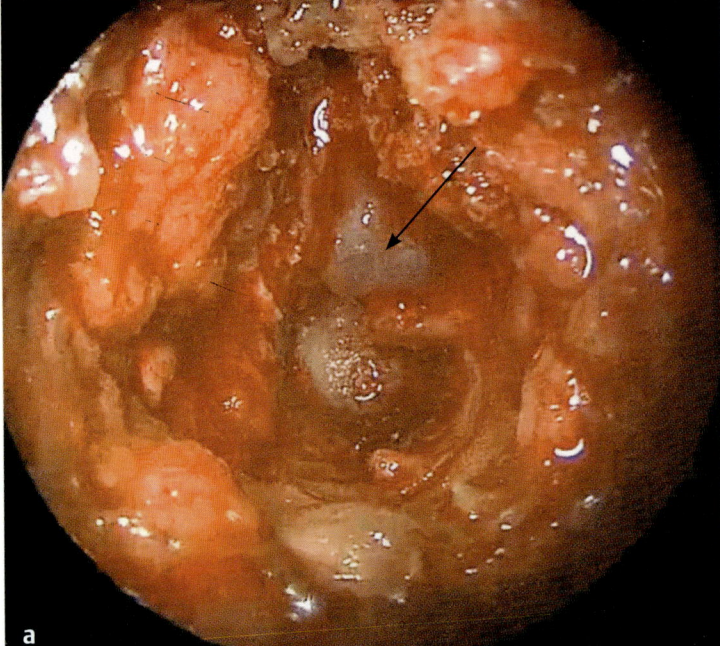

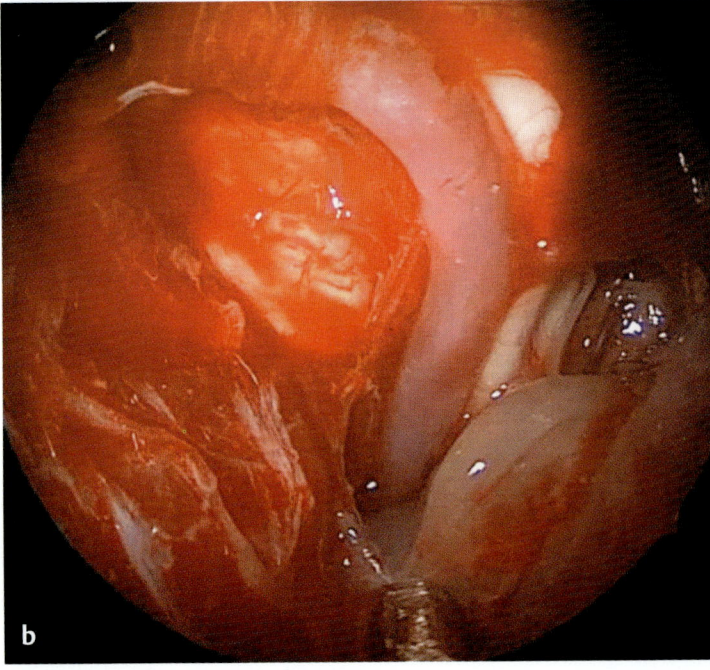

Fig. 6.14 (a) Exposure of the clival dura (*black arrow*) after drilling of the inner clival cortex. **(b)** Visualisation of the basilar artery after drilling of the clivus and tumour excision.

If craniocervical junction instability is anticipated, then occipitocervical fixation may be done prior to the surgery.

For Cranioverterbral (CV) junction tumour, an inverted posterior pharyngeal flap is raised and usually lower clivus and anterior arch of C1 is removed.

Reconstruction

Clival defect reconstruction is a bit challenging due to lack of posterior support, size of the defect, and the effect of gravity.[2] Clival surgeries obviously entails CSF leak, hence a Hadad flap needs to be harvested at the beginning of the surgery. A single-sided nasoseptal flap may be inadequate, sometimes requiring the aid of pharyngeal mucosal flap for reconstruction (**Fig. 6.15**). The flap to be harvested may be shorter than that harvested for regular cases if the lower clivus is not involved.

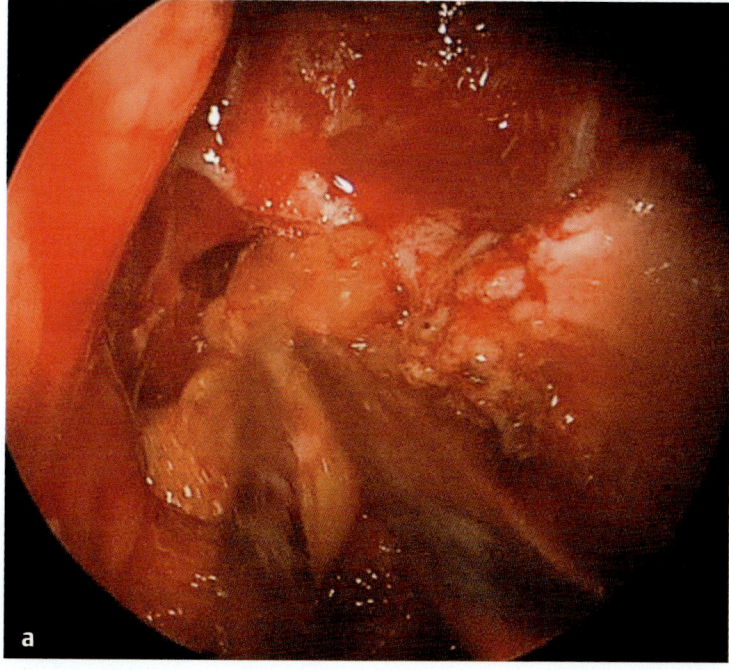

Fig. 6.15 Multilayered reconstruction of the clival defect using **(a)** underlay fat.

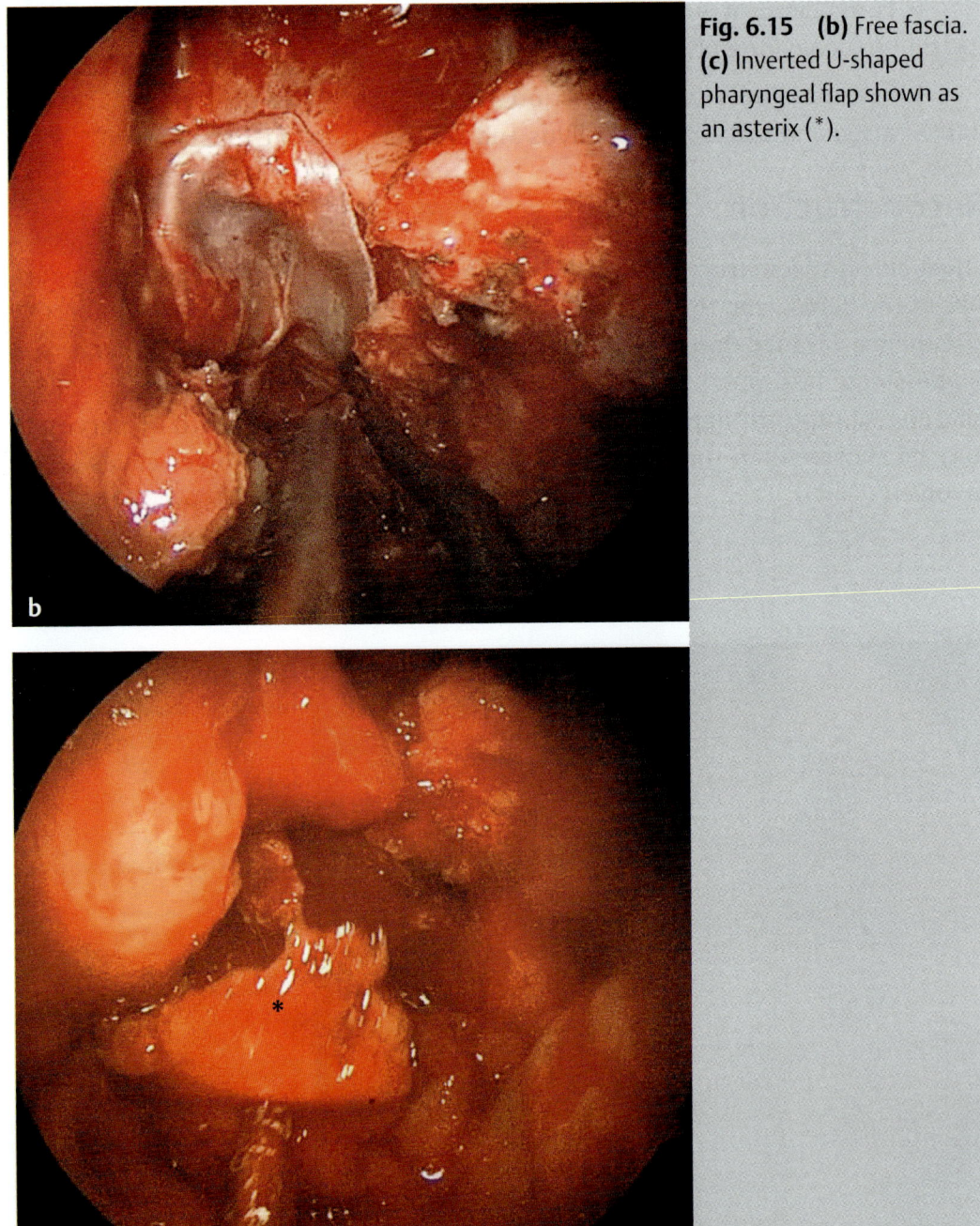

Fig. 6.15 **(b)** Free fascia.
(c) Inverted U-shaped
pharyngeal flap shown as
an asterix (*).

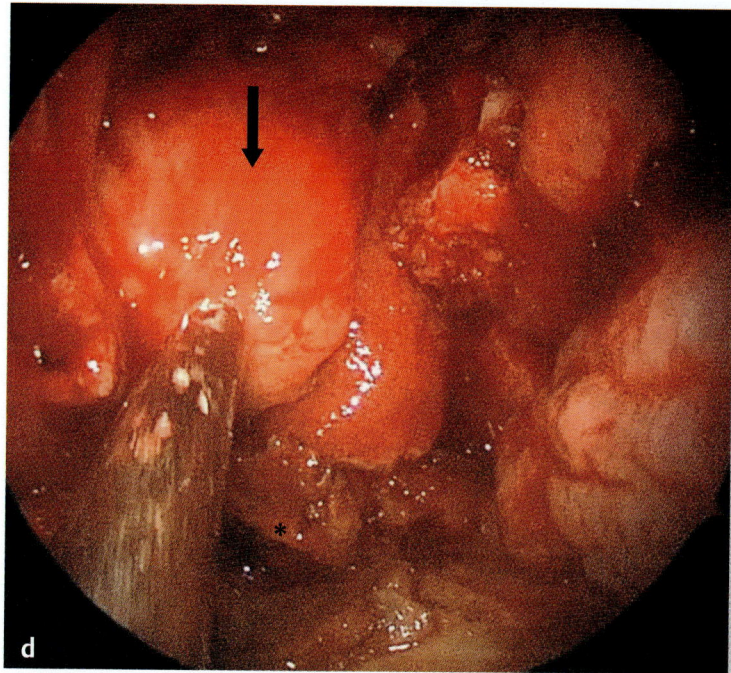

Fig. 6.15 **(d)** HB flap indicated by *thick black arrow*, is juxtaposed with the pharyngeal flap (*).

Exposure in the coronal plane is described in the very experienced groups but should remain in the domain of advanced centres and is beyond the scope of this book.

References

1. Deopujari C, Shaikh S, Shah N. Endonasal extended endoscopic skull base approaches: scope and limitations. In: Muthukumar N, Goyal V, eds. Progress in Clinical Neurosciences. Vol 32. Noida, UP: Thieme; 2017:89–102

2. Mangussi-Gomes J, Beer-Furlan A, Balsalobre L, Vellutini EA, Stamm AC. Endoscopic endonasal management of skull base chordomas. Otolaryngol Clin North Am 2016;49(1):167–182

Post-operative Care

Nishit Shah and Sai Spoorthi Nayak

Post-Operative Period

It is our post-operative protocol to keep the patient in intensive care unit (ICU) for at least a day, for monitoring of input/output, serum electrolytes, nasal discharge, if any, lumbar drain functioning (if inserted) etc.

A Foley catheter is kept in situ for monitoring the urine output. If the **urine output** exceeds 1,000 cc over 4 hours, and if serum sodium is greater than 150 mEq/L, intranasal vasopressin (IV) is administered after accounting for the intra-operative loaded fluids. Correctional measures should be taken if there is any hyponatremia.

Antibiotics are continued for a variable period ranging from three days to 5 days or more depending on the status of the patient. A broad-spectrum antibiotic like any cephalosporin is usually started in the dose of 1 g BD. This is primarily to prevent nasal infection. If a lumbar drain is used for a patient, then an aminoglycoside is added as long as the drain remains in situ, to cover anaerobic organisms. If the patient presents with foul-smelling crusts in the post-operative period, oral antibiotics may be started according to culture report.

If a **lumbar drain** has been placed, it is removed at the end of surgery if there is no cerebrospinal fluid (CSF) leak intra-operatively. If the leak is small, the drain may be removed after 24 hours. In cases where the basal cisterns have been widely opened, or the size of leak is decently wide, the drain is continued for 3 days or 72 hours at the rate of 10cc/hr. When the ventricle is widely opened, the drain may be continued for 4 to 5 days. This drain should be closely monitored. If the drain stops functioning at any point, it is advisable to remove the drain even in the immediate post-operative period. A non-functioning drain is more dangerous and is a potential threat for ascending meningitis.

In most cases, where a rescue flap has been used, we generally do not insert nasal packs at the end of surgery. The **nasal packs**, if put, are usually removed at the end of 24 to 48 hours if they have been placed for the sake of haemostasis alone. If there has been an intra-operative CSF leak, the pack is usually placed on the side of the nasoseptal flap, and is removed at the end of 4 to 5 days, depending on the leak. The patient is in bed with head elevation from 30–60 degrees.

Serum electrolytes are monitored every day for at least 3 days. It is advisable to re-evaluate the electrolytes once before discharging the patient or at 1 week following surgery. The patients are again asked to do the test at 3 weeks and inform on email or phone.

In patients having hypopituitarism pre-operatively, **hormonal replacement** is started pre-operatively itself. In patients having normal pituitary functions pre-operatively, hydrocortisone is given post-operatively for 3 days (100 mg TDS on day 1, BD on day 2, and OD on day 3). In patient having visual deficit with normal pituitary function, dexamethasone is given, pre-operatively for visual protection and continued post-operatively for 1 to 3 weeks depending on the visual recovery.

Serum cortisol levels should be checked once before discharge, at 8 am and 4 pm after being off any supplemental therapy for at least 24 hours to prevent false readings.

For a growth hormone secreting tumour, growth hormone levels checked on the morning after surgery in a fasting state should ideally be less than 2 ng/mL.

A full hormonal profile is repeated at 3 months and if abnormal, endo-crinology reference is made for long term follow up.

Post-Operative Mobilisation of Patient

Whenever there is a CSF leak observed during the surgery, it is our protocol to keep the patient in bed with head elevation gradually increased to 60 degrees over post-operative days 2-4. The patient is mobilised on day 4 or 5. That is normally the time taken for the flap/graft to primarily take up. Intracranial pressure lies in the range of 15 to 20 cm of H_2O in prone and increases to 40 cm H_2O in sitting position.[1] Over the last few years, we have been encouraging our patients to mobilise out of bed as early as possible. The head is gradually elevated from 30 to 60 degrees over post-operative days 2 to 4. The patient is allowed to walk with nasal packs in situ on day 4, and the packs are removed on day 5. Early mobilisation has not been found to have any effect on the healing of the repair site and on the contrary, the patients are more comfortable in terms of feeding and movement. In cases with intra-operative leak, the lumbar drain is left in situ for at least 24 hours for a small leak and upto 72 hours in extended surgeries with large defect and if 3rd ventricle has been opened. CSF is drained at the rate of 10 cc/h. This keeps the pressure of CSF off the repair site.

After the nasal packs are removed, the patient is mobilised out of bed and kept in the hospital for 24 hours under observation for any CSF leak.

Post-Operative Nasal Cleaning

Once the patient is fit for discharge, the patient is posted for nasal cleaning. Any crusts or fibrinous exudates in the anterior nasal cavity are cleaned using a headlight or endoscope. The nasopharynx is cleaned of all the mucinous discharge, making sure to remain low, at the level of the inferior turbinate. The purpose of this cleaning is to facilitate nasal breathing by opening up the nasal passages. At this time, the sphenoid area should not be touched or disturbed. Usually two endoscopic nasal cleanings, staged 1 week apart, are adequate. The patient is asked to visit us in case there is any nasal blockade or foul-smelling nasal discharge or any hint of CSF leak. The patient is started on saline nasal sprays immediately after pack removal. This helps reduce crust formation and makes post-operative cleaning easy. Utmost care must be taken for a patient in whom a CSF leak has been repaired during surgery, however, tiny the leak is.

Precautions, recommended in patients with CSF leak and repair, are to avoid straining at stools, avoid heavy weight lifting, and avoid flexing the neck for prolonged period as all these activities will increase the intracranial pressure. Activities that involve sudden change in atmospheric pressure such as flight travel, and scuba diving are best avoided for at least 3 weeks. Swimming in the post-operative period is contraindicated for obvious reasons. It is also advisable to avoid being in crowded places or dusty environment for the first week post-operatively so as not to catch any air-borne infections.

Follow up imaging is also routinely performed at 3 months to see adequacy of decompression or completeness of resection as per the original plan for surgery. It can alert us to any unforeseen complication and can be used for reference in further follow up.

Reference

1. Shah N, Rathore A. Step by Step CSF Rhinorrhoea. New Delhi: Jaypee; 2009:9

Surgical Complications and Their Management

C. E. Deopujari and Sai Spoorthi Nayak

In appropriately chosen cases, the complication rate of endoscopic skull base surgeries is comparable to transcranial and transnasal microsurgeries. In experienced hands, tumour removal has become increasingly safe and probably more effective.

Intra-operative Complications

Vascular Complications

The most common intra-operative complication is bleeding. It may result from the septal branch of sphenopalatine artery, cavernous sinuses, intercavernous sinuses, internal carotid artery, and very rarely from anterior cerebral artery or posterior cerebral artery, in the sagittal plane. In the coronal plane, bleeding from following arteries may be encountered: sphenopalatine artery, internal maxillary artery, or descending palatine artery.

Bleeding from the septal branch of sphenopalatine artery may occur while widening the sphenoid, as the septal branches run between the sphenoid ostium and the upper margin of the choana (**Fig. 8.1**). However, one has to be careful not to damage this vessel while raising the nasoseptal flap on the same side as

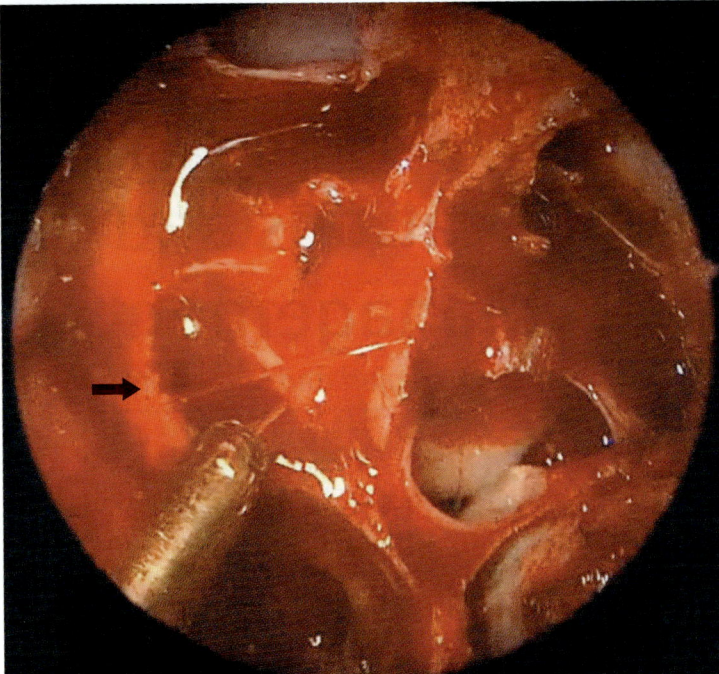

Fig. 8.1 Jet of blood seen coming from the septal branch of the sphenopalatine artery on the right (*block arrow*), after being traumatised while trying to punch the anterior wall of the sphenoid. This artery has to be preserved on the side of which the Hadad flap has to be raised.

it may jeopardise the viability of the flap. The sphenopalatine branch can also be encountered while accessing the pterygopalatine fossa. When this vessel bleeds, it is identified using suction in one hand and a cottonoid in the other. The endoscope should be held in such a way so that the jet of blood doesn't fall on the scope. Such bleeders can be easily tackled using bipolar cautery or monopolar suction cautery once identified.

Bleeding from internal maxillary artery may be encountered in transpterygoid surgeries, while accessing the pterygopalatine fossa or the infratemporal fossa. The artery is either bipolarised or is ligated using ligaclips.

For extended approaches, further chances of bleeding may be encountered while dividing the anterior intercavernous sinus which is best controlled by bipolar coagulation (**Fig. 8.2**). The coagulation and division of the sinus should be strictly in midline to avoid any damage to the inferior hypophyseal branches which supply the optic apparatus.

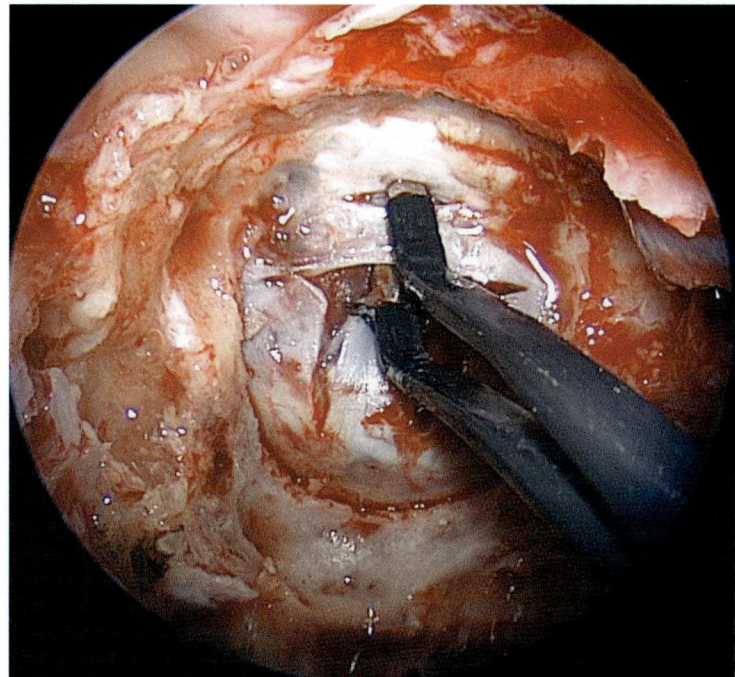

Fig. 8.2 Superior intercavernous sinus (SICS) is encountered in extended skull base cases such as transplanar or transtubercular approaches. It is cauterised strictly in the midline using vertical pistol grip bipolar forceps (See **Fig. 10.27** in chapter 10) to avoid injury to the inferior hypothalamic artery.

Bleeding at further depth is often controlled by local haemostatic agents as cauterisation tends to further damage and may even block the vessel. Gelatin sponge (Gelfoam®) is most commonly used as local haemostat. It consists of a gelatinous matrix to be directly placed over the bleeding site. However, it has to stay at the source of bleeding to provide continued haemostasis. It swells up with blood at the target site and may hamper distal vision.

Oxidised cellulose sheets or fleece (Surgicel®) is a better alternative as it works by chemical changes and does not swell up. Diffuse capillary bleeding and venous bleeding is best controlled by Surgicel and is probably a good option to use at the end of the surgery for reinforcing haemostasis.

Fibrin glue also has haemostatic properties apart from its primary use as a sealant. It is especially useful for venous bleeding from accidental injury to cavernous sinus or intercavernous sinus injuries.

Floseal® haemostatic matrix consists of a combination of gelatin granules and human thrombin. It is used in cavernous sinus bleeding as haemostasis by means of compression or cauterisation is impractical at this site. It provides a fast and effective method of haemostasis. It is injected using a special applicator exactly on the source of bleeding. It is then covered with a cottonoid for a few seconds to approximate the thrombin to the bleeding tissues. The flow of bleeding is then stemmed. The advantages of Floseal® are that it can conform to any site of bleeding, and with the help of the applicator it can reach the deepest or difficult-to-access areas. The biggest advantage of Floseal® is that it can be washed off and doesn't form a hard matrix and hamper distal vision (**Fig. 8.3**).

Carotid artery bleed is a high-pressure bleed which can immediately fill up the nasal cavity in a matter of few seconds and can readily cause instant disorientation of the surgical field. Undoubtedly, it can raise alarm and panic in the theatre. It is important not to lose one's calm in a carotid bleed and to never

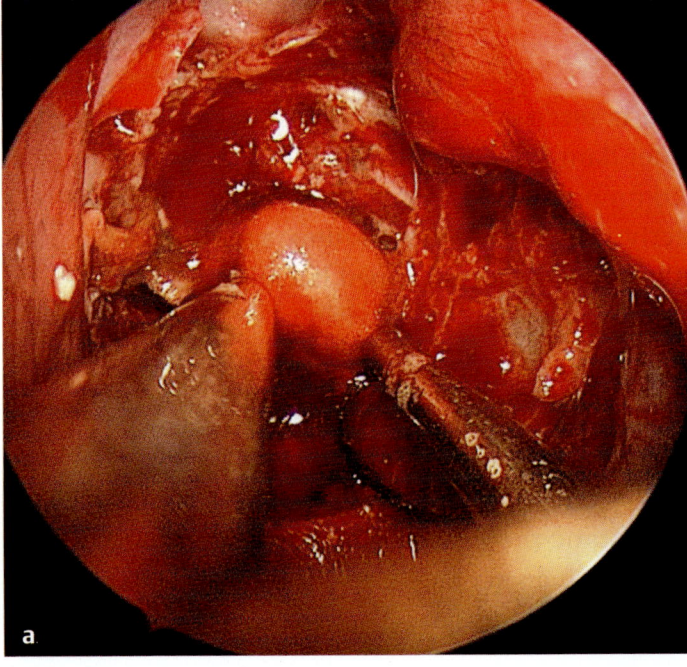

Fig. 8.3 (a) Floseal®, used for controlling left cavernous bleed, is directly applied at the target site with the help of an applicator.

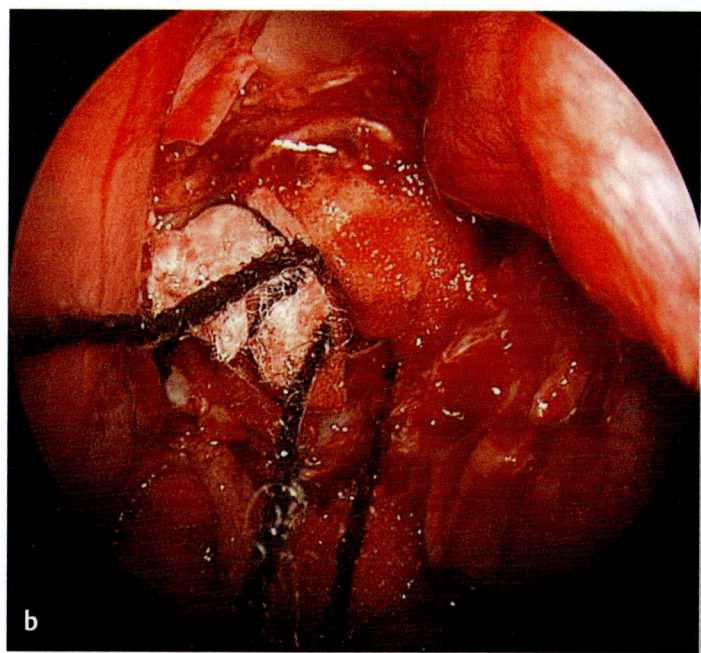

b

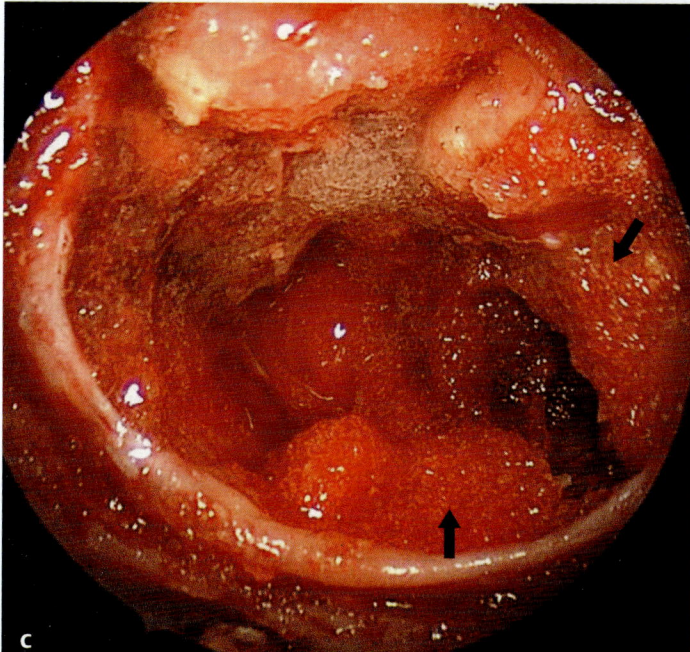

c

Fig. 8.3 **(b)** After pushing the Floseal® at the targeted site, it is approximated with the tissue with a cottonoid patty. **(c)** The sella seen clearly after the Floseal® is washed off (*black arrows*). The remnants of Floseal® are seen over the left cavernous sinus and it does not hamper distal vision.

remove the scope out of the nose. It is a good idea to use two suctions for skull base cases. The first step to do in case of such a bleed is to create more space in the nasal cavity by either doing a middle turbinectomy or inferior turbinectomy. In cases, where uninostril approaches are used, it is advisable to make a septal incision so that the second suction can be introduced from the opposite side. In most situations, binostril approach is used for skull base surgeries, so a separate septal incision may not be required. Two suctions are used, and both the suctions are triangulated to locate the site of bleed (**Fig. 8.4**).

Crushed muscle graft is the best available local haemostatic and is capable to stem the flow if applied with some pressure. For small tears, Surgicel® under pressure may prove to be adequate. It should be covered using a mucosal or connective tissue graft for further reinforcement. An interventional radiologist is called to the theatre and an intra-operative angiography is performed to look for any aneurysm, which is then tackled at the same setting. A repeat angiography is done after 1 week and after 1 month to look for development of any aneurysms.

In a bid for effective tumour removal, one has to be extremely careful not to damage important blood vessels like internal carotid artery (ICA), anterior cerebral artery, posterior cerebral artery, etc., especially in large or adherent or malignant tumours, encasing or infiltrating the blood vessels. The patient may land up in serious post-operative neurological deficits. In such situations, decision has to be taken about leaving the tumour behind to avoid catastrophic complications. Where there is an option, one can treat the residual tumour with other modalities like gamma irradiation.

Neural Complications

Any inadvertent trauma to the optic nerve while drilling the intersphenoid septations ending on the nerve, trauma to the nerve while drilling over the sella, or direct injury to the optic nerve chiasm while handling suprasellar tumours can result in post-operative blindness. Also, any damage or spasm of the ophthalmic artery can result in visual complications. Vision may be completely lost or may be worsened in a pre-existing visual loss.

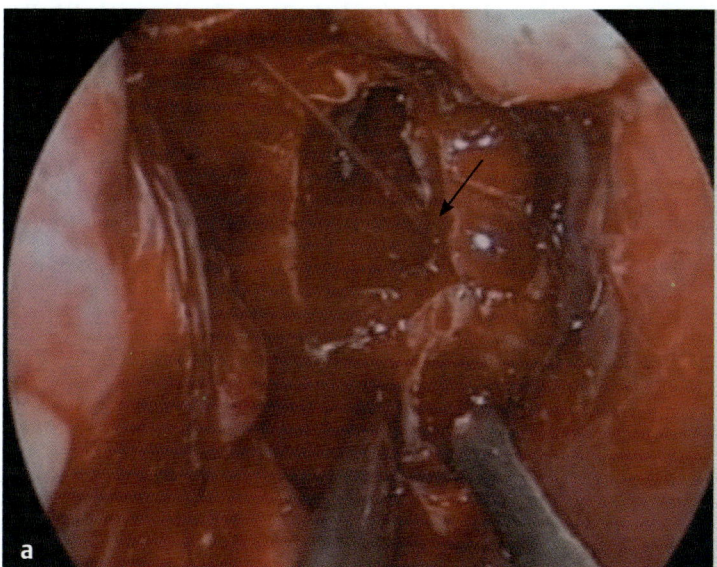

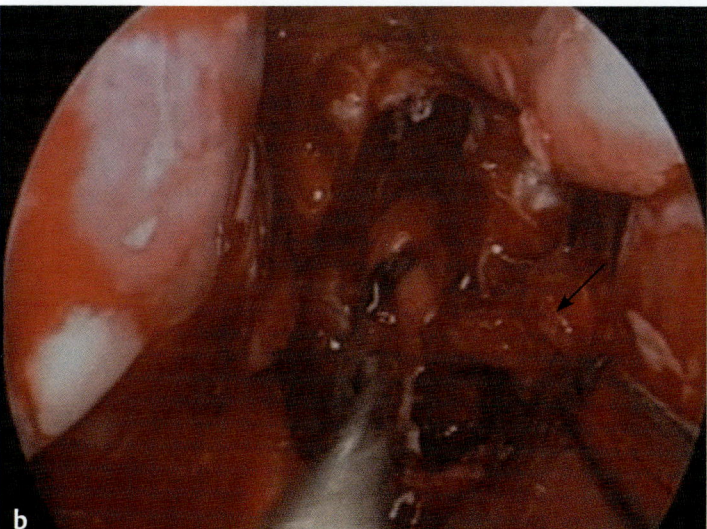

Fig. 8.4 **(a)** Bleeding from the left clival carotid artery (*black arrow*). **(b)** Bleeding from the carotid artery is stemmed with muscle patch with pressure (*black arrow*).

Extensive compression over or manipulation in the cavernous sinus can result in trauma to the III, IV, VI, and V1 nerves which course along its lateral wall. Patient may develop post-operative diplopia/ophthalmoplegia with III, IV, or, more commonly, VI nerve gaze palsy or ptosis.

Overenthusiastic packing of the sella may put pressure over these nerves and can also result in temporary ophthalmoplegia. Overzealous packing to control the bleeding in the venous gulf area most commonly will result in post-operative VI nerve palsy as the VI nerve runs its horizontal course just posterior to the venous gulf.

The treatment is essentially to conserve these patients by giving them intravenous (IV) corticosteroids to reduce the neural oedema. Rarely, the patient may have to be taken back to the theatre to remove any excessive packing to decompress the nerve. Of course, this decision needs to be taken according to the surgical team discussion. The conservative option may be tried first for a couple of days with close monitoring of the vision and eye movements. Should this method fail, the surgical option may be chosen safely.

CSF Leak

In extracapsular dissection, the tumour removal is more complete, but the chance of CSF leak is slightly more. In intracapsular dissection of tumours, the chance of CSF leak is less if the surgeon is careful enough not to injure the diaphragm sellae. In intradural tumoural extension, chance of a CSF leak is always present. CSF leak is identified by continuous clear flow of fluid, (intra-operatively mixed with blood)(**Fig. 8.5**), which is usually pulsatile due to the transmitted pulsations of the brain. It may reduce after a while depending on the intracranial pressure but never stops completely. Upon noticing a leak, it is mandatory to identify the site and close it in the same sitting, at the end of the tumour removal.

A small rent in the diaphragm can be easily plugged with fat. It can be then reinforced with fascia, nasoseptal flaps, free mucoperiosteal flaps, glue, etc., depending on the size of the rent. The morbidity associated with a CSF leak

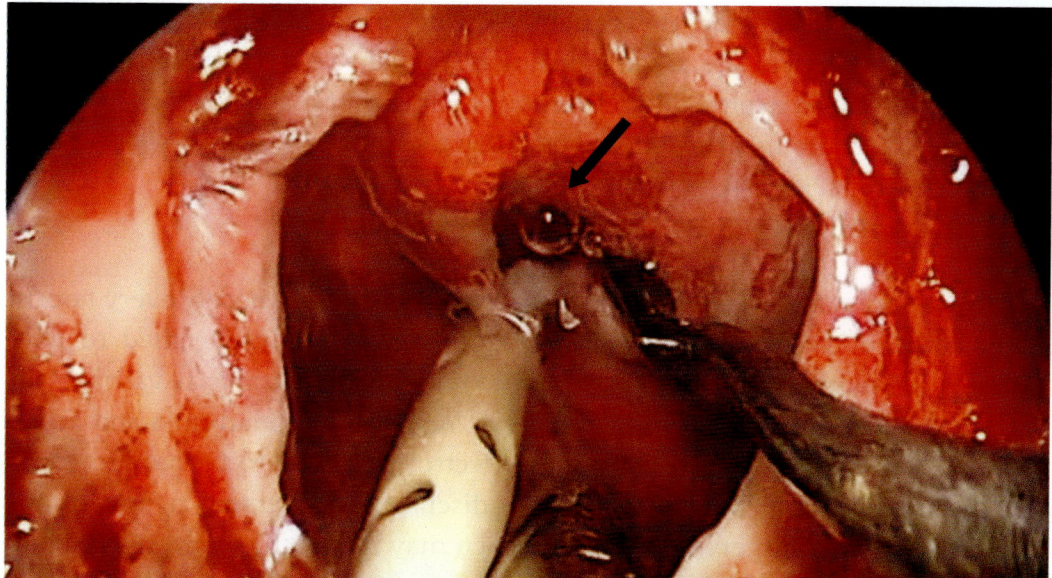

Fig. 8.5 CSF leak from a dural rent (*black arrow*) following extracapsular dissection of craniopharyngioma.

repair is always more than a clean case. The patient is asked to have bed rest for a period of 5 days to avoid the slightest chance of CSF leak recurring. Generally, the patient may or may not have a lumbar drain.

Immediate Post-operative Complications

Bleeding

In the recovery room, patient may develop bleeding, within 24 hours of surgery, due to inadequate haemostasis or packing, sudden rise in blood pressure, or due to any bleeding tendencies in the patient. Minor bleeding may be controlled by nasal packing. If the bleeding continues in spite of packing, or if the bleeding seems to be arterial, then the patient may be taken back to the theatre to re-explore the surgical site. If the bleeding is from the sella, then the repair area should be lifted and explored for cavernous or any arterial bleed. Once the site is identified, adequate measure should be taken to control the bleed.

Diabetes Insipidus and Hyponatremia

In the post-operative period, the urine output is monitored closely every hourly. If the urine output exceeds over 200 mL/h, the patient is deemed to have diabetes insipidus (DI). This can be settled by giving intranasal vasopressin. Persistent DI or increased urine output may result in hyponatremia and has to be corrected accordingly. Hence, serum electrolytes need to be monitored on post-operative day1, 3, and at the time of discharge. Conversely, hyponatremia is often seen with surgery in this area which may be due to syndrome of inappropriate anti-diuretic hormone (SIADH) or cerebral salt wasting syndrome. Apart from serum sodium values, urinary sodium values and serum osmolarity help in treating these patients more effectively. Underlying cortisol deficiency has to be corrected.

CSF Leak

Utmost care must be taken for a patient in whom a CSF leak has been repaired during the surgery, however, tiny the leak is. It is our protocol to keep the patient in bed generally for a period of 5 days. That is normally the time taken for the graft to primarily take up. Flaps with a vascularised pedicle require 48 to 72 hours for uptake. In some cases, where vascularised flaps have been used for reconstruction, patients may be mobilised early.

In the immediate post operative period, there may be clear watery discharge from the nostrils, in spite of a good reconstruction. If the nasal packs are in situ, one could assume that the watery discharge could be the saline trickling from the packs. If the discharge keeps decreasing with each passing day, the patient is just managed conservatively with complete antibiotic coverage for meningitis prophylaxis. However if there is watery discharge in the absence of nasal packs, or immediately after pack removal (i.e., after 4-5 days), one has to be cautious and suspect CSF leak. If the discharge persists or increases with conservative management, the patients need to be taken back to the theatre for re-exploration and closure of the leak site at the earliest.

Meningitis

Meningitis can occur in patients who have undergone skull base surgery in the presence of a nasal infection or in the post-operative period where aseptic precautions have not been maintained. As mentioned earlier, a non-functioning drain can also serve as a source of ascending infection.

Delayed Post-Operative Complications

Nasal Complications

Patient may present with nasal infection, purulent nasal discharge, and nasal crusting, which need to be treated with regular nasal cleaning and post-operative antibiotics. Patient may also present with post-operative nasal blockage, this may be due to nasal crusting or synechiae (**Fig. 8.6**).

Panhypopituitarism

Any damage to the normal gland or the pituitary stalk can result in permanent hypopituitarism. The patient may then require lifelong hormonal supplements.

Delayed CSF Leaks and Fistula

Although a rare complication, delayed CSF leaks are attributed to displacement of the graft or ischaemia of the graft. A computed tomography (CT) in conjunction with nasal endoscopic examination help in detecting any displacement of flap. Presence of pneumocephalus near the repair area is highly suggestive of

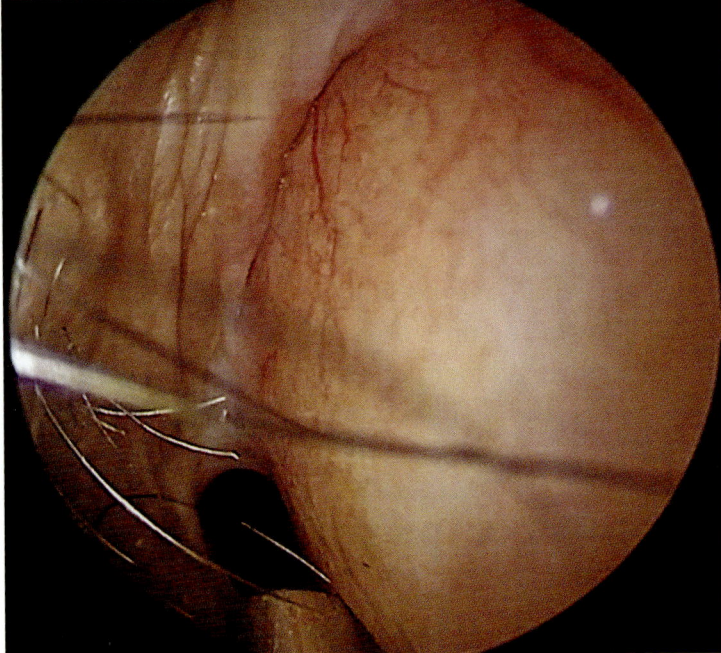

Fig. 8.6 Anterior synechiae between the septum and the lateral wall on the right side formed post-operatively.

a CSF fistula. In case of low flow leaks, a lumbar drain is introduced and kept in situ for 3 to 5 days and started on IV antibiotics for meningitis prophylaxis. Should this conservative method fail, the patient is taken up for re-exploration for a CSF fistula and repaired. In case of high-pressure leaks, the patient is immediately taken up for re-exploration in the theatre. It is imperative to look for ischaemia of the graft and flaps used for reconstruction and that fresh materials are used for re-repair the second time.[1]

References

1. Horowitz PM, DiNapoli V, Su SY, Raza SM. Complication avoidance in endoscopic skull base surgery. Otolaryngol Clin North Am 2016;49(1):227–235

Decision Making in Endonasal Skull Base Surgery

Sai Spoorthi Nayak and C. E. Deopujari

Endoscopic endonasal surgery is a very versatile approach for most skull base tumours. Endoscopy provides a panoramic view and offers the ability to look around in corners as compared to a microscope, which gives a tunnel vision. The most important principle in endonasal surgery is to avoid crossing the plane of important neurovascular structures especially cranial nerves.[1] An endonasal approach gives direct and easy access to the midline cranial base lesions without inadvertently damaging the more lateral neurovascular structures. Although most cases can be tackled endonasally, a proper risk–benefit ratio for every patient must be charted by the surgical team. Just because a lesion can be accessed endonasally does not mean that it has to be tackled by that approach (**Table 9.1**).

Table 9.1 Ideal case candidates for endoscopic approach versus transcranial approach

Endoscopic approach	Transcranial approach
Sella tumour	Large suprasellar tumour, little sellar component
Widened sella	Small sellar window
Sellar-suprasellar tumour with vertical or posterior lie of the tumour	Fairly anterior tumour or crossing mid-pupillary lines
Sellar–suprasellar tumour communicating with a wide neck	Sellar–suprasellar tumour connected with a narrow neck
Extradural tumour	Extensive intradural extension

Sellar and suprasellar masses with major portion of the tumour being in the sella and the sphenoid and little suprasellar extension are ideal cases. However, large suprasellar tumours with minimal parasellar extension are tumours which can be easily tackled endoscopically. Middle skull base tumours with parasellar extension, going lateral to the carotid pose a threat to the carotid as well as the cranial nerves running along the lateral wall of the cavernous sinus, when endoscopic approach is employed. Anterior skull base lesions with lateral extension crossing the mid-pupillary line are tumours which cannot be approached endoscopically. Transorbital approaches are, however, making it possible to address these lateral tumours as well.

For an endonasal trans-sphenoid approach, the most important corridor for access is formed by the sella. Hence, the width of the sella forms an important determining factor for ease of endonasal approach. Tumours with major suprasellar component and little sellar and sphenoid component are not easy/ ideal candidates for endonasal approach. Patients having a sellar–suprasellar lesion but with a narrow sella and a wide suprasellar component are difficult candidates for endoscopic surgery (**Fig. 9.1**) This is especially true if there is a normal pituitary gland present. A sella widened by the tumour is not only thin and can be easily drilled, but also provides a wider window to access the suprasellar portion (**Fig. 9.2**). The width of the sella is seen pre-operatively on computed tomography (CT) scan paranasal sinus (PNS) coronal or axial cuts.

In some cases, where the suprasellar component of the tumour is large, the surgeon may opt for a staged surgery. The sellar tumour is removed endoscopically in the first sitting leaving some suprasellar portion untouched. The surgeon waits for a few months for the suprasellar component to descend into the sella which is determined by a repeat magnetic resonance (MR) scan. Once the tumour descends adequately, the second surgery is performed. If the tumour fails to descend down, then transcranial route is employed.

The lie of the tumour also determines the ease of endonasal surgery. Tumours with anterior extension or lie pose a challenge for endonasal access. Vertical tumours with a slight posterior inclination are favourable for endoscopic removal (**Fig. 9.3**).

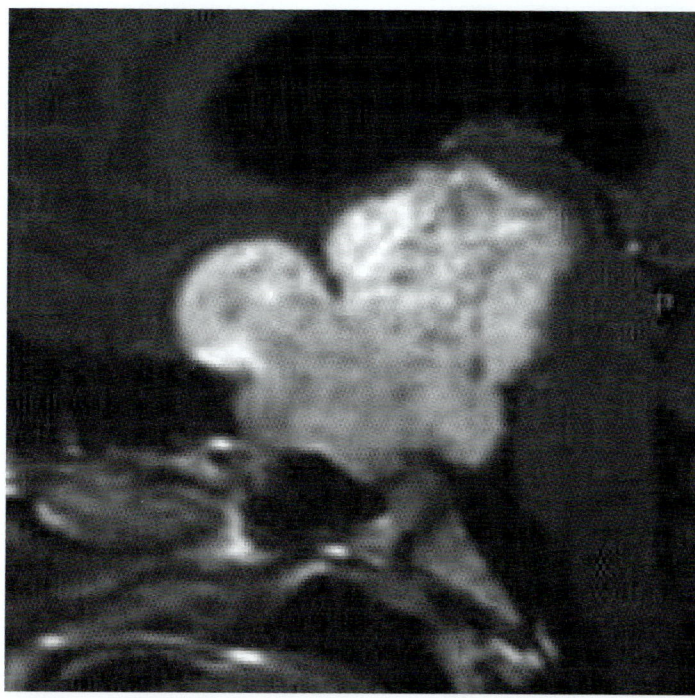

Fig. 9.1 T1 Sagittal MRI image of a sellar–suprasellar lesion (craniopharyngioma) having a small sellar and a huge suprasellar component compressing the midbrain. For teams with inadequate experience, such surgical candidates may not be suitable for endoscopic approach alone and warrant a combined endonasal and transcranial procedure. On the other hand, experienced teams may employ extended approach for endonasal excision of the same tumour.

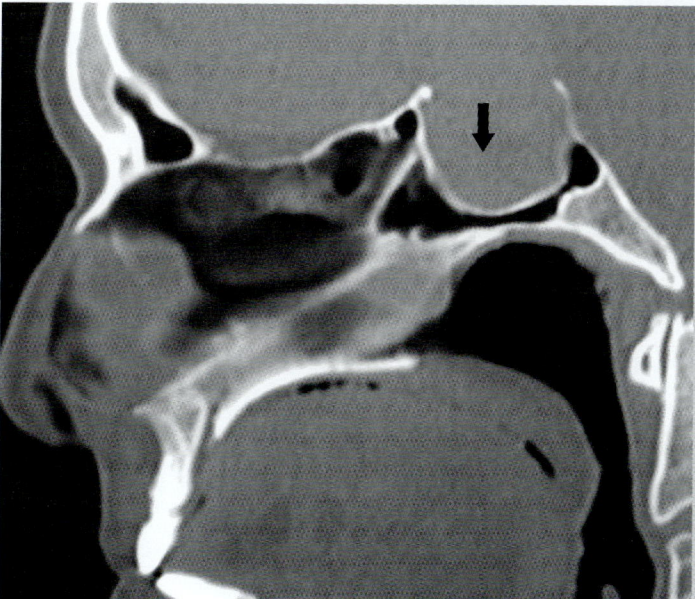

Fig. 9.2 Sagittal CT bone window scan of a patient with sella widened (*black arrow*) by the tumour (in this case a pituitary macroadenoma).

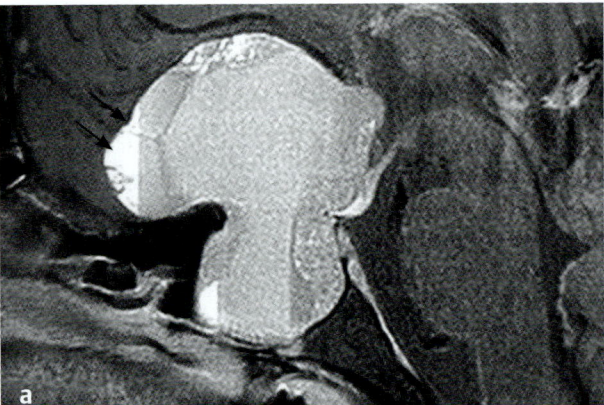

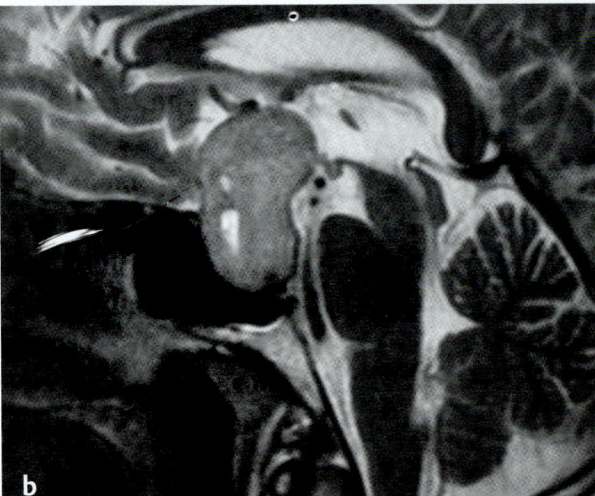

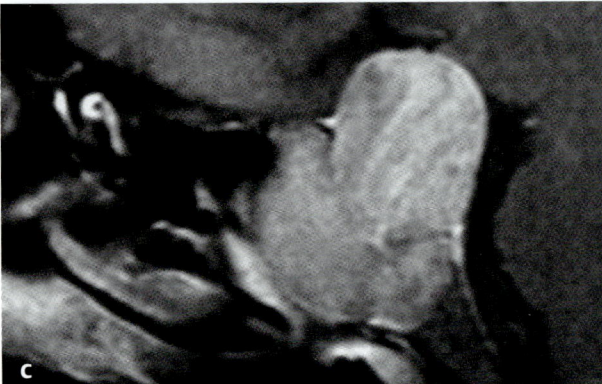

Fig. 9.3 **(a)** Tumours with considerable anterior extension (two *thin black arrows*) pose a challenge to use straight endoscope. In such cases, tuberculum and the planum sphenoidale have to be drilled considerably. **(b, c)** Tumours having a straight suprasellar component with a vertical or posterior axis can be addressed easily via endoscopic approach.

Not all sellar tumours may have a suprasellar portion communicating with a wide neck. Sometimes, the suprasellar portion happens to be multilobulated, or even the suprasellar portion may be attached to the sellar portion with a narrow neck (**Fig. 9.4**). In such cases, the sellar tumour may come off easily, but it may be rather difficult to dissect the suprasellar tumour through the narrow neck. It may be a good idea to go for combined approach for such cases. The sellar portion may be dissected via endonasal route and the suprasellar portion via transcranial route.

Tumours with extensive intradural extension and large suprasellar tumours, which require intradural dissection may be well excised via transcranial route (**Fig. 9.5**).

Even petrous apex lesions (**Fig. 9.6**) can be tackled using trans-sphenoid endoscopic approach provided the lesion is causing an indentation on the wall or present within the sphenoid sinus.

The ENT and neurosurgeon must sit together and discuss the pros and cons of all available routes of surgery. The final decision must be taken keeping the patient in mind. The route with the least morbidity and optimum exposure that allows maximum tumour removal should be chosen. At every step of the surgery, decisions are taken whether to proceed with tumour removal or not. If the risk is greater than the benefit, surgery must stop. For example, if the tumour is encasing the carotid in a non-secretory tumour, it may be advisable to leave the lateral tumour alone. On the other hand, in case of a chordoma, we may proceed with tumour removal as chordoma does not respond to any other modality of treatment. This decision also depends on the experience of the team and the backup of the institute in terms of interventional radiologist, intensivist, radiotherapist, endocrinologist, etc.

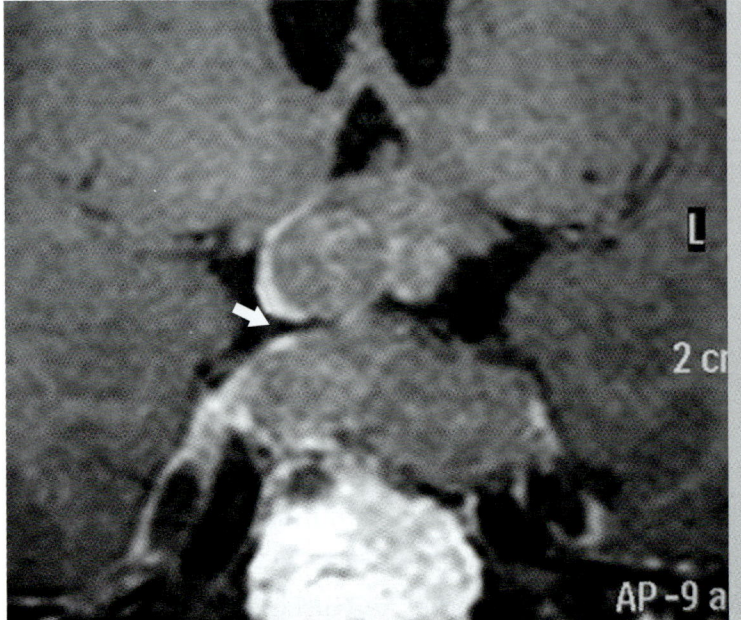

Fig. 9.4 Tumours having multilobed suprasellar component. The lobes may be connected by a narrow neck (*white block arrow*). In such cases, removal of the entire tumour via endoscopic approach may be difficult since blind manoeuvring of the instruments through the narrow window may be disastrous. Hence, such cases often require a combined transcranial and endoscopic approach.

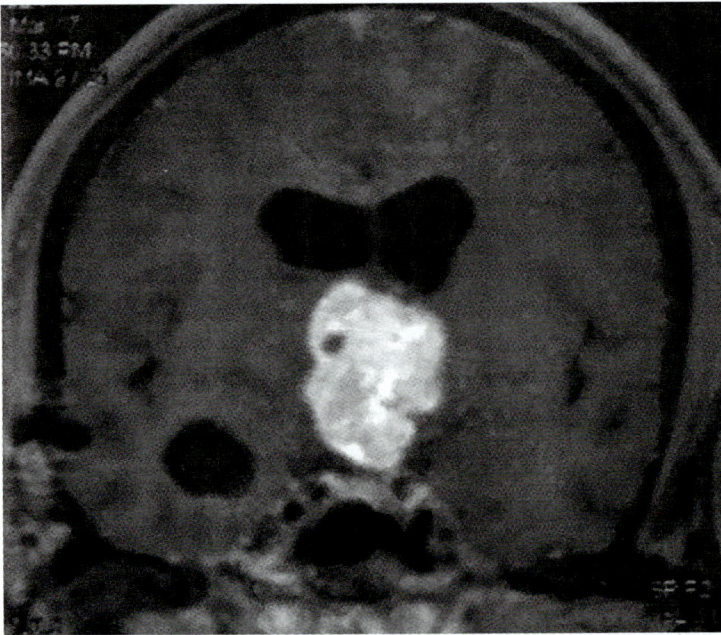

Fig. 9.5 Tumours with large suprasellar component with intradural extensions require intradural dissection. These tumours may well be approached via transcranial route.

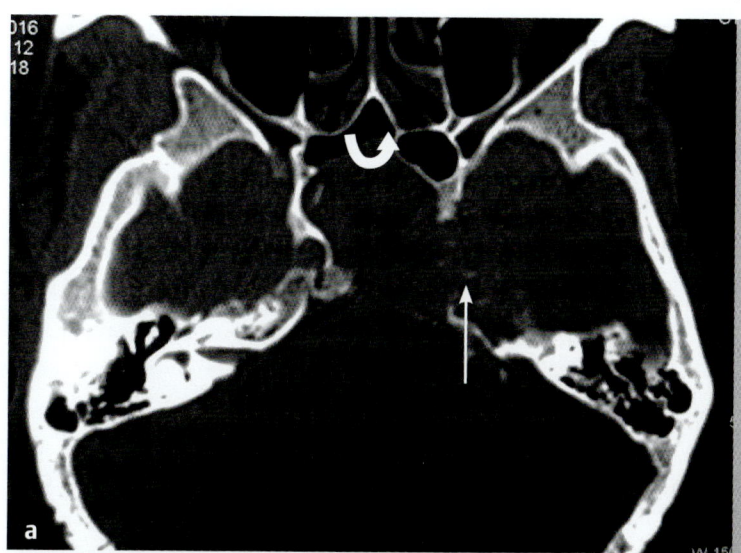

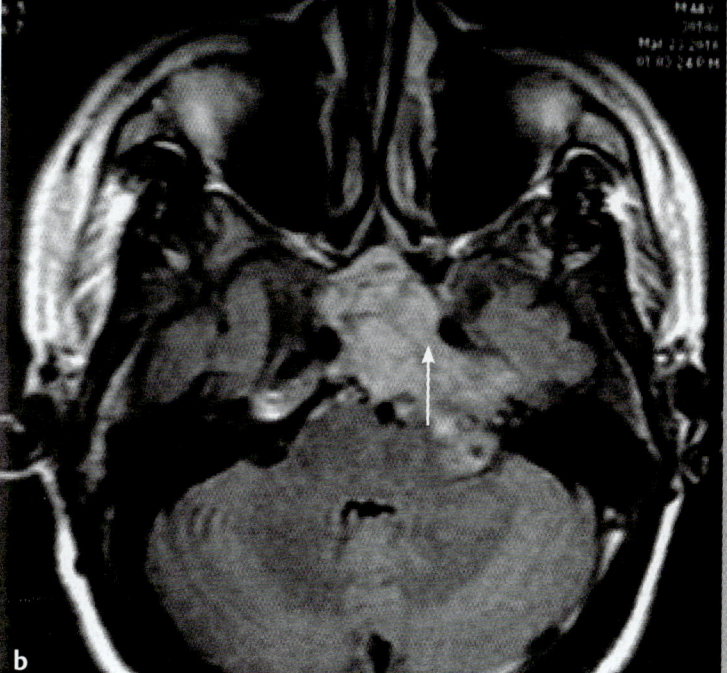

Fig. 9.6 (a) CT images and **(b)** MR images of lesion arising from the left petrous apex (*straight white arrow*), occupying the sphenoid sinus and causing a bulge/indentation on its posterior wall (*curved white arrow*). The entire tumour was excised completely via endoscopic approach and turned out to be a schwannoma on post-operative histopathology report.

Reference

1. Kassam AB, Gardner PA. Endoscopic approaches to skull base. Prog Neurol Surg 2012;26:21–26

10 Instruments Commonly Used in Endoscopic Skull Base Surgery

Nishit Shah and Sai Spoorthi Nayak

Instrument 1: Nasal Packing Forceps

Nasal packing forceps (**Fig .10.1**) are used for the following:

- Packing and decongestion of the nasal cavity.
- Placing flap, fascia, and Gelfoam.
- Reversing of the reverse flap through the posterior septectomy.
- Placing sinus packs.

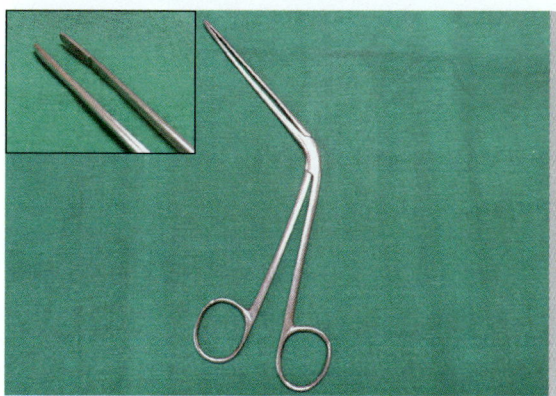

Fig. 10.1 Nasal packing forceps.

Instrument 2: Freer's Elevator

It has a blunt rounded end and a sharper curved end. The rounded end could be used to raise mucoperichondrial or mucoperiosteal flaps, whereas the sharper end is useful for elevating the flap tethered at the mucoperichondrial–periosteal junction (**Fig. 10.2**).

Used for the following:

- Out-fracturing of turbinates.
- Elevation of mucoperiosteal/ mucoperichondrial flap.
- Demarcation and medialisation of ST for posterior ethmoidectomy.
- Elevation of sphenoid mucosa.

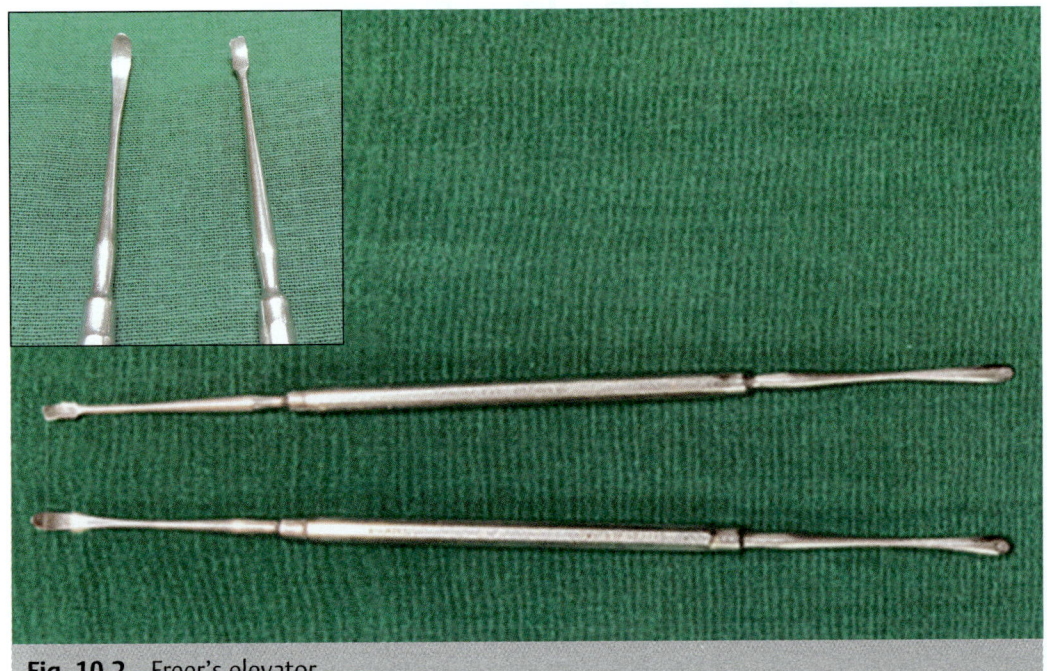

Fig. 10.2 Freer's elevator.

Instrument 3: Electrosurgical Needle Cautery

It is essentially an electrosurgical needle cautery electrode; its tip is bent to 45 degrees roughly for convenience of nasal mucosal incisions (**Fig. 10.3**).

Used for the following:

- Making nasal flap incisions.
- Coagulation of a point bleeder arising from the bone.

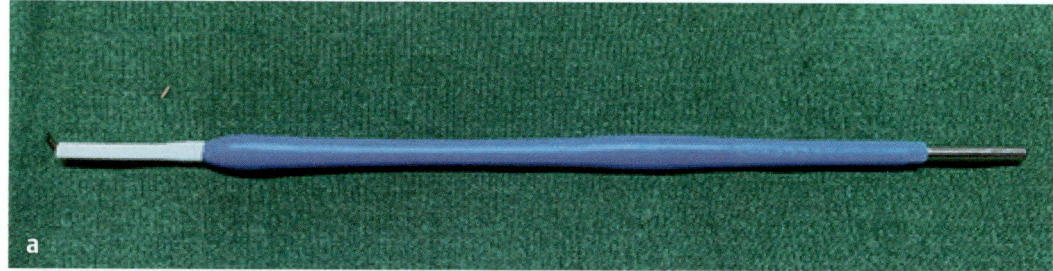

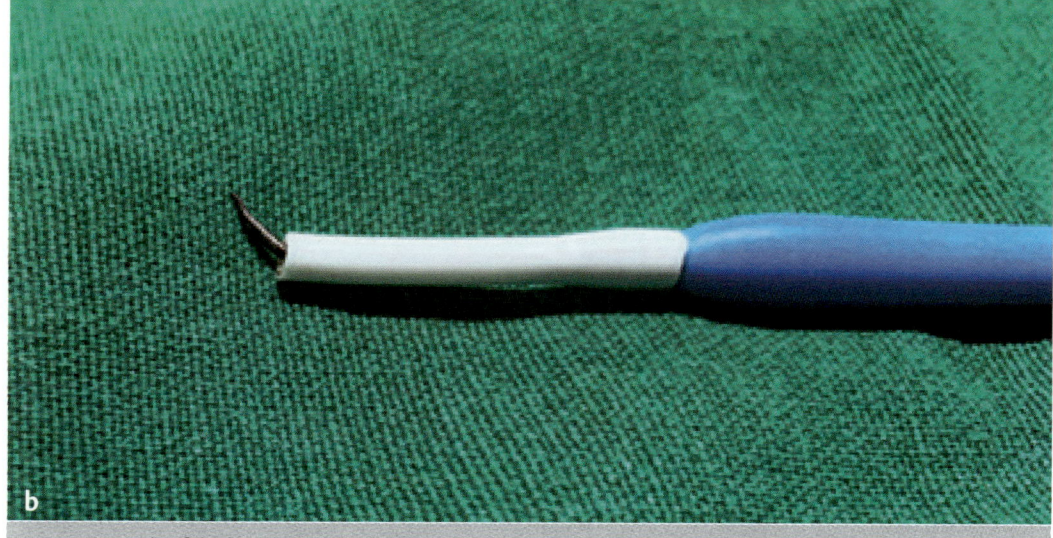

Fig. 10.3 **(a, b)** Electrosurgical needle cautery.

Instrument 4: Luc's Forceps

Luc's Forceps (**Fig. 10.4**) are used for the following:

- Posterior septectomy.
- Removal of anterior sphenoid wall.

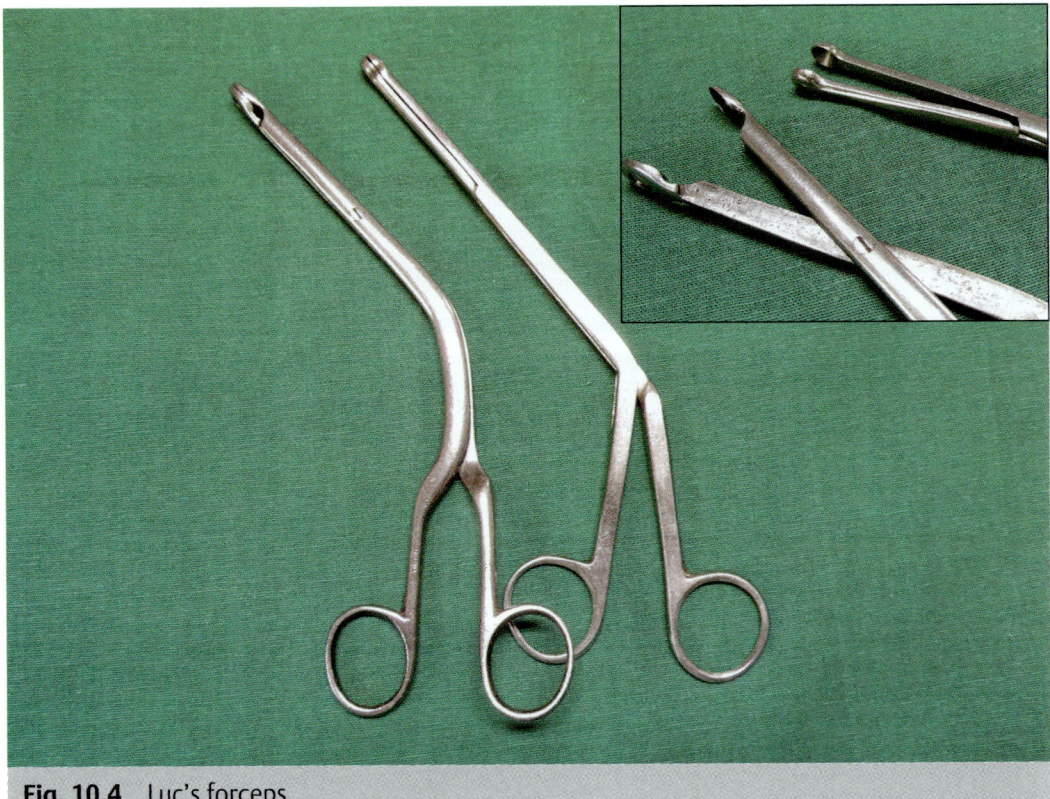

Fig. 10.4 Luc's forceps.

Instrument 5: Straight Ethmoid Forceps

Straight ethmoid forceps (**Fig. 10.5**) are used for the following:

- Posterior septectomy.
- Removal of bone chips.
- Stripping of sphenoid mucosa.

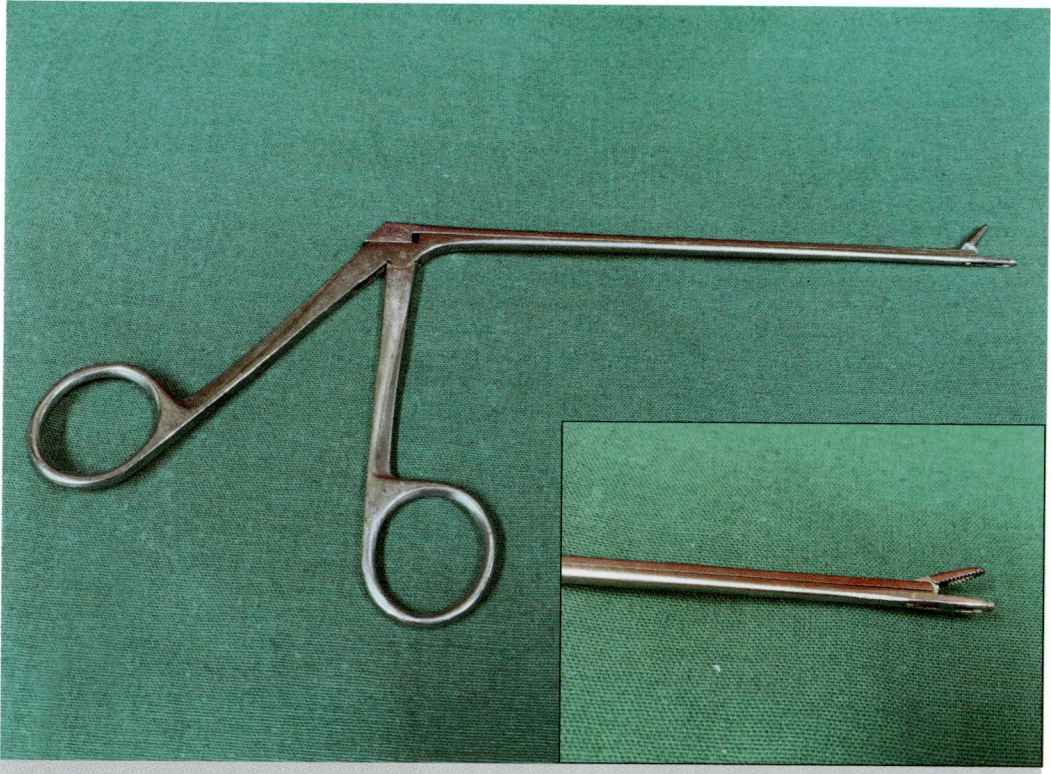

Fig. 10.5 Straight ethmoid forceps.

Instrument 6: Upward Ethmoid Forceps

Upward ethmoid forceps (**Fig. 10.6**) are used for the following:

- Removing bony spicules or pieces situated at an angle.
- Stripping of mucosa from the upper sphenoid.

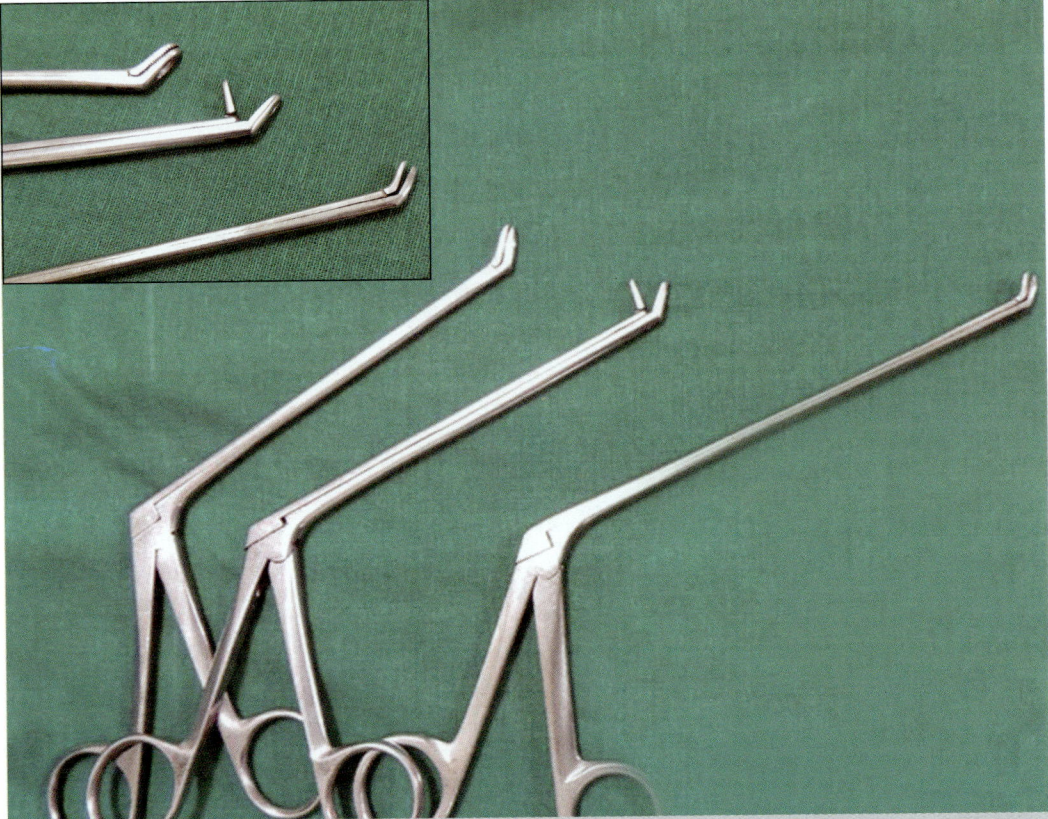

Fig. 10.6   Upward ethmoid forceps.

Instrument 7: Downward Ethmoid Forceps

Downward ethmoid forceps (**Fig. 10.7**) are used for the following:

- Stripping mucosa from the floor of the sphenoid.

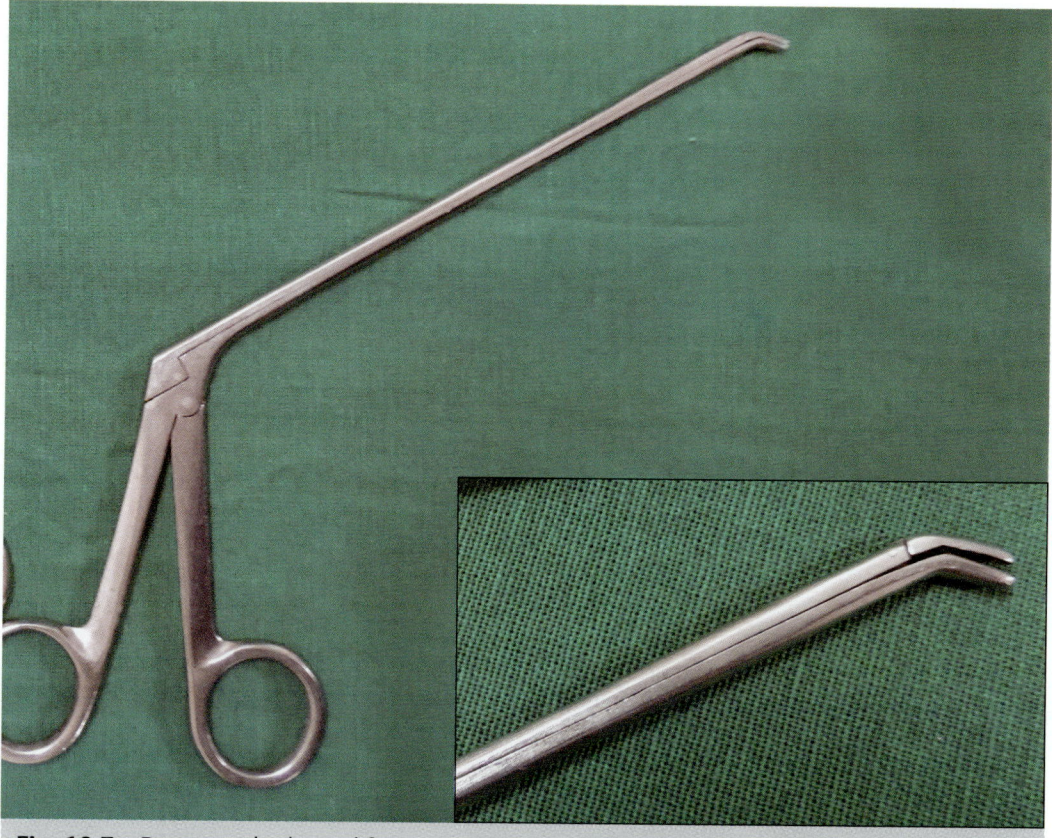

Fig. 10.7 Downward ethmoid forceps.

Instrument 8: Drill 3-mm Diamond/Cutting

Drill 3–4mm rough diamond (**Fig. 10.8**) is used for most of the bone work in the sella and sphenoid.

- Drilling of the anterior sphenoid wall from the sphenoid ostia.
- Drilling of sphenoid keel.
- Drilling of intersphenoid septations and pterygoid plates.
- Sellar drilling.

3 mm cutting drill is where maximum bone work is required, for example, drilling over the clivus.

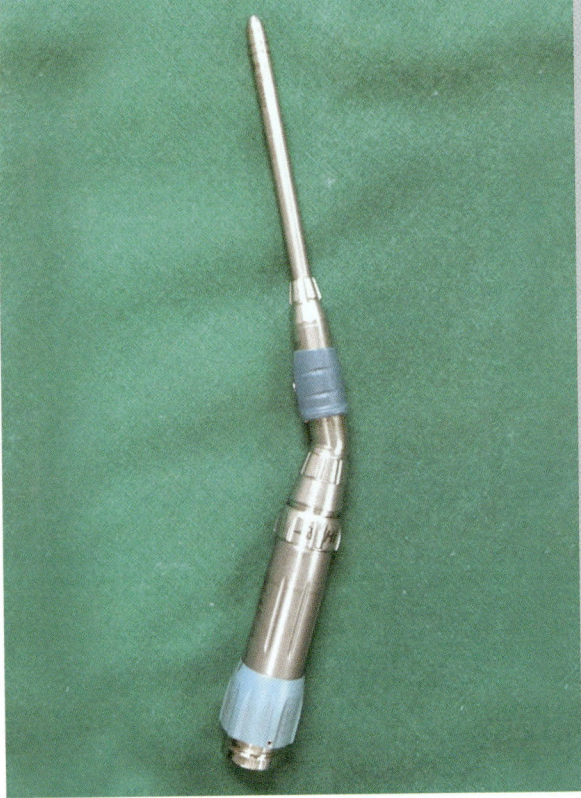

Fig. 10.8 Drill 3-mm diamond/cutting. Hand-piece of drill on which 3–4 mm diamond or cutting drill bits are loaded.

Instrument 9: Osteotomes

Osteotomes (**Fig.10.9**) are used for the following:

- Shoulder osteotomies of sphenoid.
- Posterior septectomy.

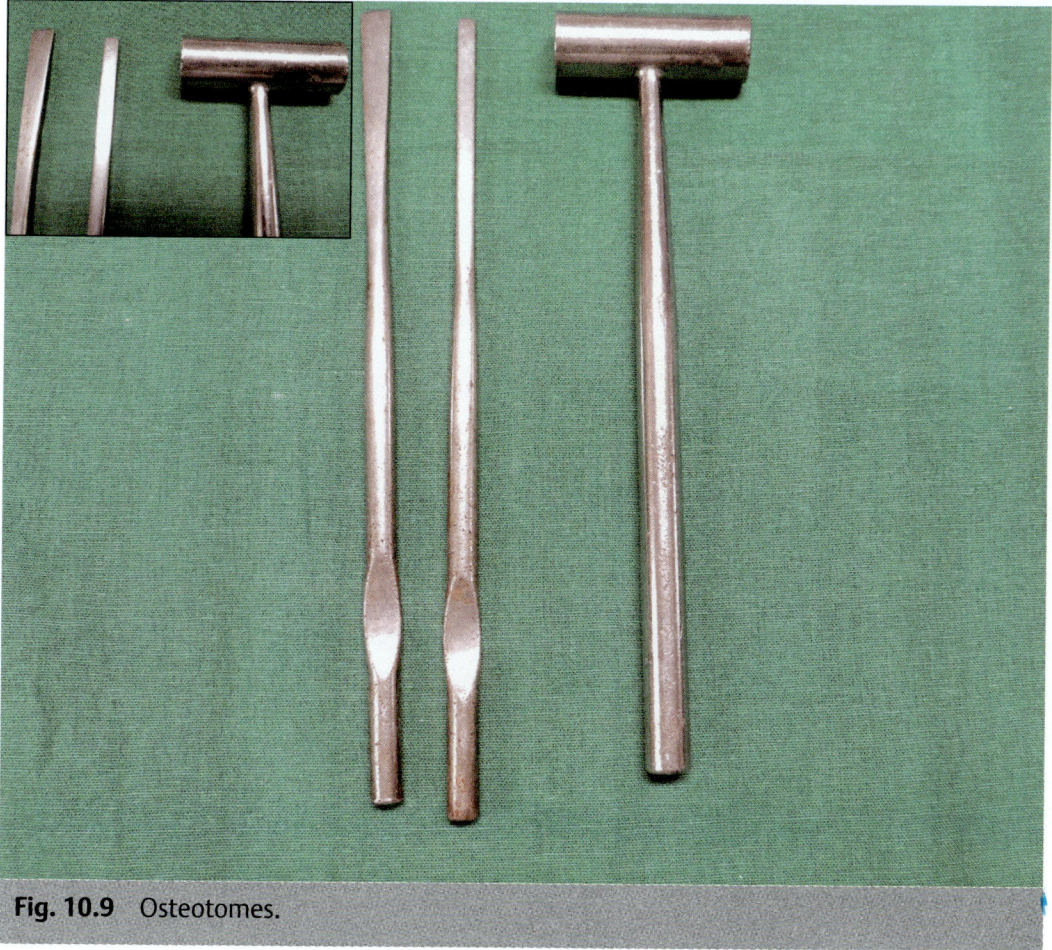

Fig. 10.9 Osteotomes.

Instrument 10: Turbinectomy Scissors

Turbinectomy scissors (**Fig. 10.10**) are used for the following:

- Middle turbinectomy.
- Superior turbinectomy.
- Conchoplasty.

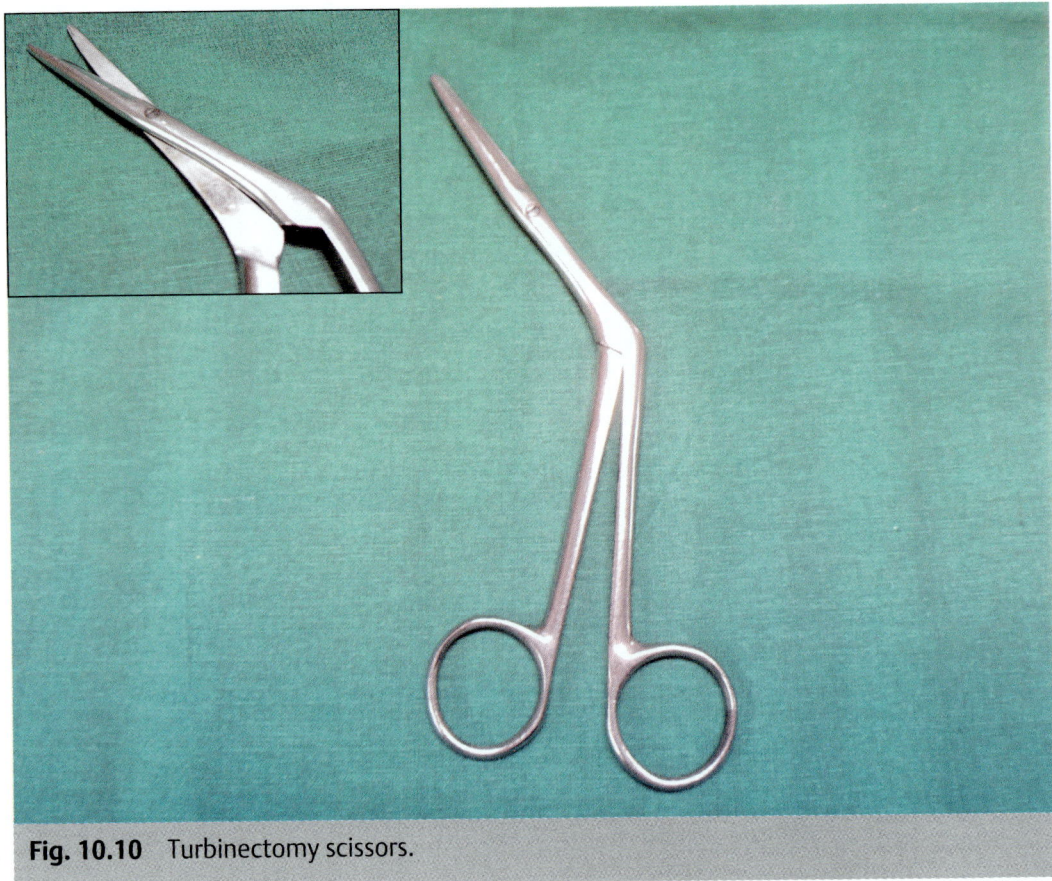

Fig. 10.10   Turbinectomy scissors.

Instrument 11: Through-Cut Forceps

Through-Cut forceps (**Fig.10.11**) are used for the following:

- Removal of intersphenoid septations (ISS).
- Cutting thin bony septations.
- Through and through cutting of mucosa when stripping is not required.

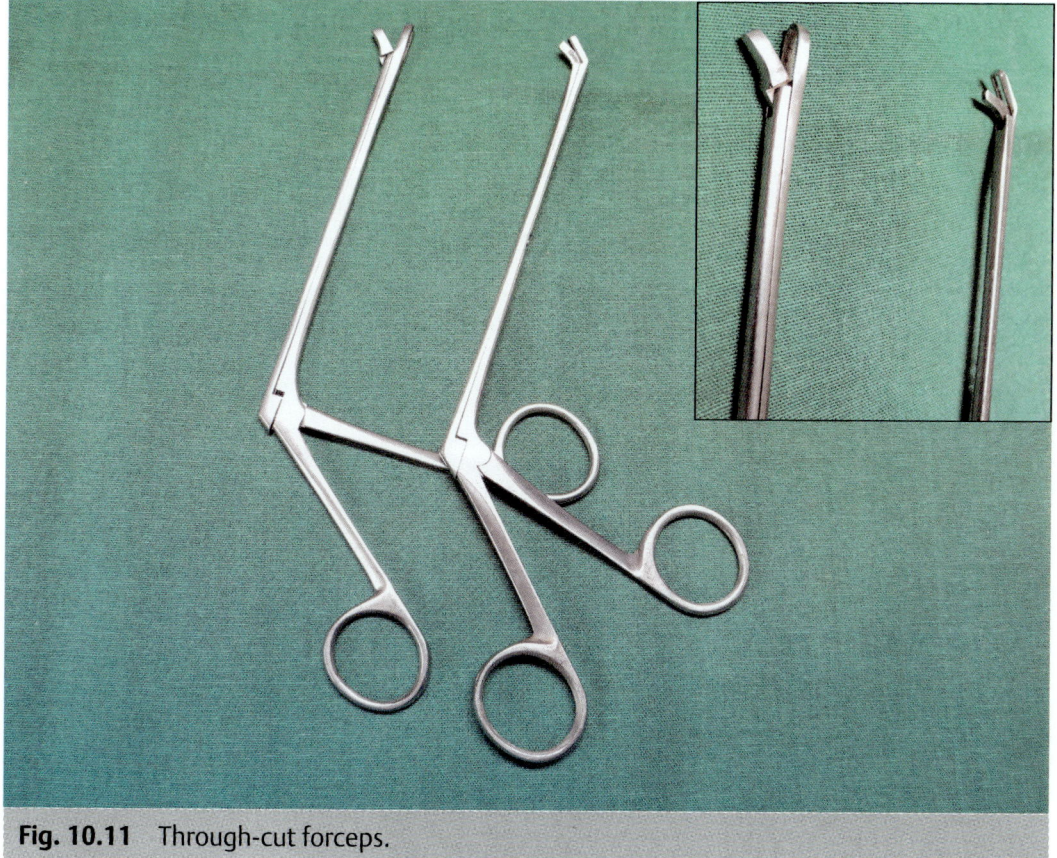

Fig. 10.11   Through-cut forceps.

Instrument 12: Straight Suction (Keyhole)

Keyhole suctions are very useful as controlled suctioning can be achieved, especially during placement and repositioning of flaps and grafts during skull base reconstruction. Control over the the pressure on the suction is varied by the amount of occlusion of the keyhole (**Fig. 10.12**).

Used for the following:

- Suctioning in the nasopharynx and the sphenoid.
- No. 1 suction-—suctioning in sella—helps in reconstruction of sella defect.
- Mucosal stripping.

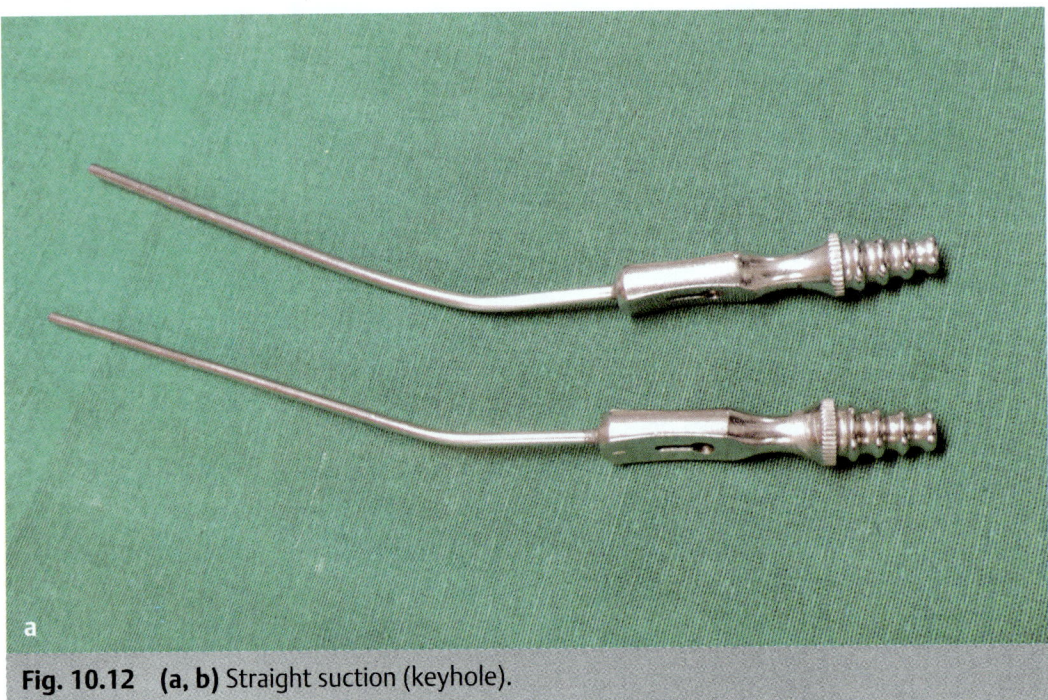

Fig. 10.12 **(a, b)** Straight suction (keyhole).

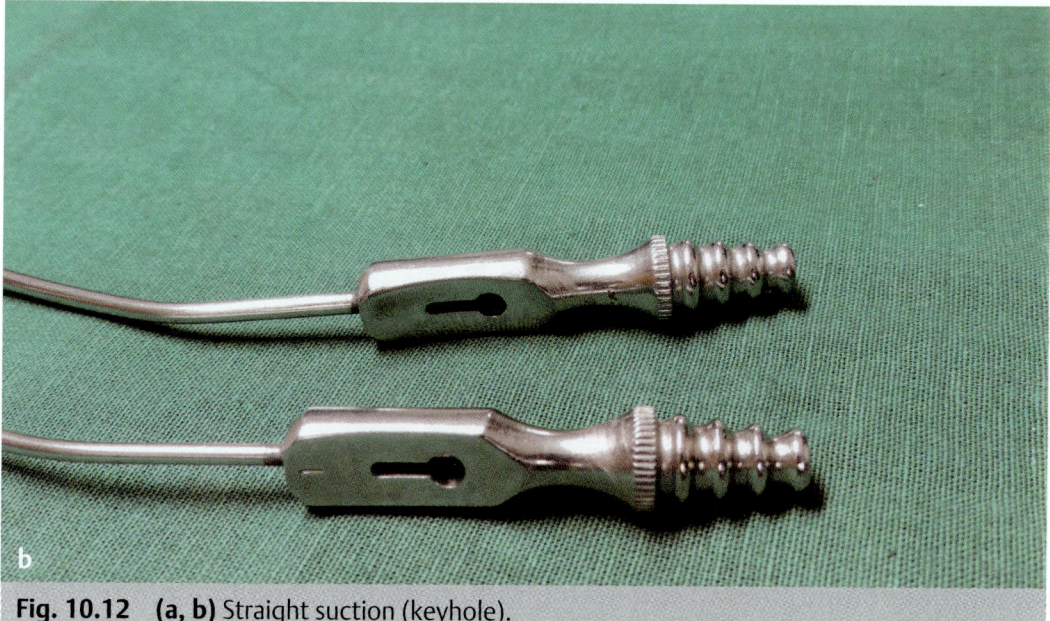

Fig. 10.12   (a, b) Straight suction (keyhole).

Instrument 13: Kerrison's Rounger (Punch)

Upward and downward.

90 and 45 degrees.

Kerrison's rounger punch comes in various sizes: 1-, 2-, and 3 mm (**Fig 10.13 a, b**).

It is used for the following:

- Opening of sella.
- Punching of sella margins.
- Punching of lateral margins of anterior wall of sphenoid.
- Punching of septations between posterior ethmoids and sphenoid.

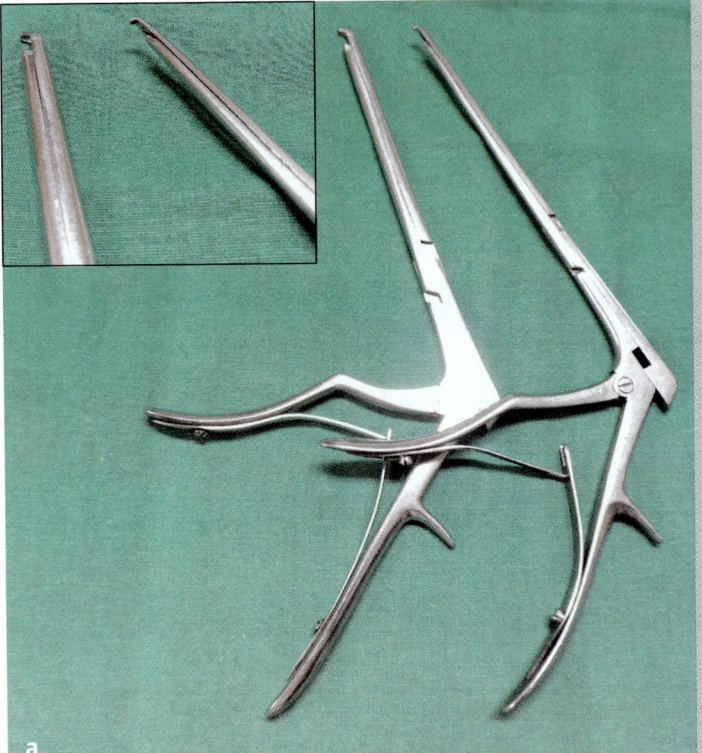

Fig. 10.13 **(a)** Downward Kerrison's punch 45 degrees. **(b)** Upward Kerrison's punch 90 degrees.

a

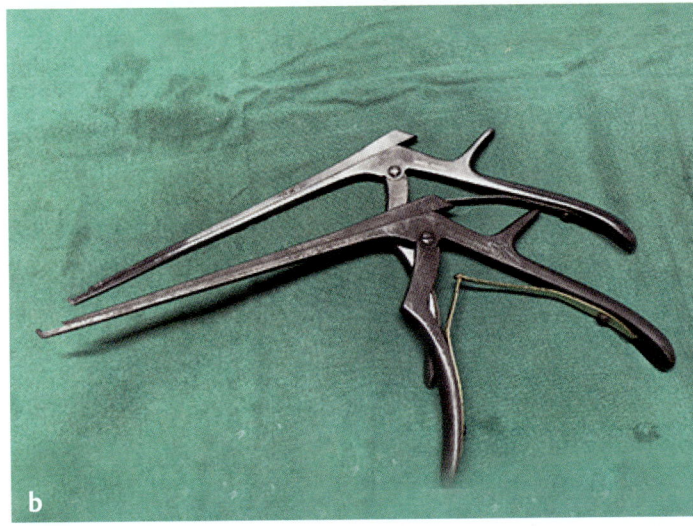

b

Instrument 14: Stamberger Mushroom Sphenoid Punch

Uses of sphenoid punch (**Fig. 10.14**) are as follows:

- To widen the sphenoid ostium.
- To punch out bony chips from the anterior face of sphenoid.

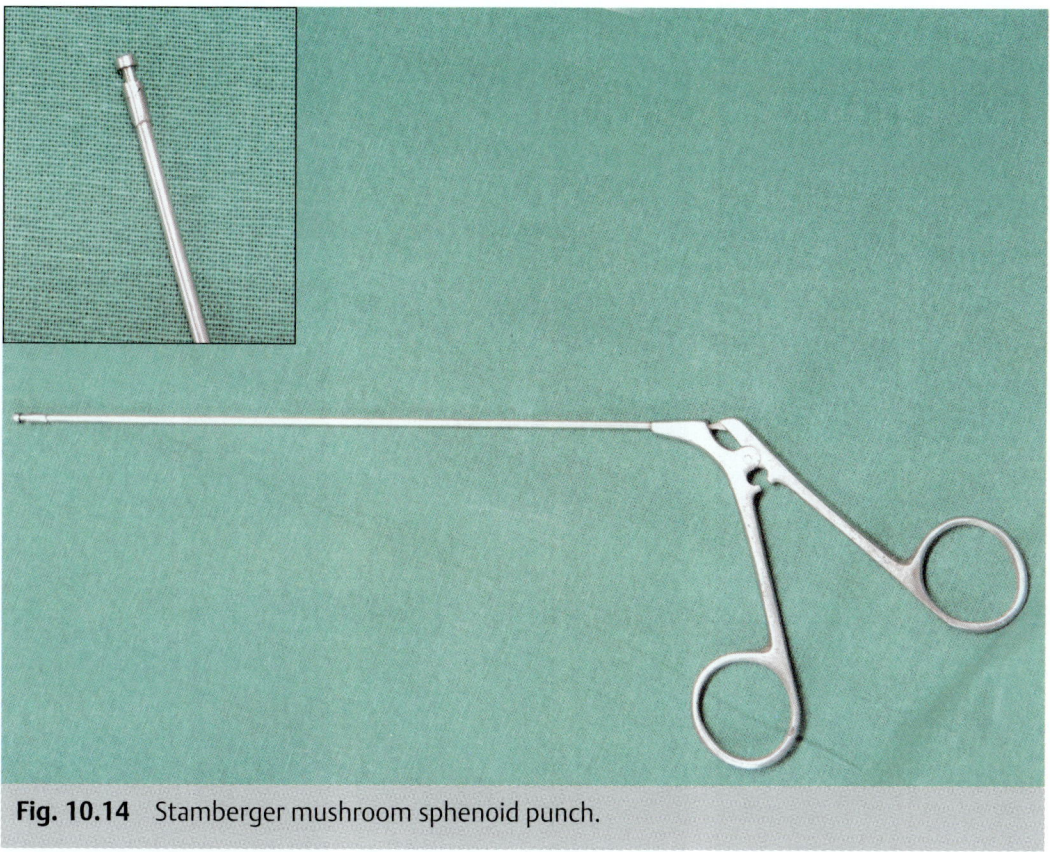

Fig. 10.14 Stamberger mushroom sphenoid punch.

Instrument 15: Cappabianca Retractable Dural Knife

Since the tip if this instrument is retractable, the chances of nasal mucosal trauma during its introduction is nil. This is of great advantage to beginners (**Fig. 10.15**).

Used for the following:

- Dural incision.

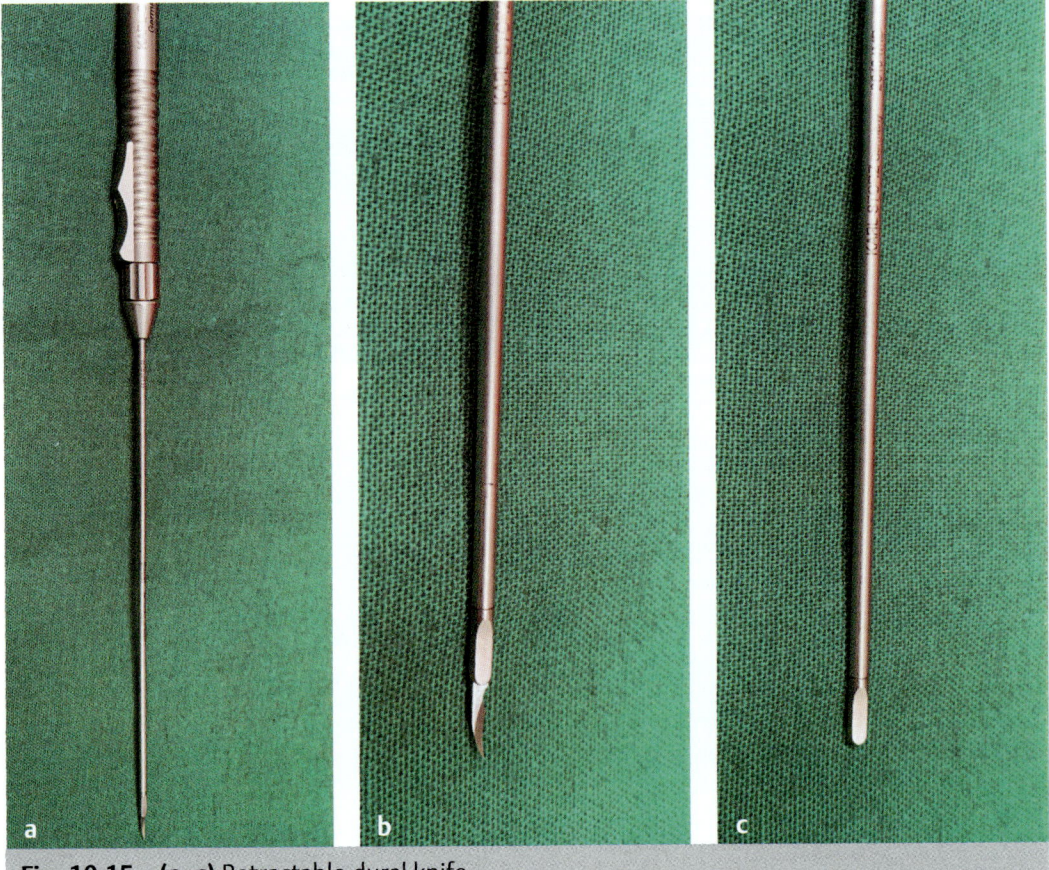

Fig. 10.15 **(a–c)** Retractable dural knife.

Instrument 16: Disc Dissector

Disc dissectors (**Fig. 10.16**) are used for the following:

- Elevation of thinned out sella bone.
- Elevation of dural flap.

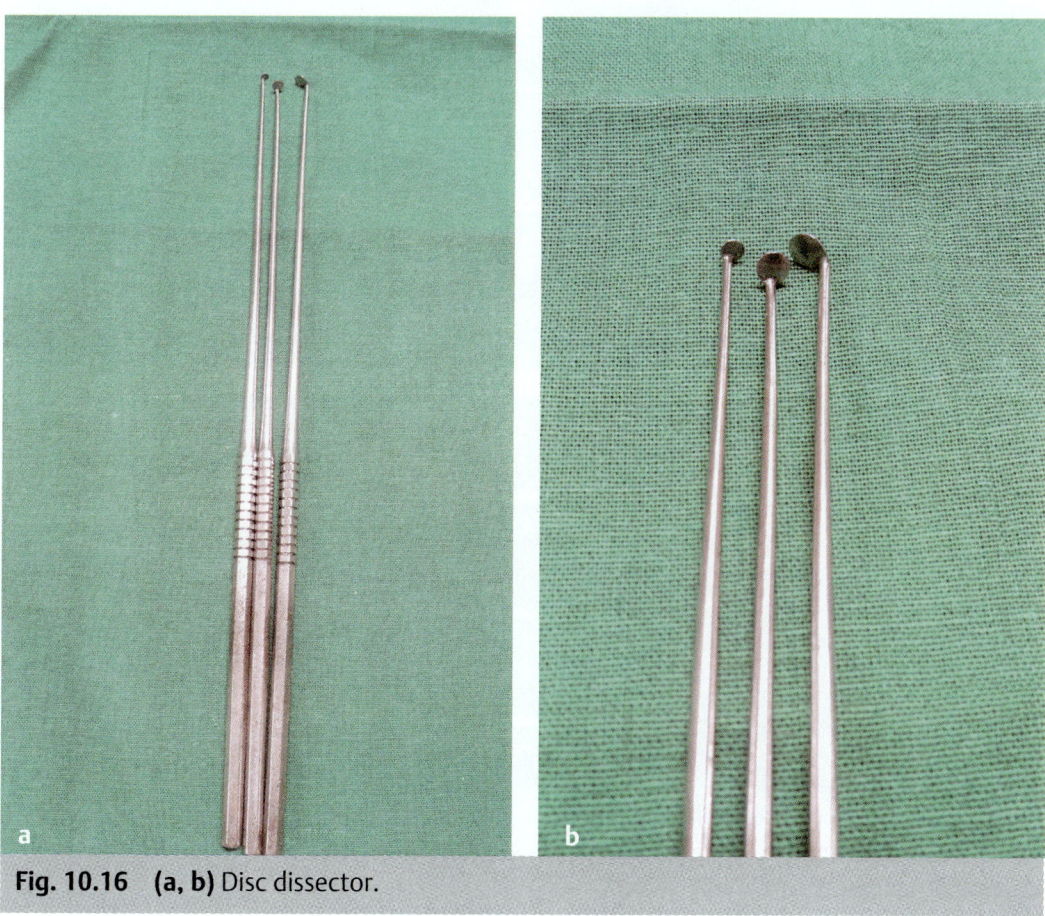

Fig. 10.16 (a, b) Disc dissector.

Instrument 17: Curved Suction

This instrument (**Fig.10.17a, b**) is used for the following:

- Debulking tumour in suprasellar region.

- Debulking of lateral tumour nodule.

- Non keyhole curved suction is used for providing continuous irrigation while drilling, or to clearout a bloody field, or to clear the lens of the scope.

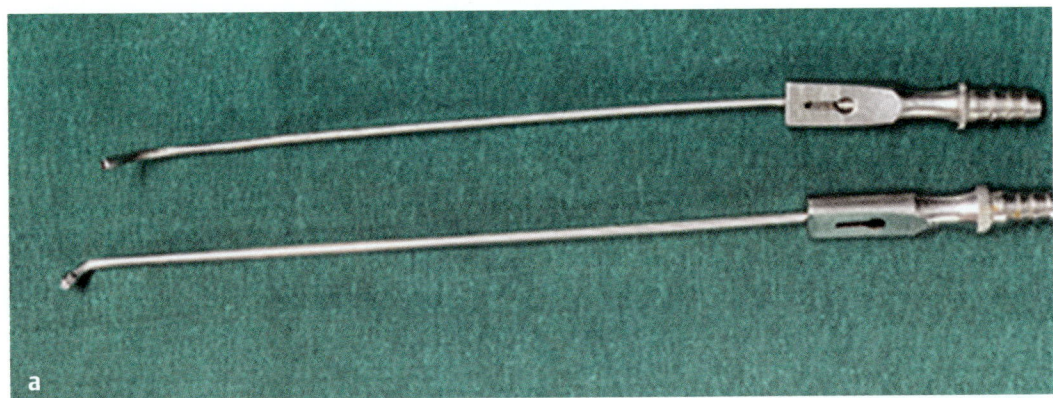

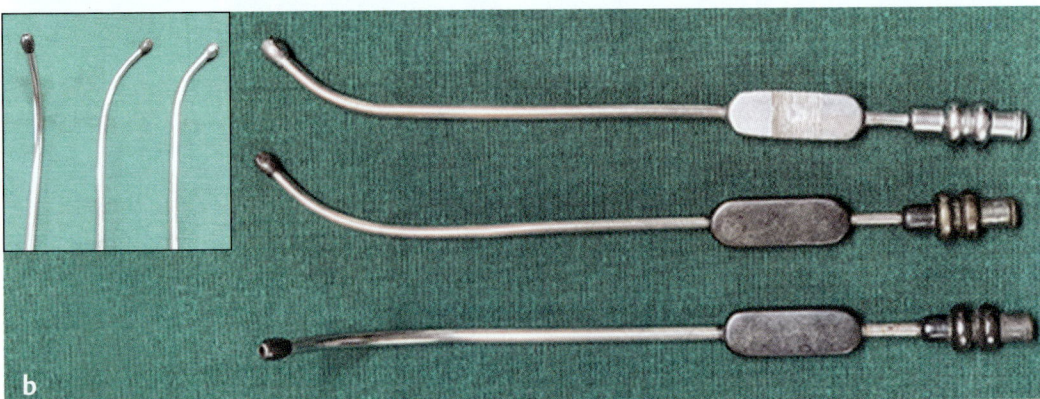

Fig. 10.17 (a) Curved keyhole suction 1 mm. (b) Curved keyhole and non-keyhole suction 1- and 2 mm. The non-keyhole suction can be used for irrigation and washing out of loose fragments of dissected tumour.

Instrument 18: Ring Curette

Ring Curettes (**Fig. 10.18**) are used for the following:

- Debulking sellar and suprasellar tumours which do not break easily or are firm.

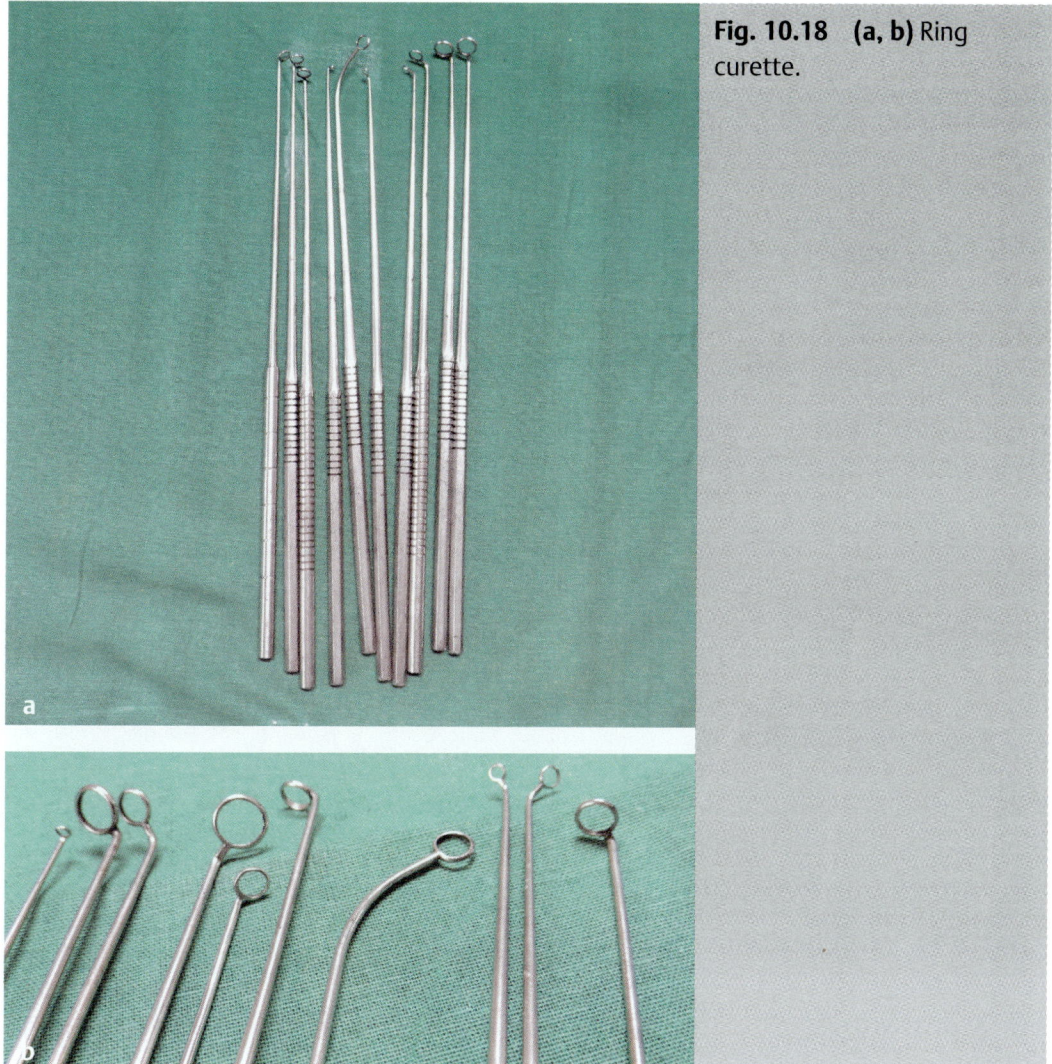

Fig. 10.18 **(a, b)** Ring curette.

187

Instrument 19: Tumour Removal Forceps

Straight and upward (**Fig. 10.19**). Tumour removal forceps are used for the following:

- Tumour debulking and removal.
- Biopsy of lesion.

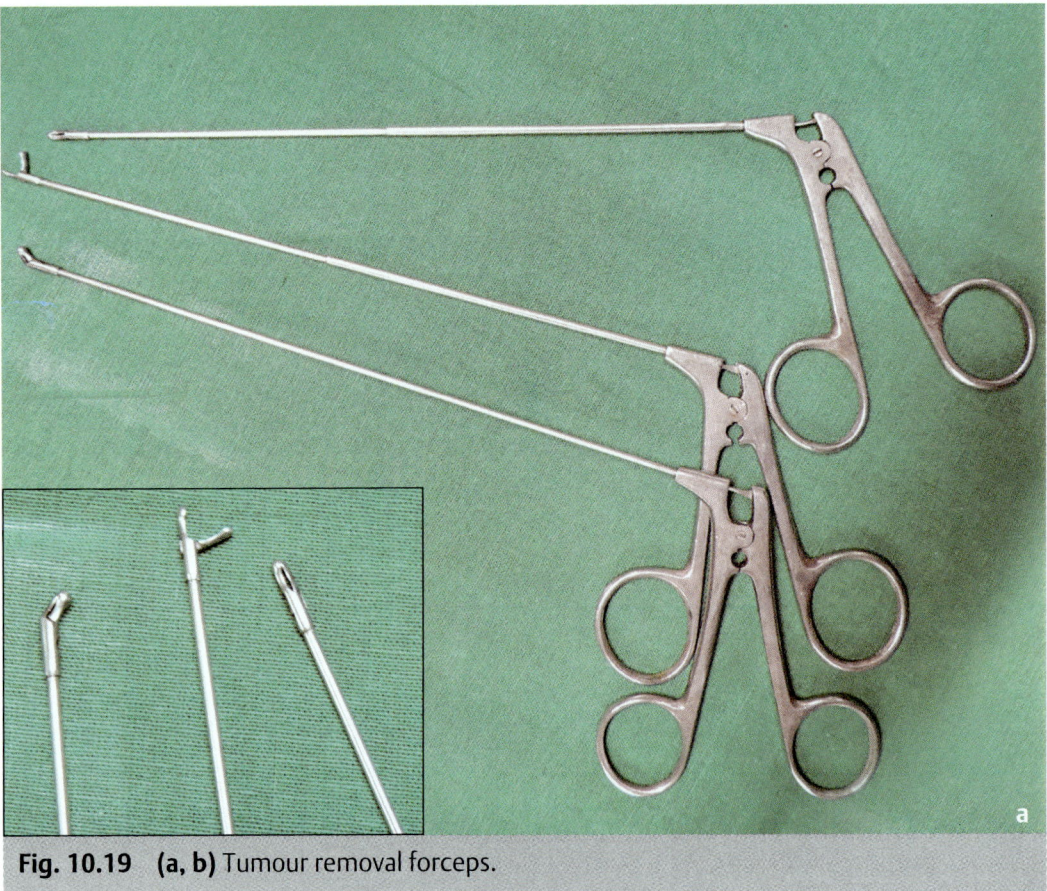

Fig. 10.19 (a, b) Tumour removal forceps.

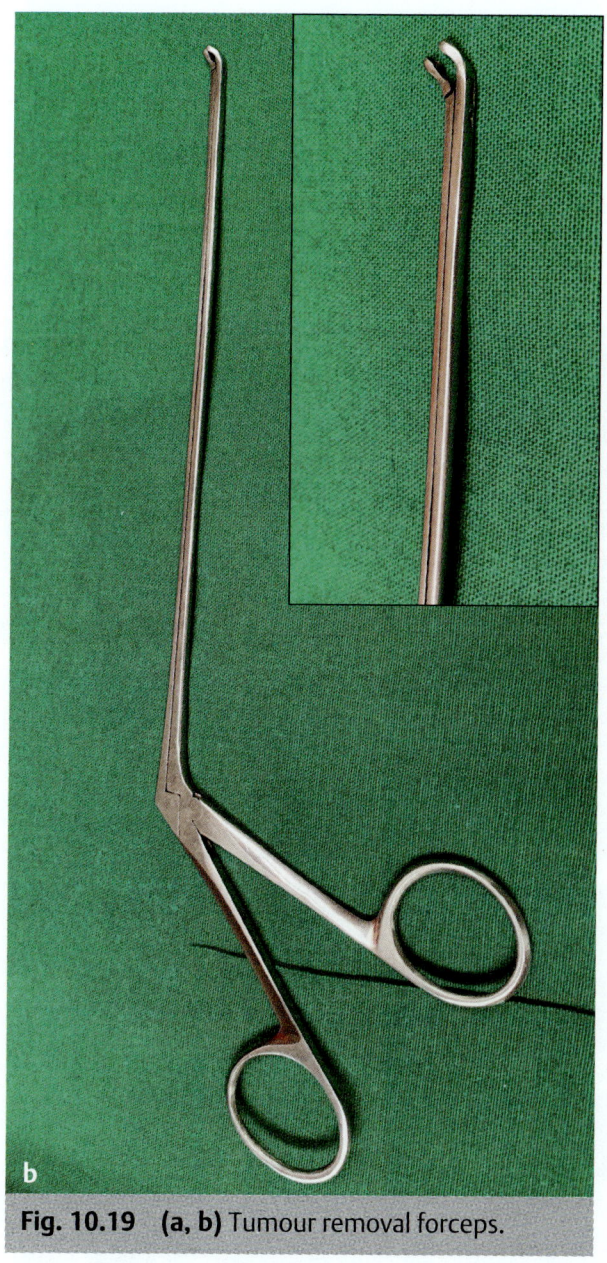

b

Fig. 10.19 (a, b) Tumour removal forceps.

Instrument 20: Amin Suction

Amin suction (**Fig. 10.20**) is used for the following:

- Fine malleable suction for tumour dissection as well as for suction in small interfaces.

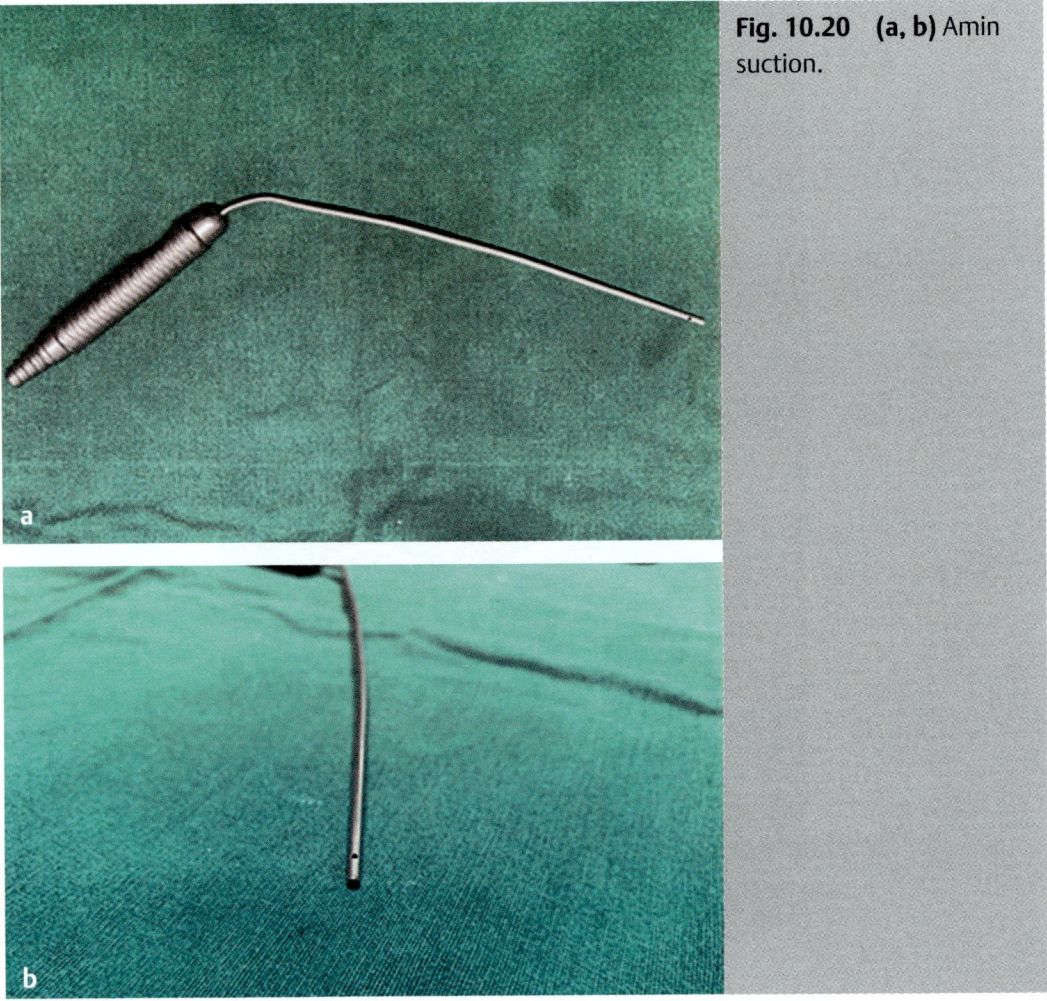

Fig. 10.20 **(a, b)** Amin suction.

Instrument 21: Silver (Malleable) Dissector

Silver (malleable) dissectors (**Fig. 10.21**) are used for the following:

- Counter-traction of flaps during reconstruction.
- Assisting by placing fat, Gelfoam.
- Malleable, so the curvature can be adjusted to desired angle.

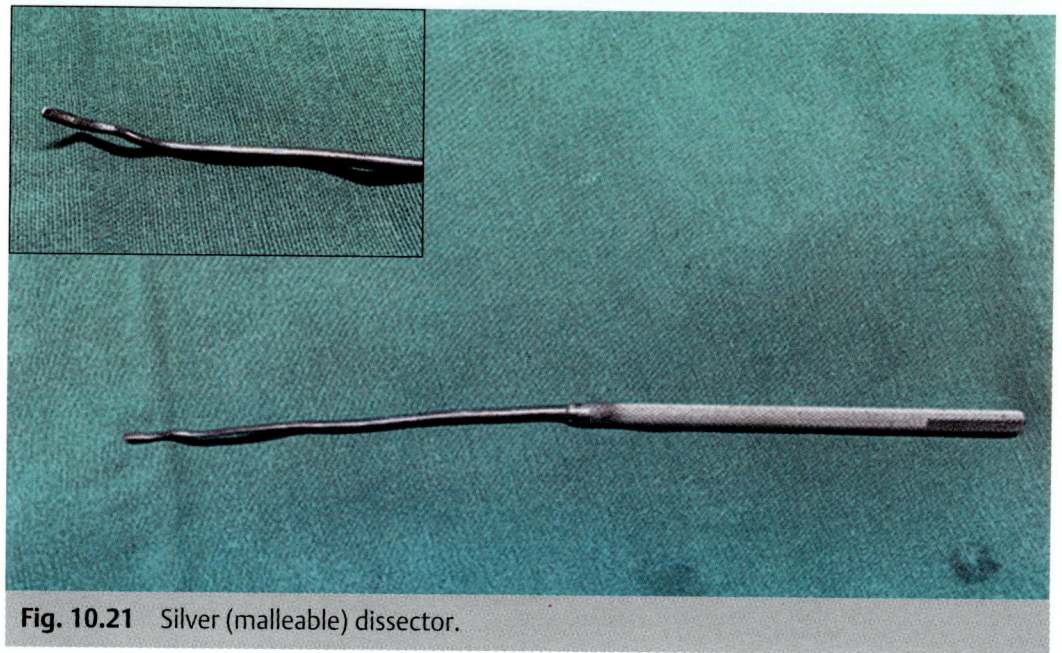

Fig. 10.21   Silver (malleable) dissector.

Instrument 22: Rotatable Dural Scissors

Rotatable dural scissors (**Fig. 10.22**) are used for the following:

- Extending the dural incision to desired shape and pattern.

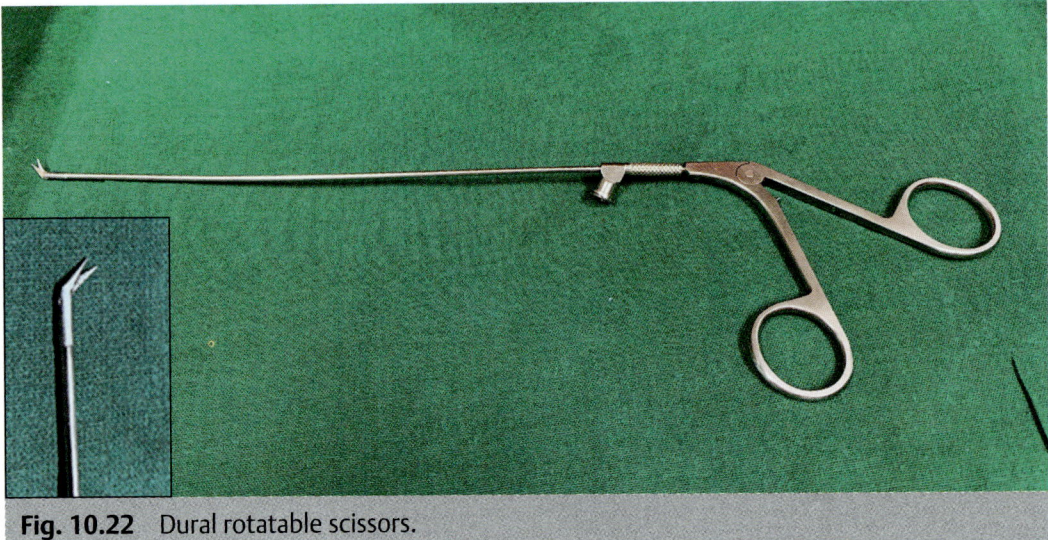

Fig. 10.22   Dural rotatable scissors.

Instrument 23: Endoscopic Scissors

Endoscopic scissors (**Fig. 10.23**) are used for the following:

- Cutting through small bony septations.
- Superior turbinectomy.

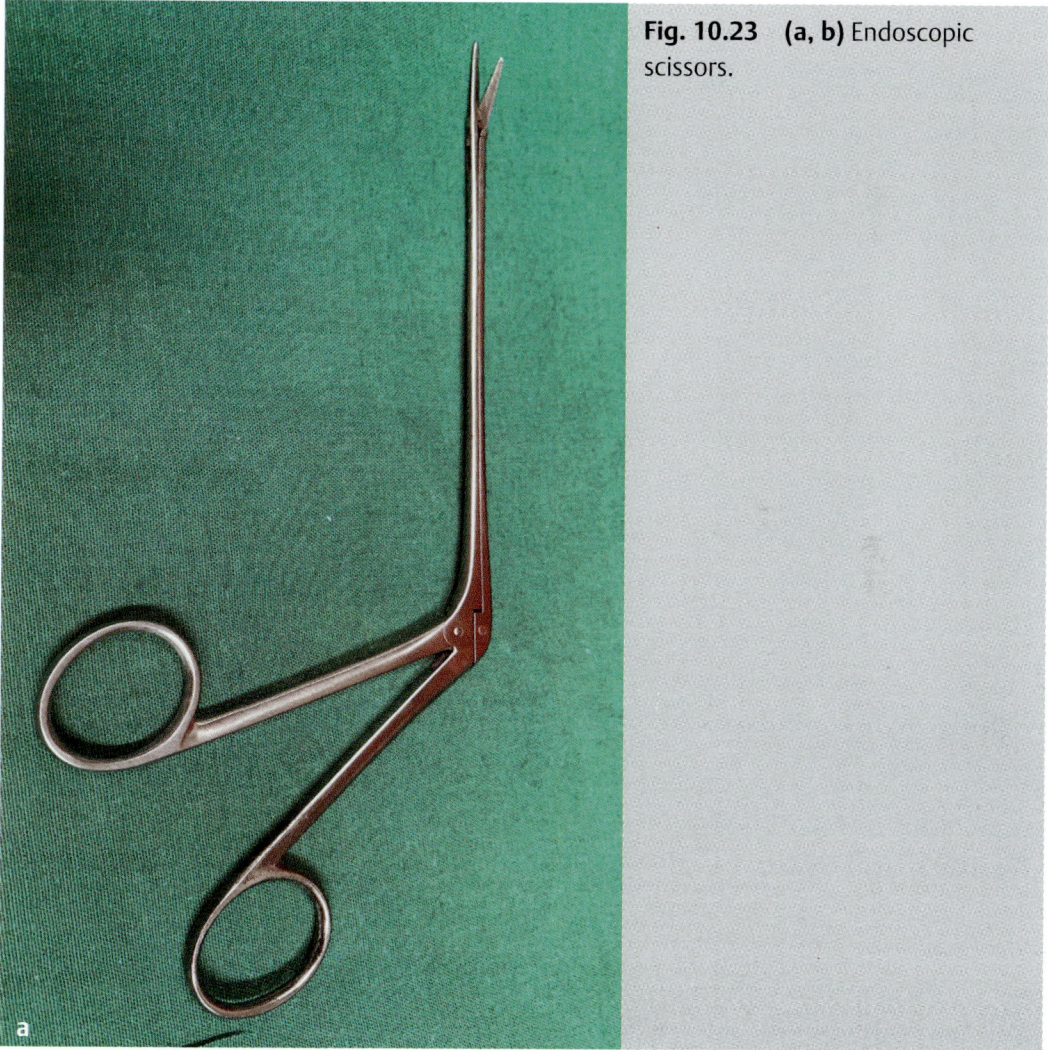

Fig. 10.23 **(a, b)** Endoscopic scissors.

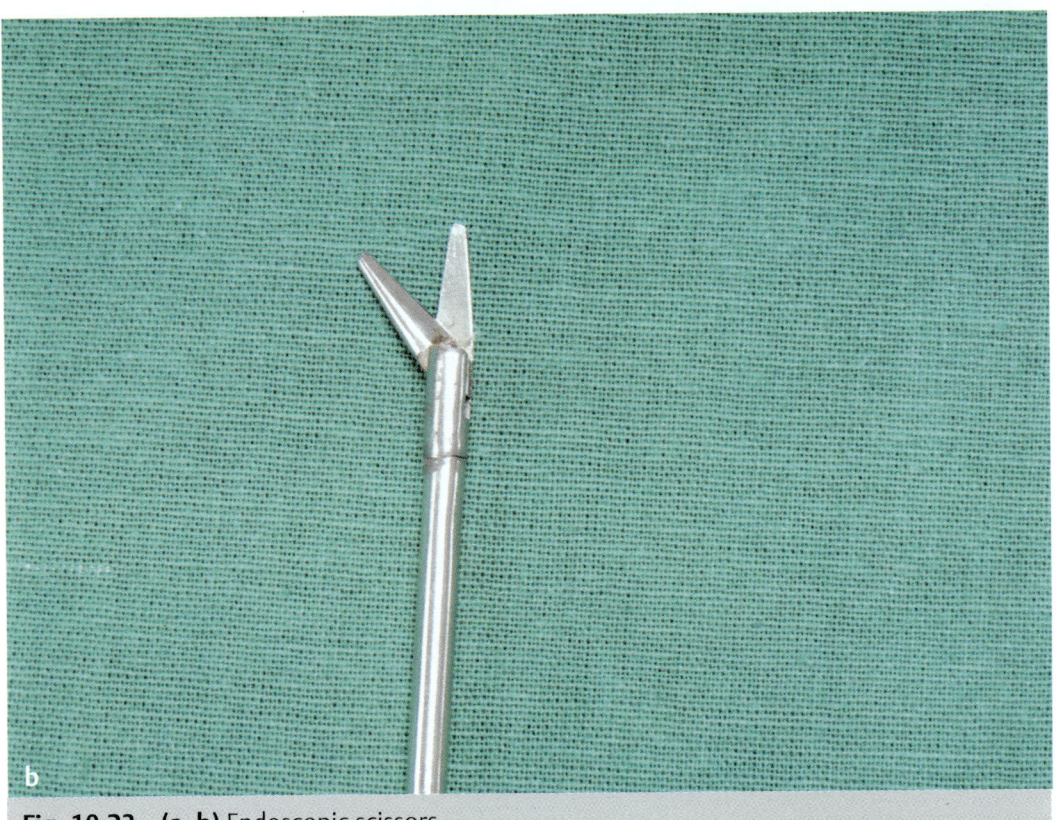

b

Fig. 10.23 **(a, b)** Endoscopic scissors.

Instrument 24: Backbiting Forceps

Backbiting forceps (**Fig. 10.24**) are used for the following:

- Removing anterior cartilage from the bony–cartilaginous junction.
- Removing posterior ethmoid septations/lateral sphenoid margin.

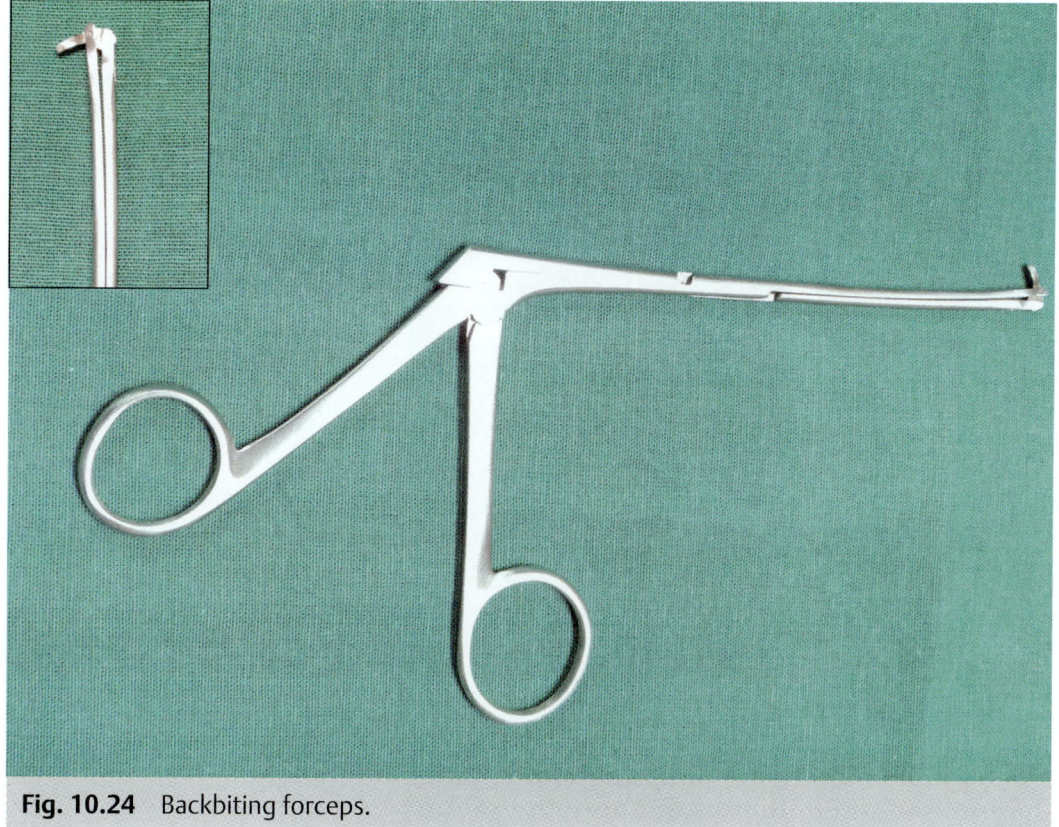

Fig. 10.24 Backbiting forceps.

Instrument 25: Ball Probe

Ball probe (**Fig. 10.25**) is used for the following:

- Elevation of the rescue flap anteriorly.
- Elevation of capsule/firm to hard tumour like chordomas.
- Elevation of sella bone flap.
- Looping of the internal maxillary artery (IMA) for ligation/cauterisation.

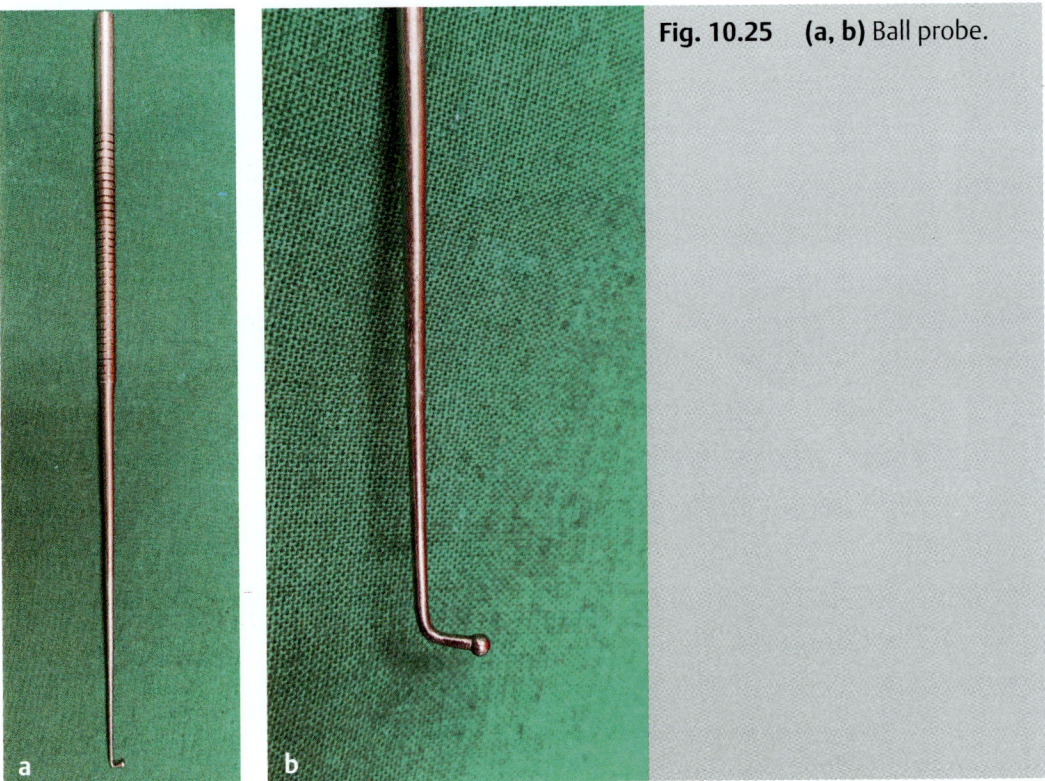

Fig. 10.25 **(a, b)** Ball probe.

Instrument 26: Fine Dissector

Fine dissectors (**Fig. 10.26**) are used for the following:

- Elevation of sellar bone flap.
- Extracapsular tumour dissection.

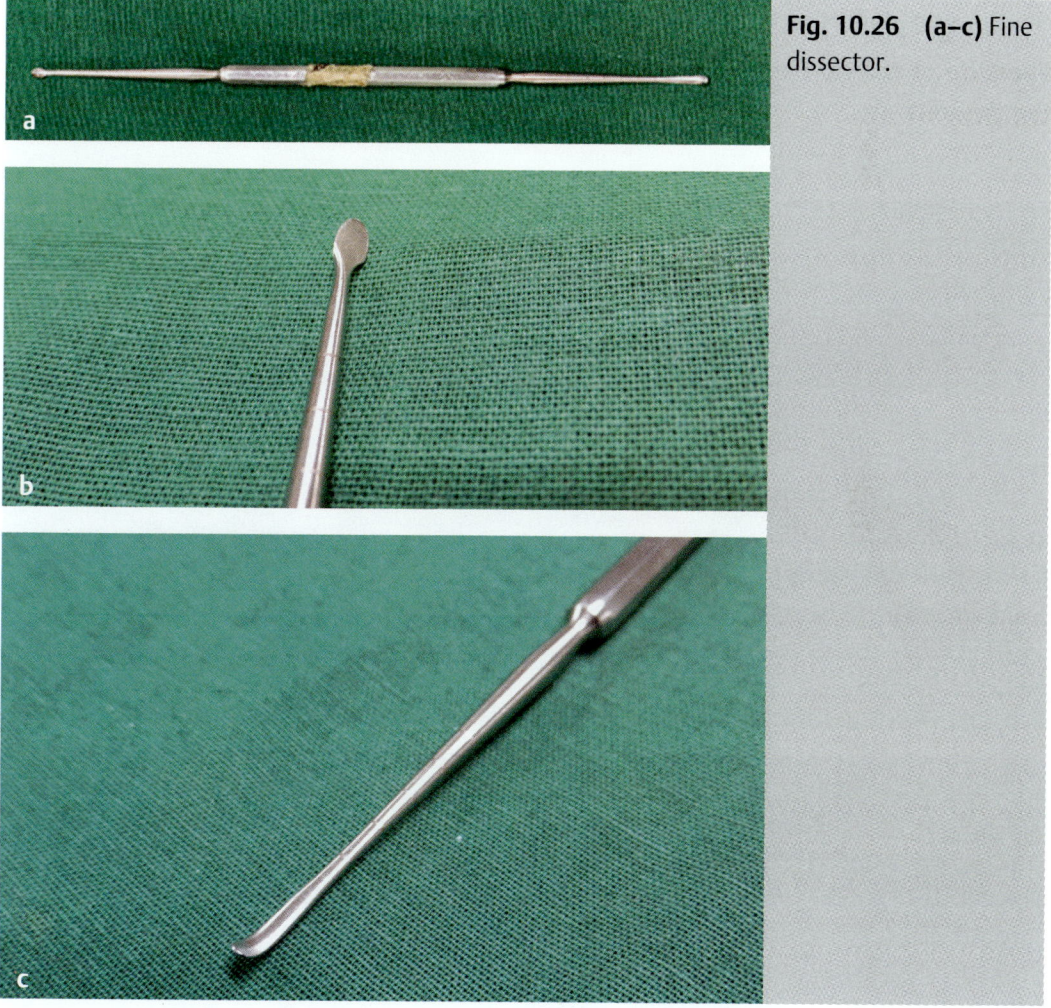

Fig. 10.26 (a–c) Fine dissector.

Instrument 27: Endoscopic Bipolar Forceps (Pistol Grip)

Endoscopic bipolar forceps (piston grip) (**Fig. 10.27**) are used for the following:

- Cauterisation of sphenopalatine artery, septal branch of the sphenopalatine artery (using horizontal forceps).
- Cauterisation of the superior and inferior intercavernous sinuses (using vertical forceps).

The side of the tip can be rotated from the distal end and adjusted according to the desired site.

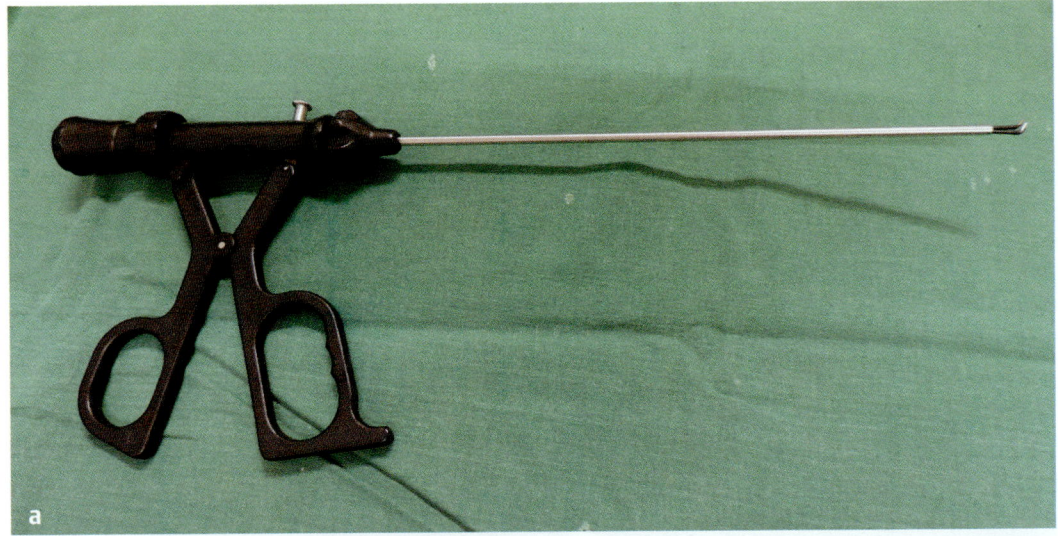

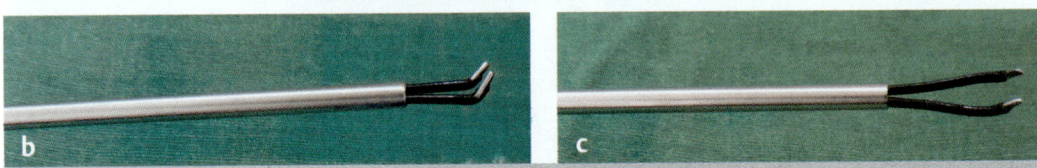

Fig. 10.27 **(a)** Endoscopic bipolar forceps (pistol grip). **(b)** Vertical forceps. **(c)** Horizontal forceps.

Instrument 28: Insulated Monopolar Suction Cautery

Monopolar suction cautery (**Fig. 10.28**) is basically an endonasal suction which is insulated all over except at its tip. It is used for controlling bleeders in the nasal cavity which aren't situated at an angle. Due to potential dissipation of thermal energy, its use is strictly prohibited inside the sphenoid, or over cribriform plates or any cranial base close to any neurovascular structure.

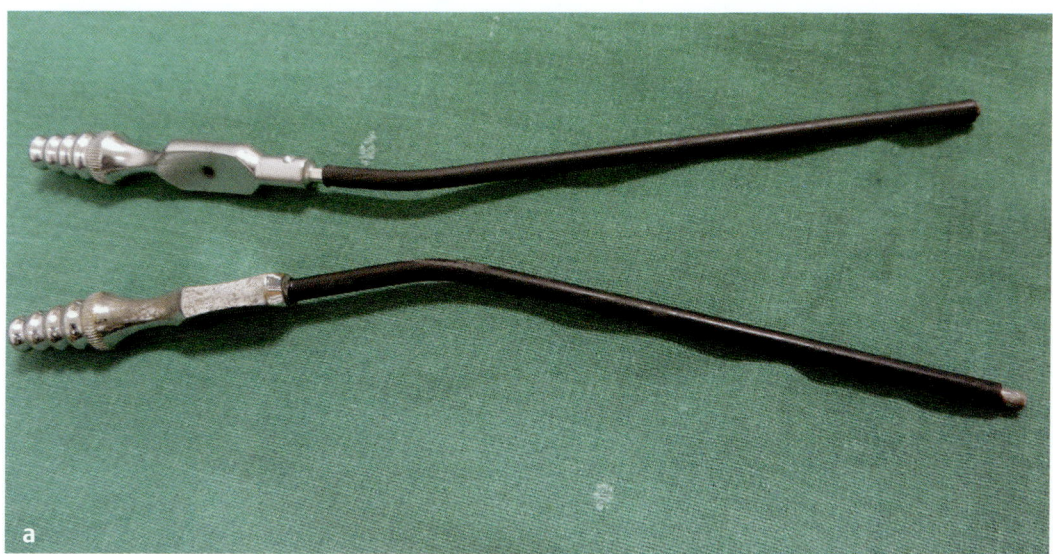

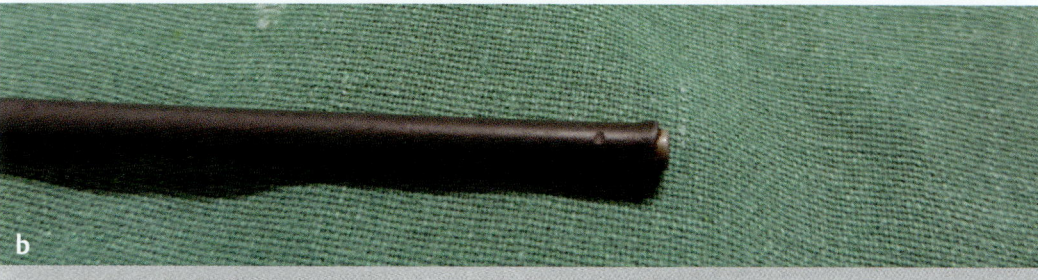

Fig. 10.28   (a, b) Monopolar suction cautery.

11 | Case Reports

Nishit Shah and C. E. Deopujari

Case 1

A 50-year-old patient presented with history of headache and visual disturbances.

Pre-Operative Scans (Fig.11.1)

Because of the anterior extension of the tumour, an extended transplanar approach was employed and the tumour was completely excised. Cerebrospinal fluid (CSF) leak was inevitable, hence, a lumbar drain was inserted pre-operatively. The sella defect reconstruction was done by fat, glue, and the Hadad flap. The post-operative magnetic resonance (MR) images are shown in **Fig. 11.2**.

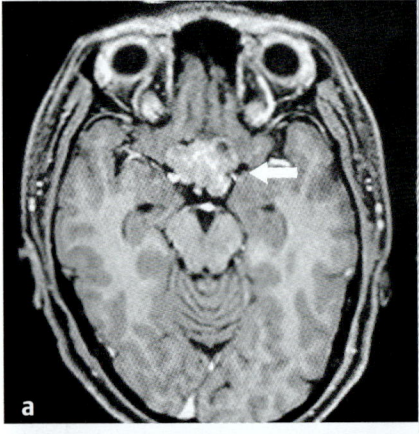

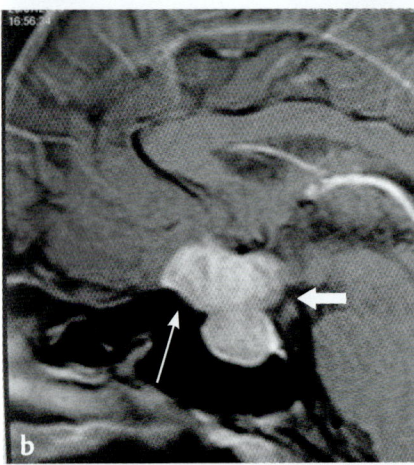

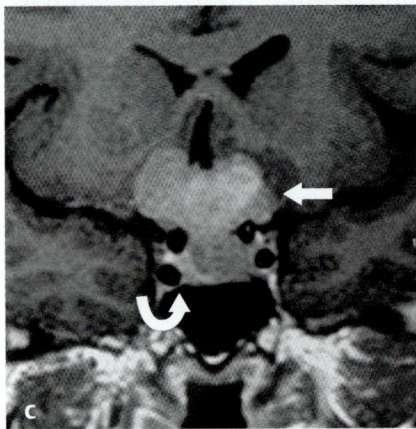

Fig. 11.1 **(a-c)** T1-weighted MRI scans revealed a giant pituitary adenoma (*block arrow*) with anterior extension (*thin white arrow*) **(b)**. The lesion is hypointense to the normal gland which is seen pushed to the right (*curved white arrow*) **(c)**. The heterogeneity best seen on axial view **(a)** is probably due to internal haemorrhages or cystic degeneration.

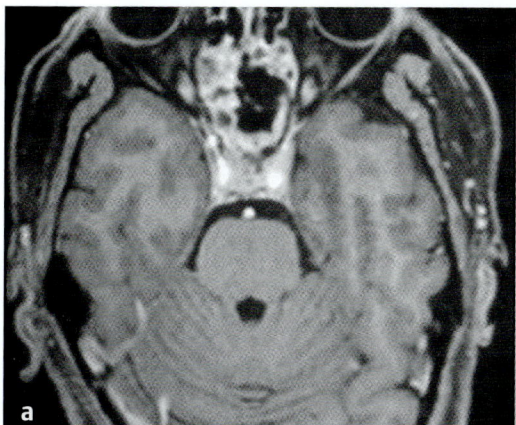

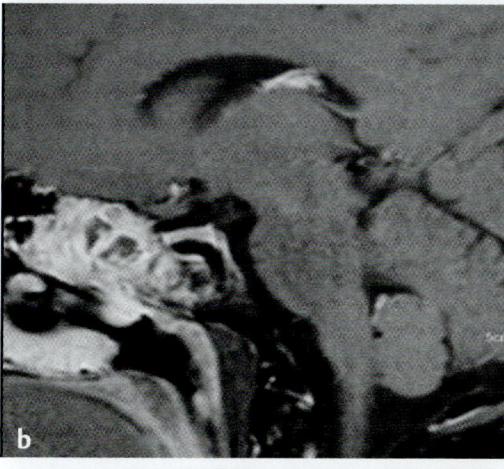

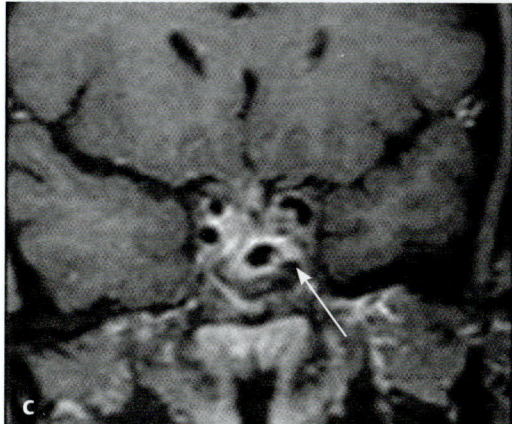

Fig. 11.2 **(a, b)** Post-operative MRI images showing complete excision of the tumour. **(c)** Sella packed with reconstruction material (*thin white arrow*).

Case 2

Pre-Operative MRI Images (Fig. 11.3)

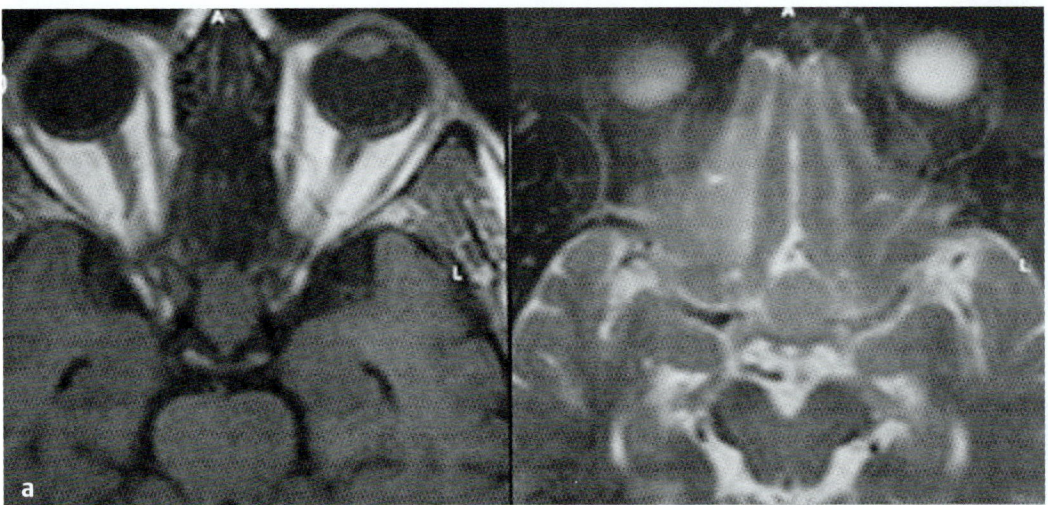

Fig. 11.3 **(a)** Planum sphenoidale meningioma seen on axial (T1W and T2W), coronal (T1W). **(b)** Sagittal (T1W) MR images. **(c)** The lesion is isointense on T1 and T2.

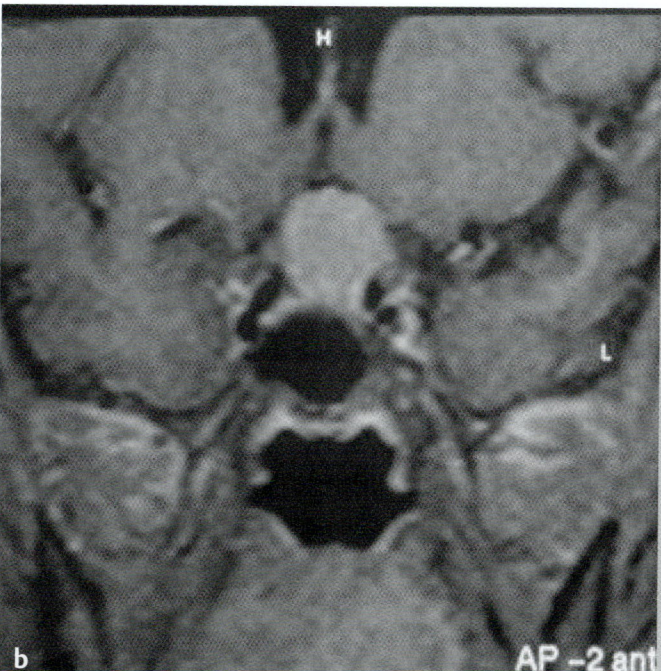

Fig. 11.3 (b) The carotids are mildly displaced laterally with inter-ICA distance of over 12 mm. **(c)** Sagittal image shows an enhancing dural tail (*thin white arrow*). The normal pituitary gland (*block white arrow*) is seen separately below the meningioma. Note that the sphenoid sinus has pre-sellar type of pneumatisation.

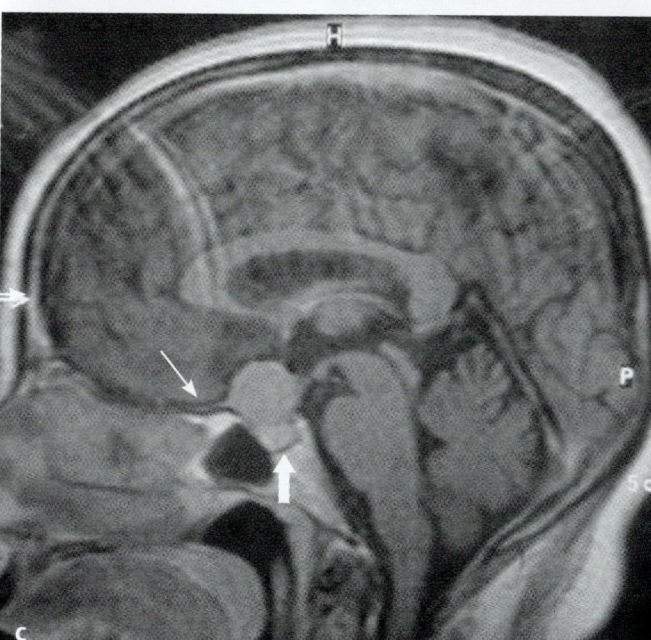

205

CT Brain + Angiography (Fig. 11.4)

This planum meningioma could be completely excised via an extended endoscopic transplanar route. Because of the pre-sellar pneumatisation of the sphenoid, and the location and the nature of the lesion, neuro-navigation system was used in this case as a considerable amount of bony drilling over the sella, tuberculum, and planum was anticipated over a narrow inter-carotid distance.

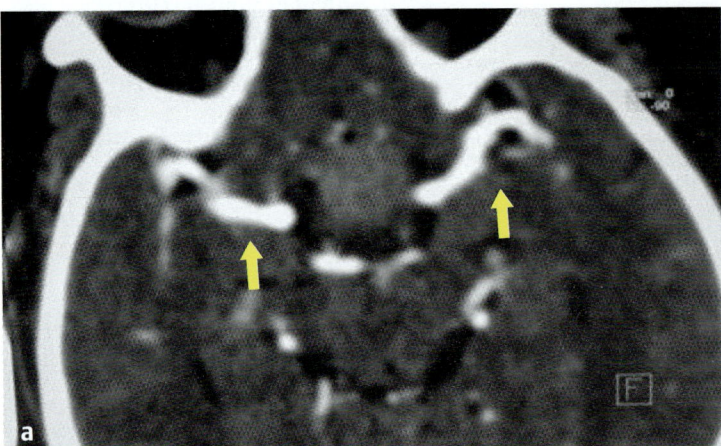

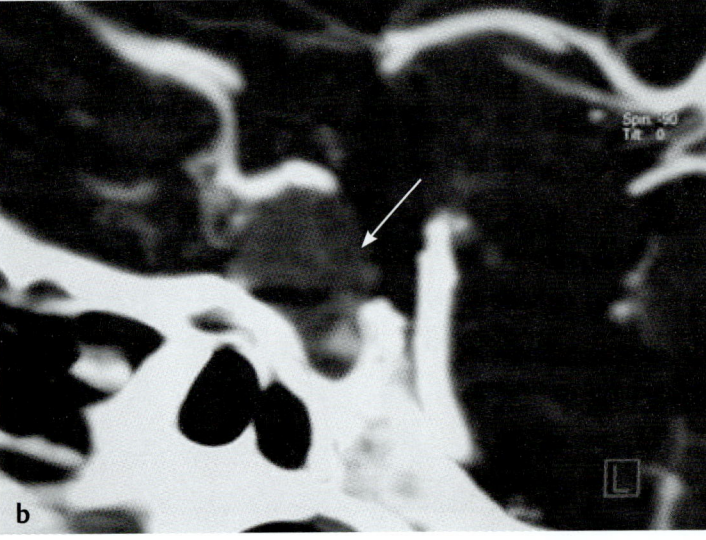

Fig. 11.4 **(a)** Axial and **(b)** sagittal view of CT angiogram of the planum meningioma (*thin white arrow*). Anterior cerebral artery is marked by *yellow arrows*.

Intra-Operative Images (Figs. 11.5–11.10)

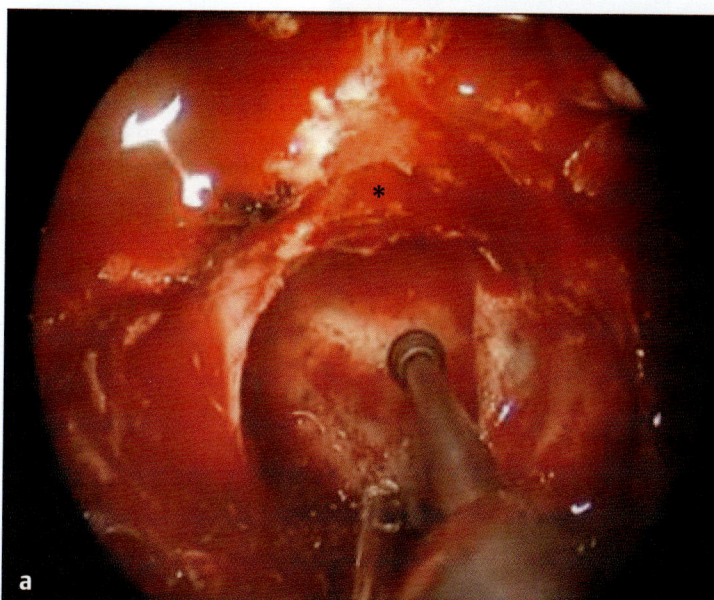

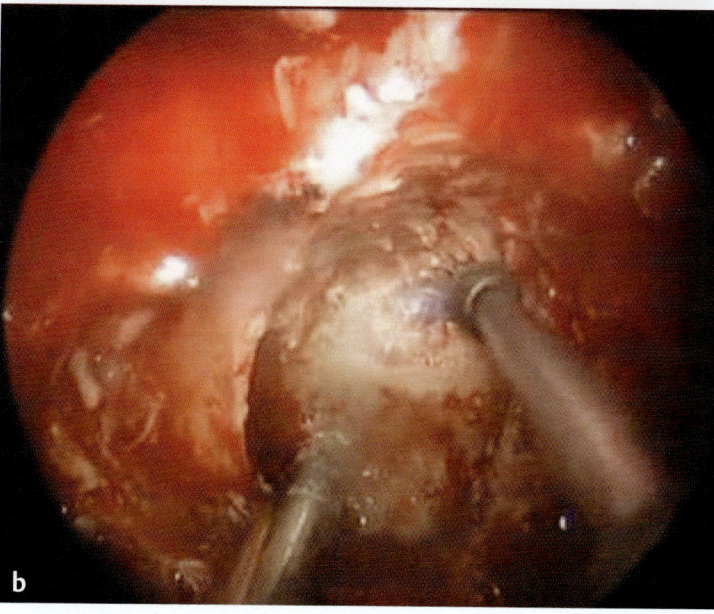

Fig. 11.5 **(a)** Intra-operative picture of drilling of the sella (*). **(b)** The blue lining thus seen is the sellar dura. Note: that the sella bulge is not seen prominently as the sphenoid pneumatisation in this case is pre-sellar.

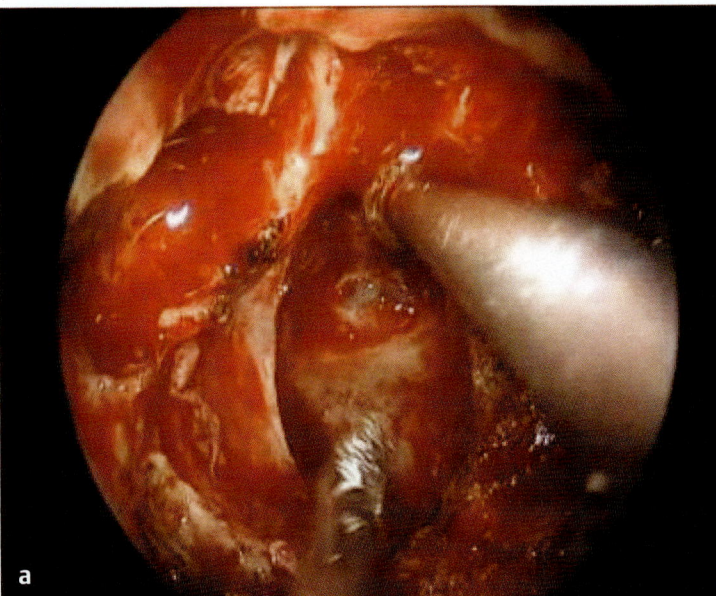

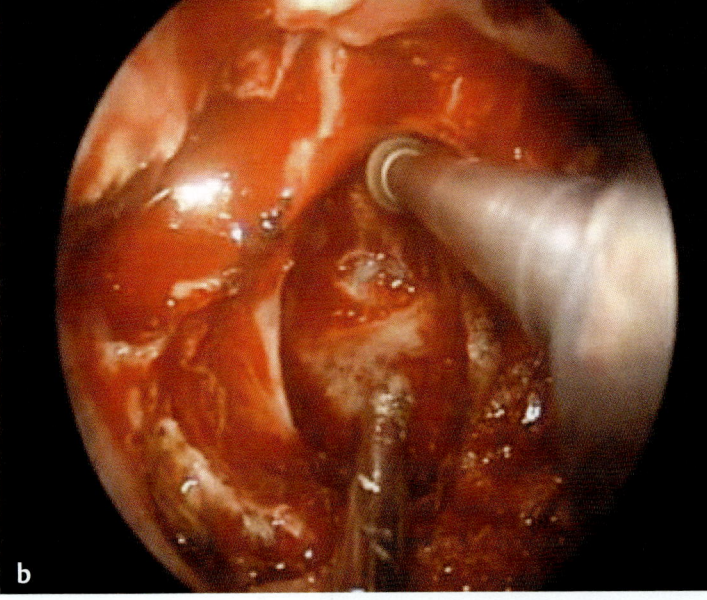

Fig. 11.6 After the sella is defined, the drilling is then continued onto the **(a)** tuberculum and the **(b)** planum sphenoidale. The carotids are kept in the visual field at every point.

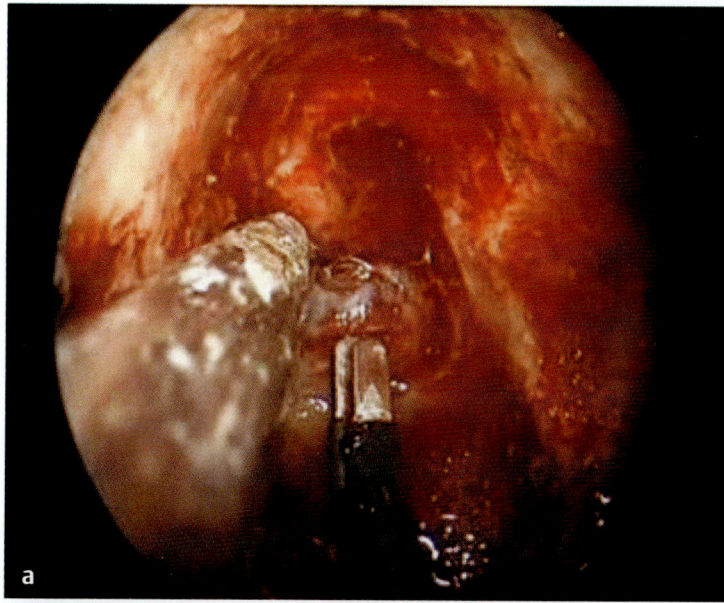

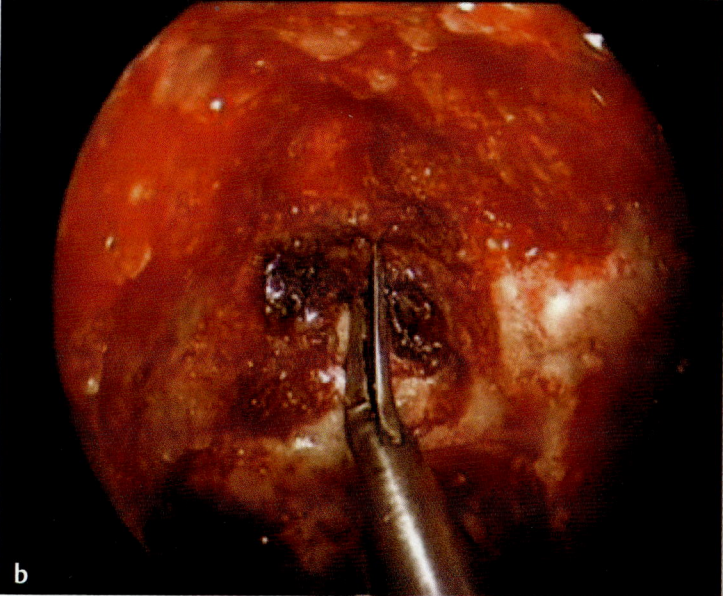

Fig. 11.7 **(a)** The superior intercavernous sinus being cauterised (using vertical bipolar forceps). **(b)** Cut (using angled dural scissors).

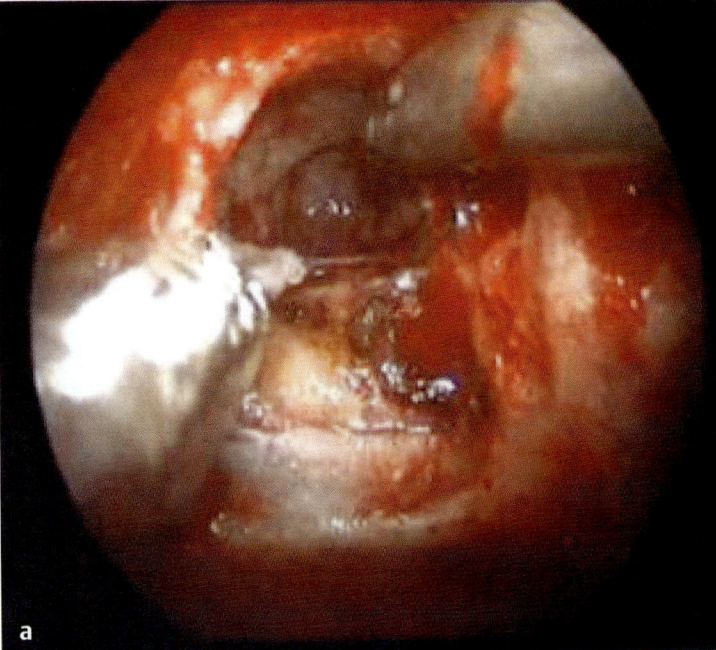

Fig. 11.8 Excision of the tumour from the suprasellar space using various blunt instruments such as **(a)** curved olive-tip suction, **(b)** ring curette.

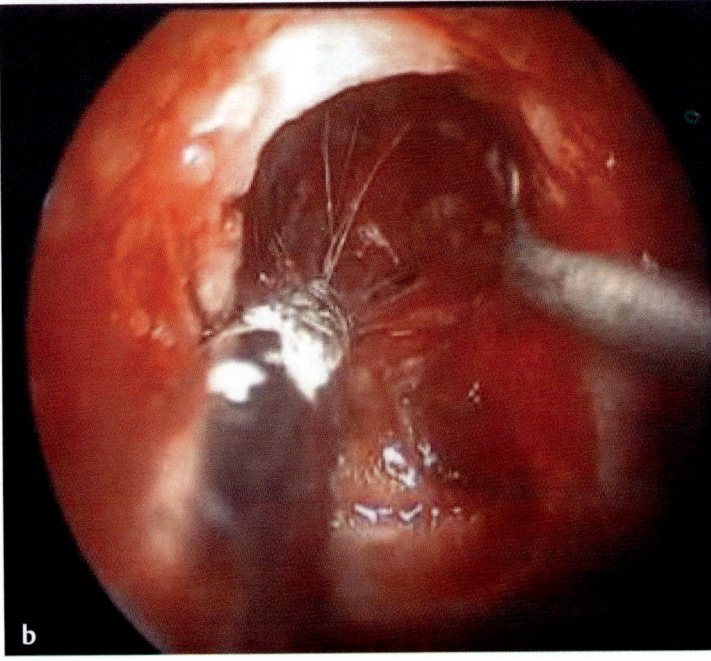

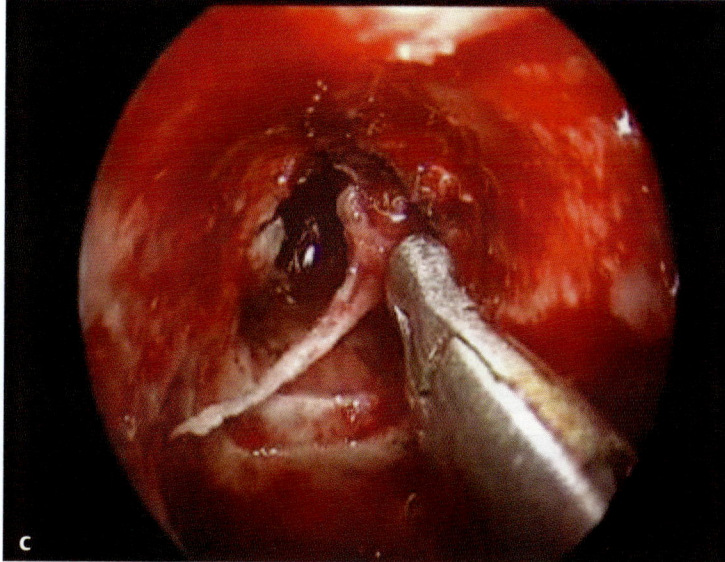

Fig. 11.8 (c) Blakesley's upward tumour forceps.

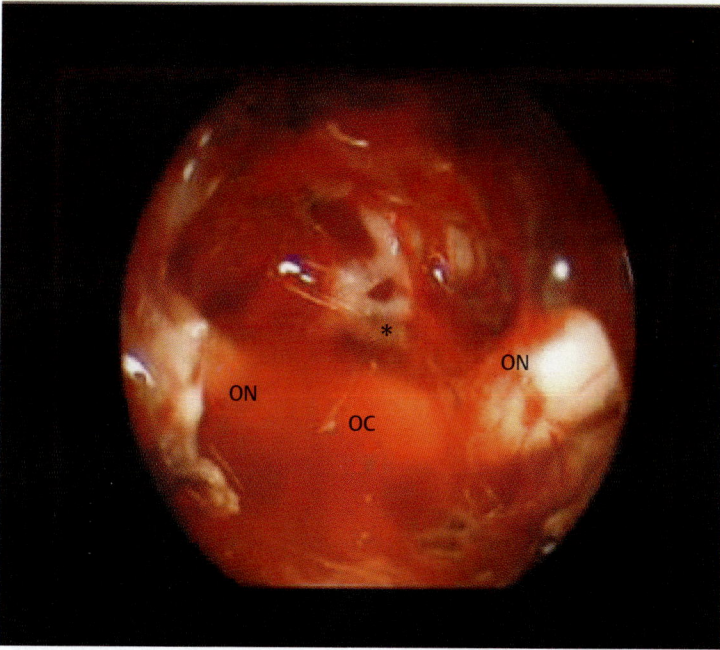

Fig. 11.9 Visualisation of the suprasellar space after complete excision of the meningioma. ON, optic nerve; OC, optic chiasm; (*), anterior communicating artery.

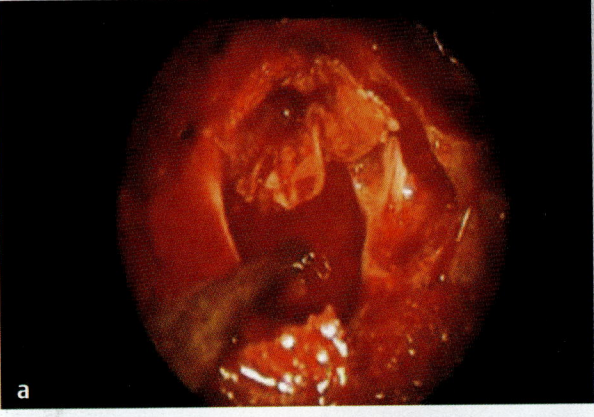

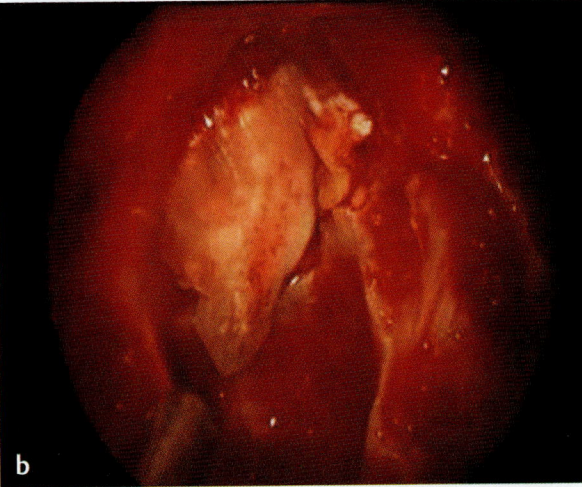

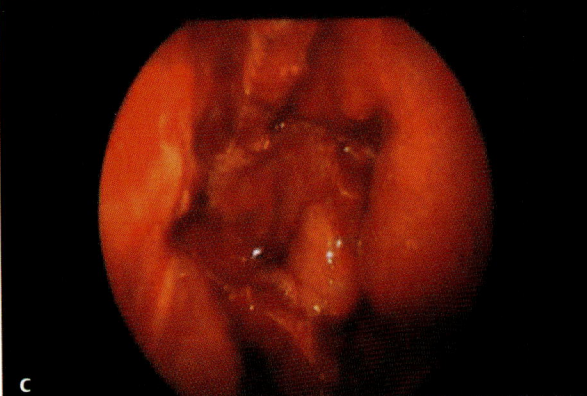

Fig. 11.10 **(a)** Reconstruction of the planar defect using overlay free fascia harvested from the lateral thigh. The free fascia is directly in contact with the bone. **(b)** A free bone obtained from the anterior wall of the sphenoid. **(c)** The Hadad flap are used to reinforce the reconstruction.

Post-Operative Scans (Figs. 11.11, 11.12)

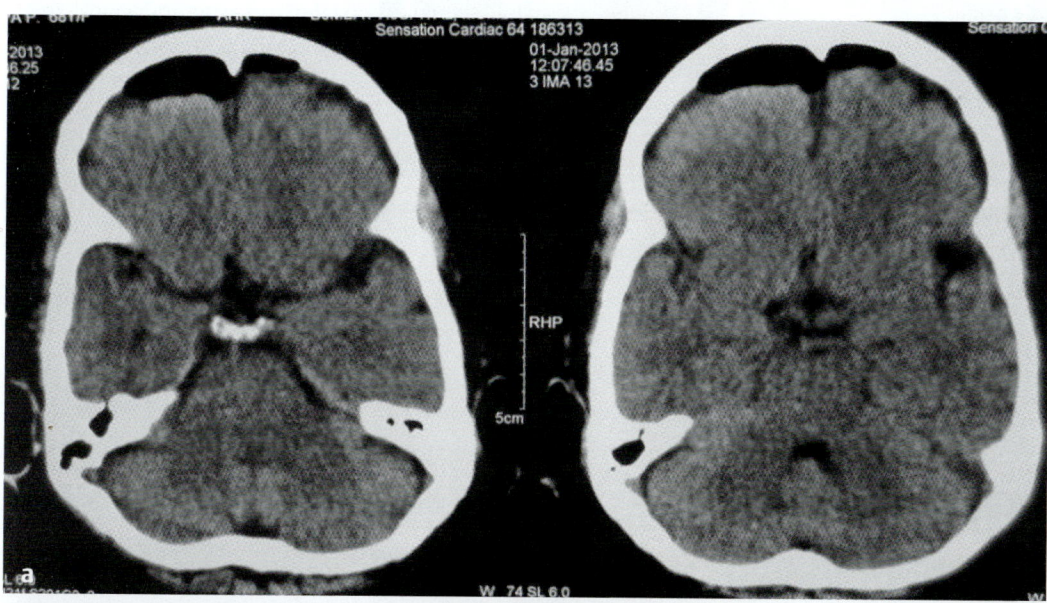

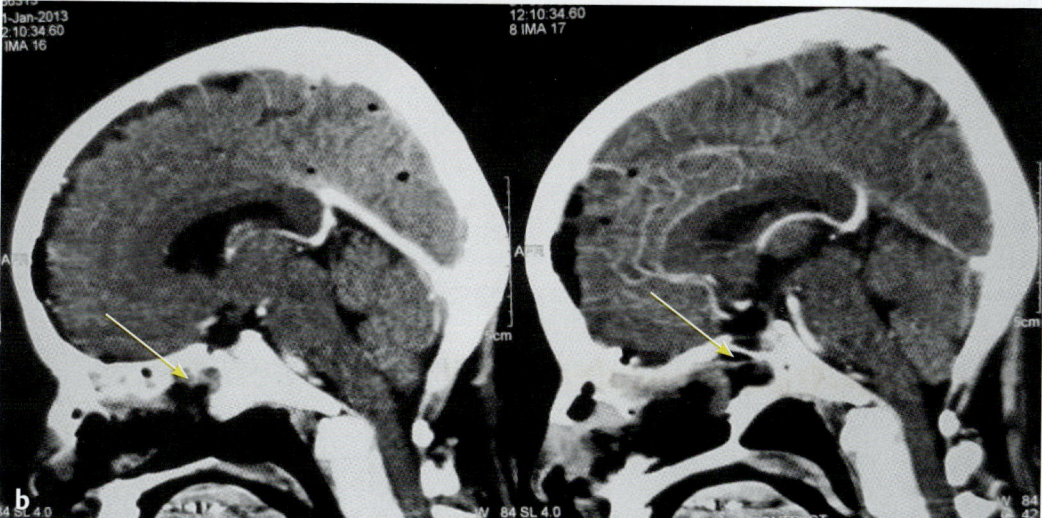

Fig. 11.11 **(a, b)** Post-operative CT angiography showing complete excision of the tumour, indicated by *yellow arrow*.

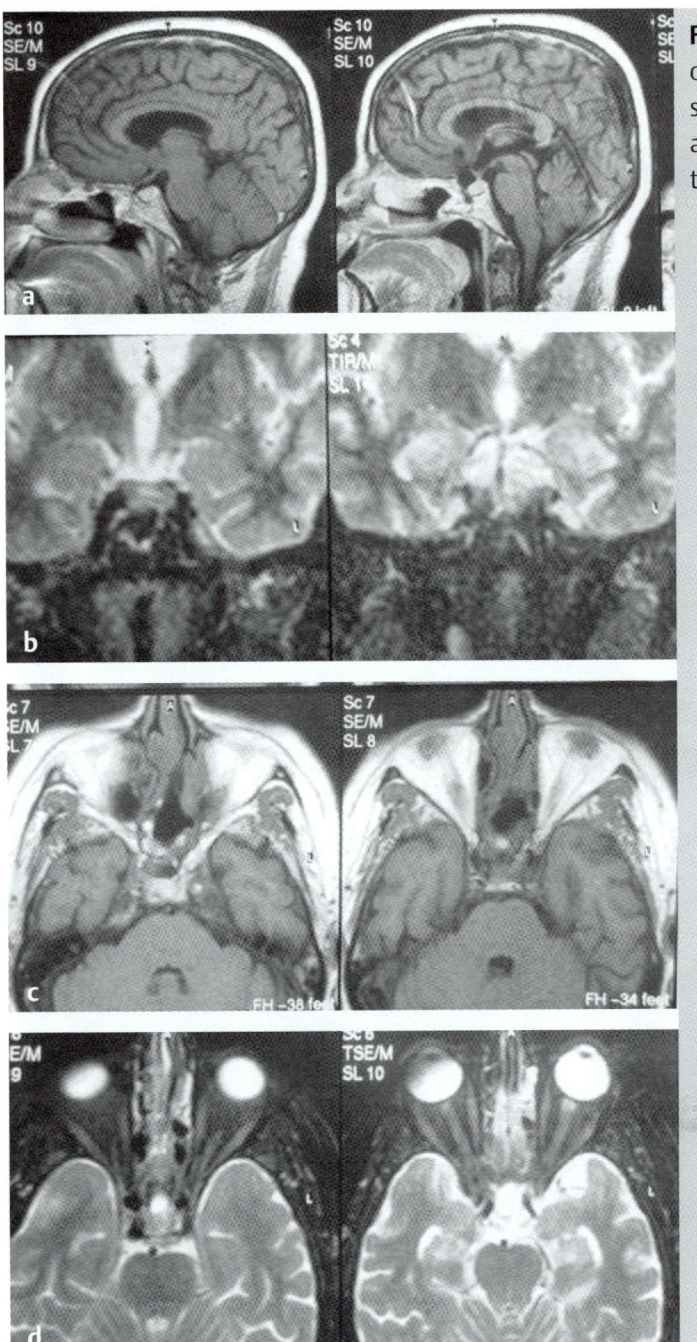

Fig. 11.12 (a-d) Post-operative T1 and T2 MRI scans in sagittal, coronal, and axial plane after endonasal transplanar surgery.

Case 3

Pre-Operative Scans (Fig. 11.13)

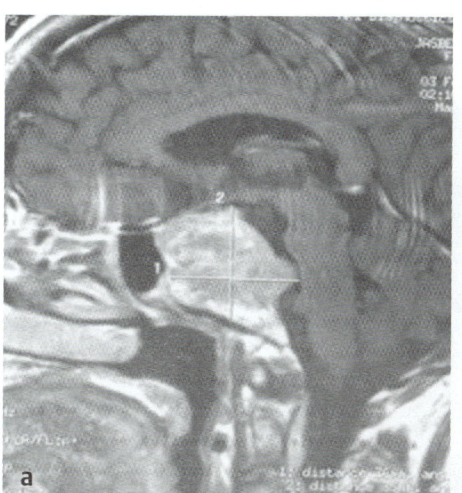
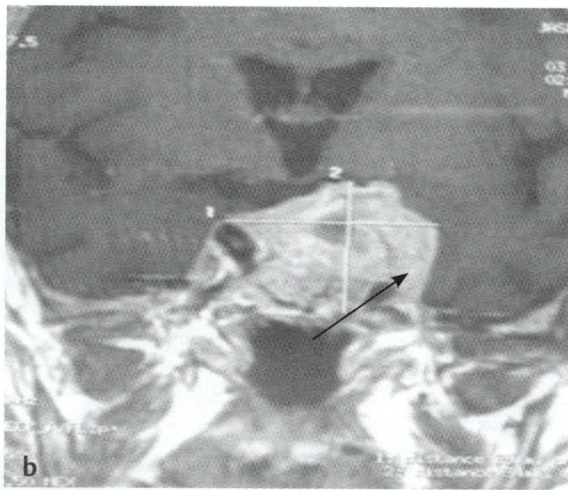

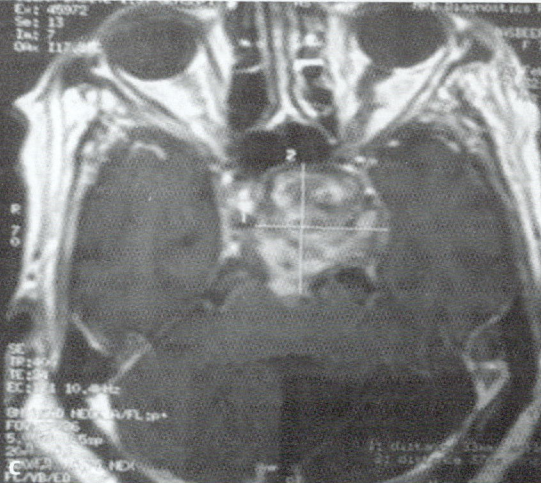

Fig. 11.13 Sagittal **(a)**, coronal **(b)** and axial **(c)** T1w MR images showing a clival chordoma occupying the upper two-thirds of the clivus as seen in **(a)**, with coronal MR image showing extension into the left cavernous sinus **(b)** lateral to the carotid (*arrow*).

Intra-Operative Images

This lesion was excised via the transclival approach, with the help of neuro-navigation system to assess and confirm the posterior limits of the tumour dissection **Figs. 11.14–11.17.**

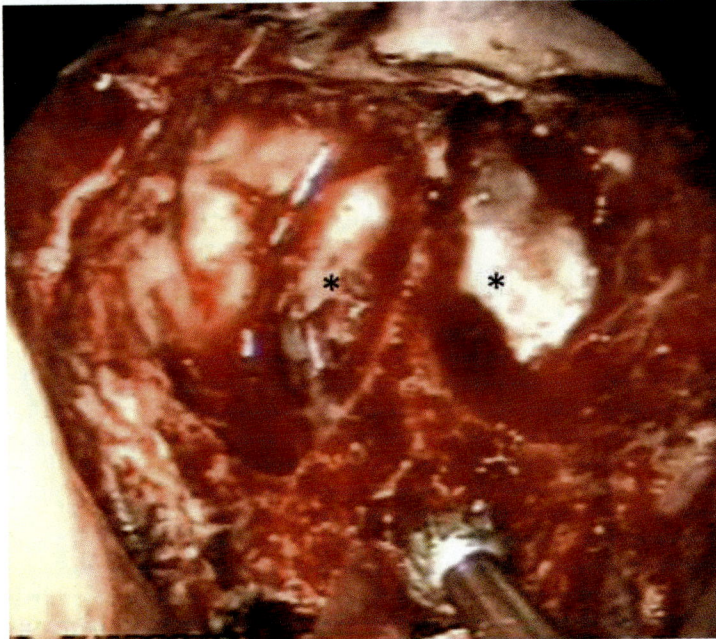

Fig. 11.14 Intraoperative pictures showing drilling of the clivus. The tumour is seen bulging into the sphenoid sinus (*).

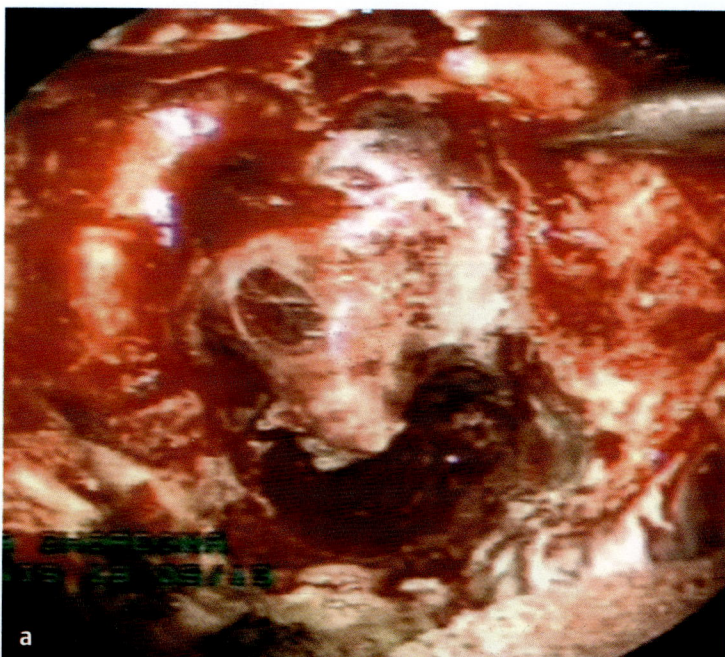

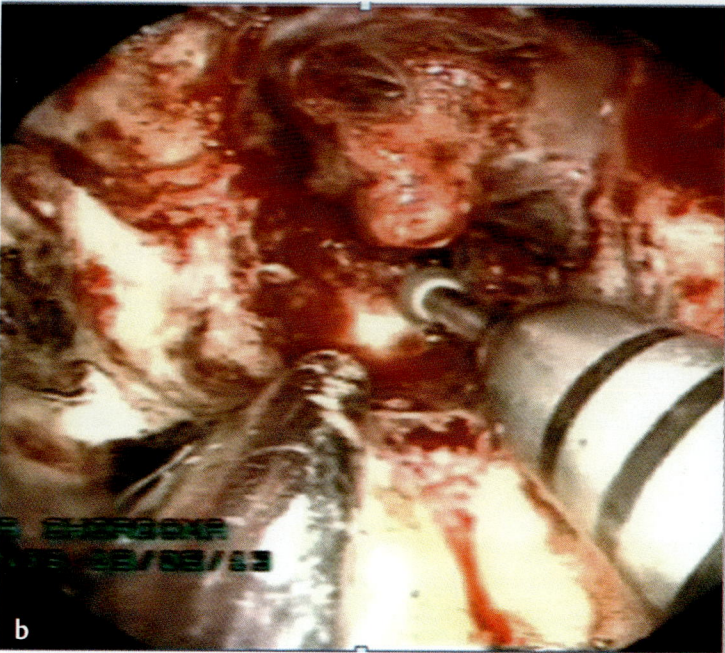

Fig. 11.15 **(a)** After the exposure of the upper clival part of the chordoma, **(b)** the lower two-third portion of the clivus is being drilled.

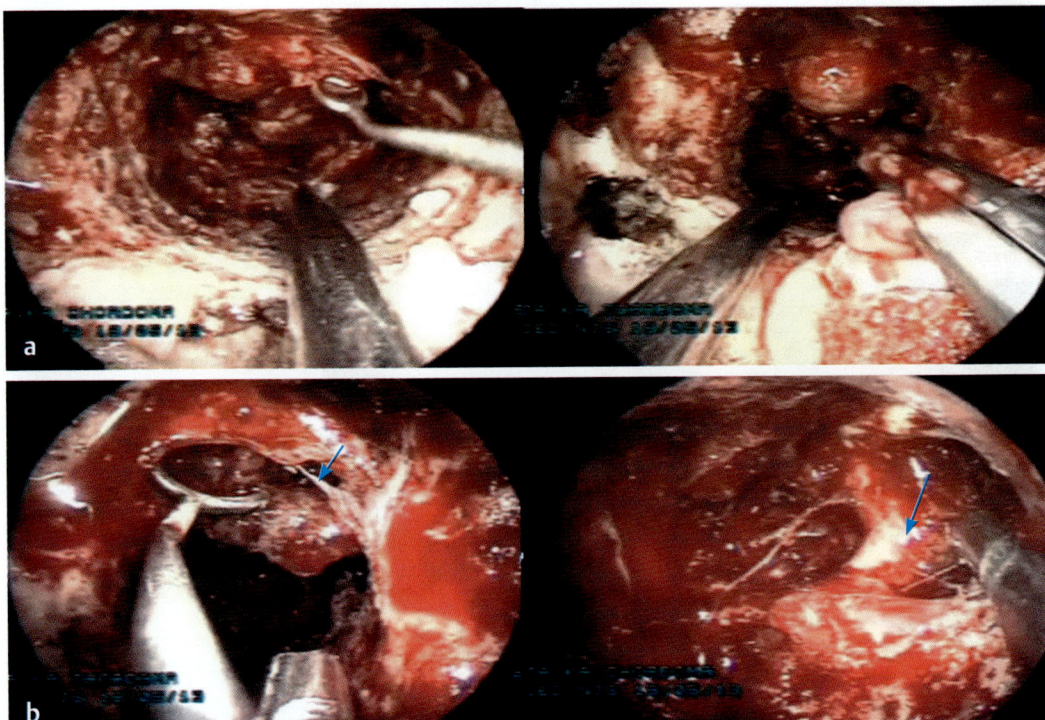

Fig. 11.16 **(a)** Excision of the clival chordoma using ring curette and tumour forceps. **(b)** Lateral extension of the tumour, beyond the carotid (*blue arrow*) is being dissected using a ring curette.

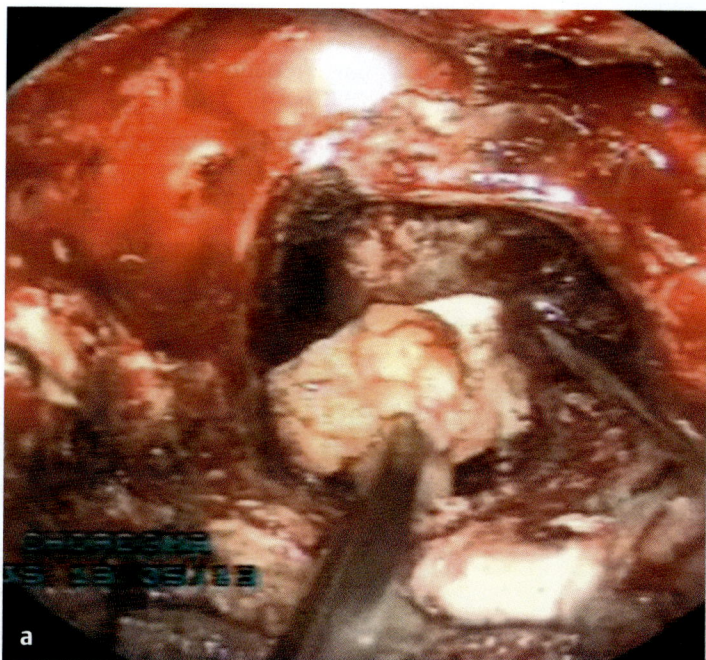

a

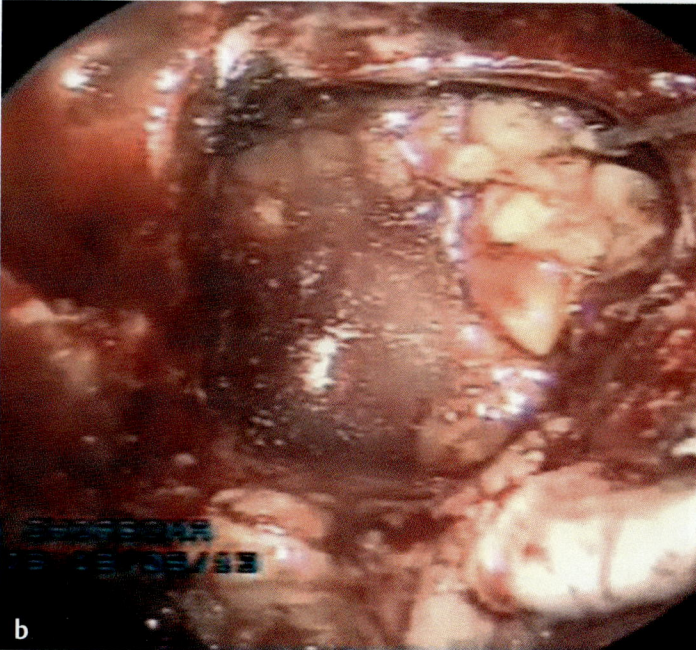

b

Fig. 11.17 Reconstruction of the clival defect using **(a)** underlay fat, **(b)** glue and **(c)** overlay free mucoperiosteal flap. While placing the overlay flap, it is mandatory to remove all the intervening mucosa/glue between the flap and bone.

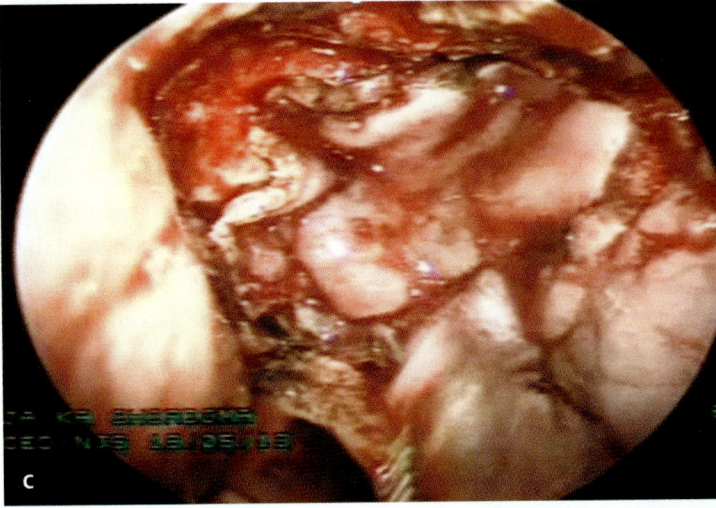

Fig. 11.17 **(c)** overlay free mucoperiosteal flap. While placing the overlay flap, it is mandatory to remove all the intervening mucosa/glue between the flap and bone.

Post-Operative Scans (Fig. 11.18)

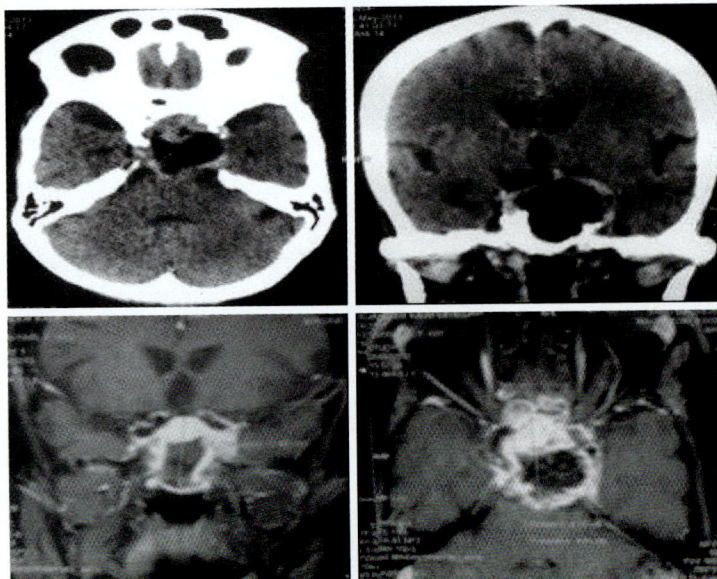

Fig. 11.18 Post-operative CT and MR images showing complete excision via transclival approach.

Case 4

Recurrent Craniopharyngioma

A 60-year-old woman presented with blurring of vision in right eye since 6 months. She gave past history of loss of vision in left eye since 2007 when she was operated for transcranial excision of craniopharyngioma.

On examination, right eye finger counting was 2 feet and left eye vision was absent. Her hormonal profile was normal.

Pre-Operative Scans 2007 (Fig. 11.19)

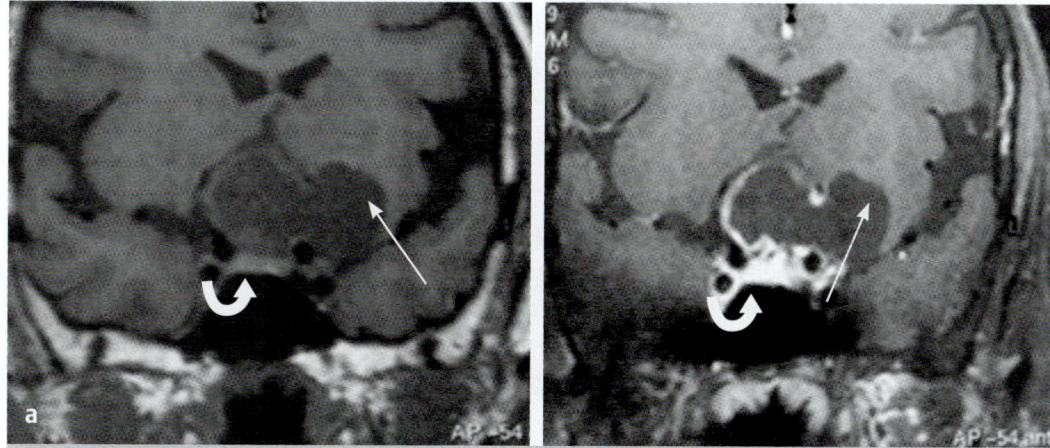

Fig. 11.19 **(a,b)** Pre- and post-contrast images of completely suprasellar lesion in coronal and sagittal view. Extension of the tumour is seen lateral to the carotid (*straight white arrow*) and the sellar portion of the tumour (*curved arrow*) is practically nil. Hence, transcranial route was employed for excision of this lesion, which turned out to be craniopharyngioma.

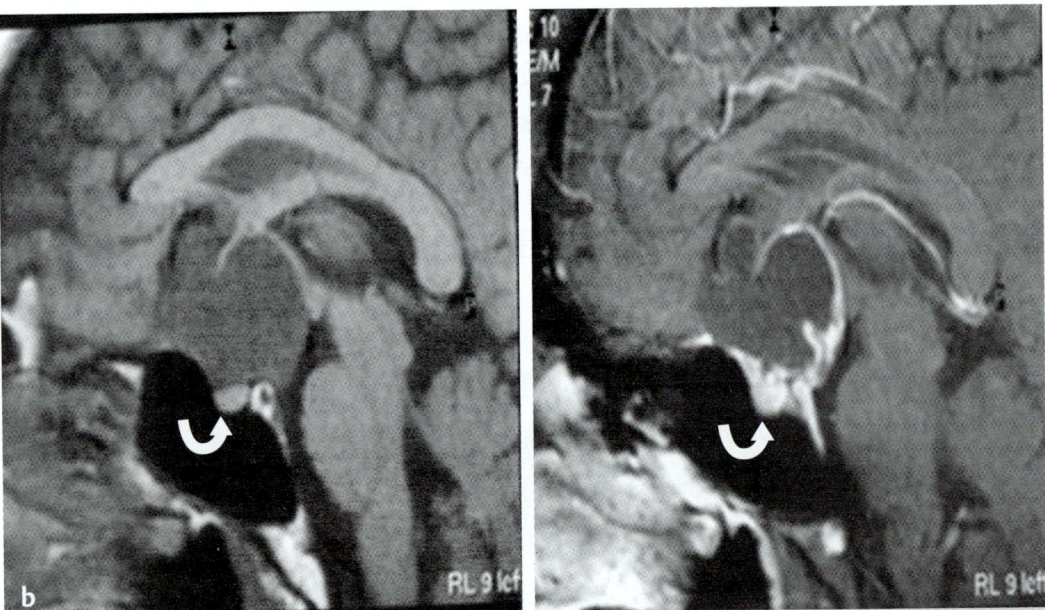

Fig. 11.19 **(a,b)** Pre- and post-contrast images of completely suprasellar lesion in coronal and sagittal view. Extension of the tumour is seen lateral to the carotid (*straight white arrow*) and the sellar portion of the tumour (*curved arrow*) is practically nil. Hence, transcranial route was employed for excision of this lesion, which turned out to be craniopharyngioma.

Post-Operative Scan 2007 (Figs.11.20–11.22)

The patient did not follow up after the first surgery and presented directly after 10 years with the following scans and decreased vision in the right eye.

The second surgery was performed via endonasal transtubercular approach.

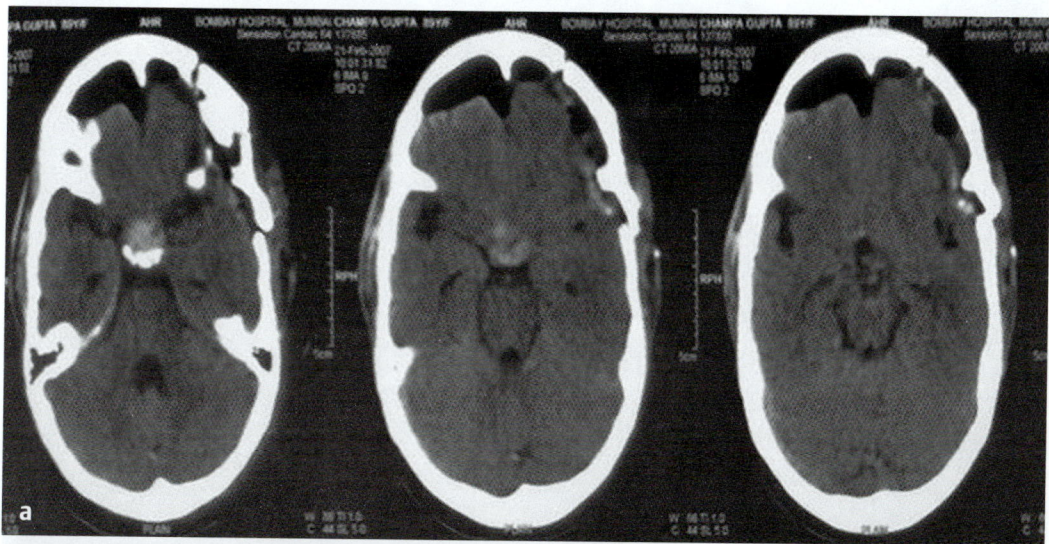

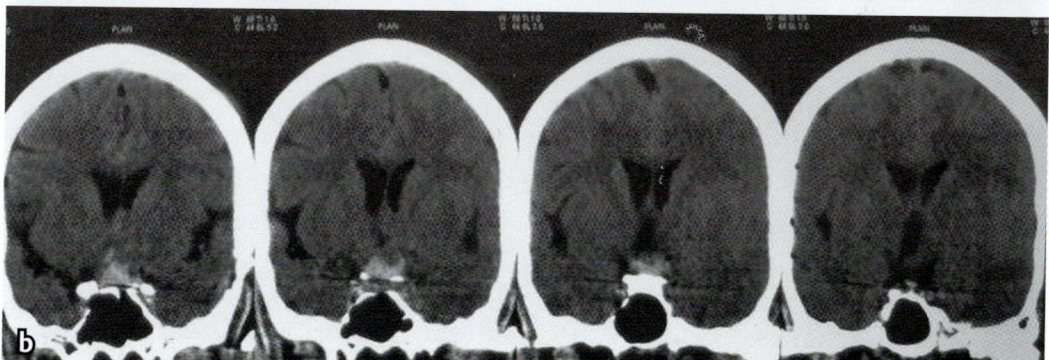

Fig. 11.20 **(a,b)** Post-operative CT images of the above patient following transcranial excision of the craniopharyngioma, demonstrating complete excision of the tumour.

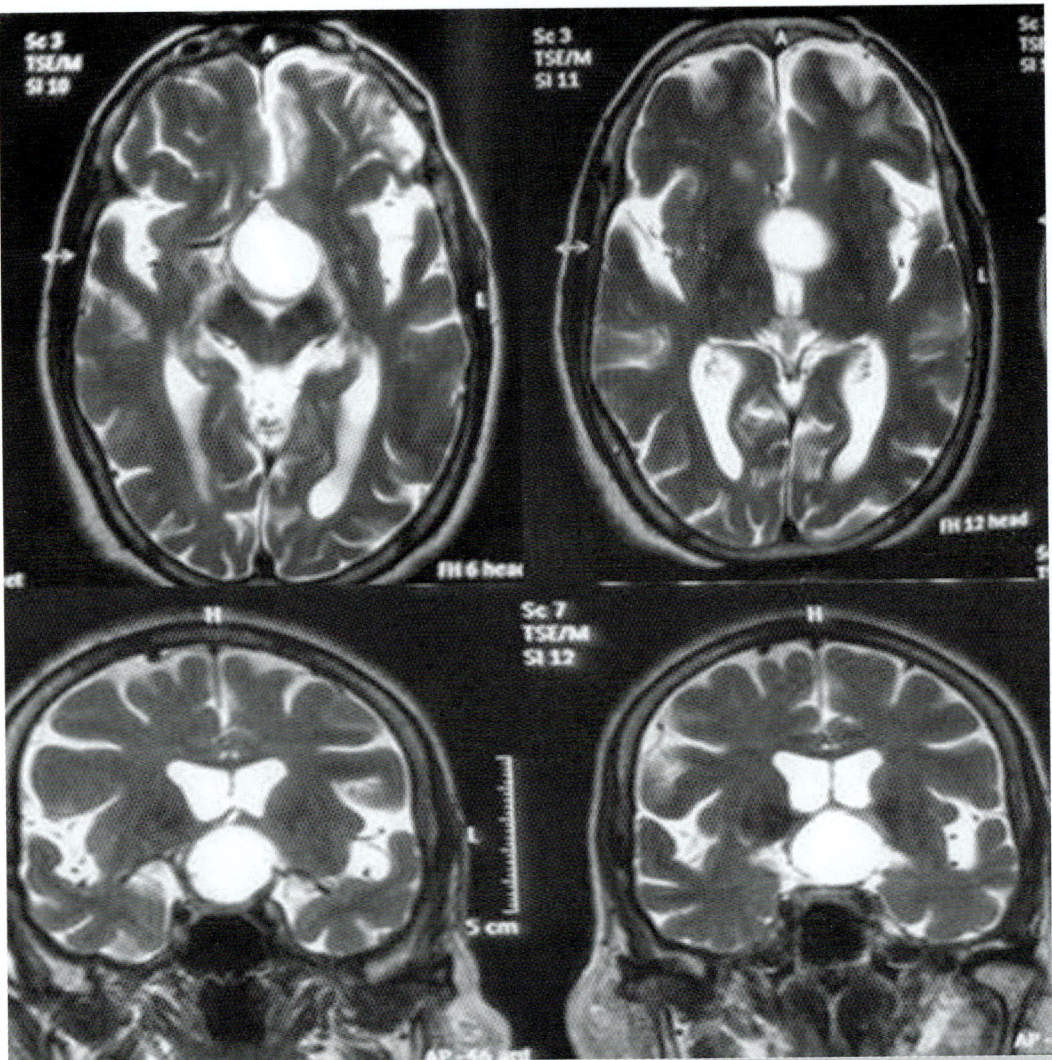

Fig. 11.21 Pre-contrast T2W images of the recurrent suprasellar craniopharyngioma.

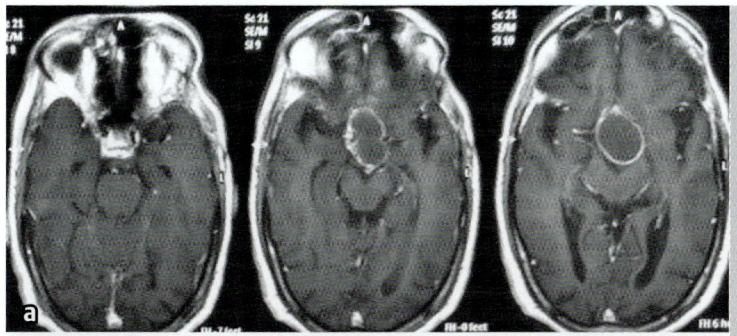

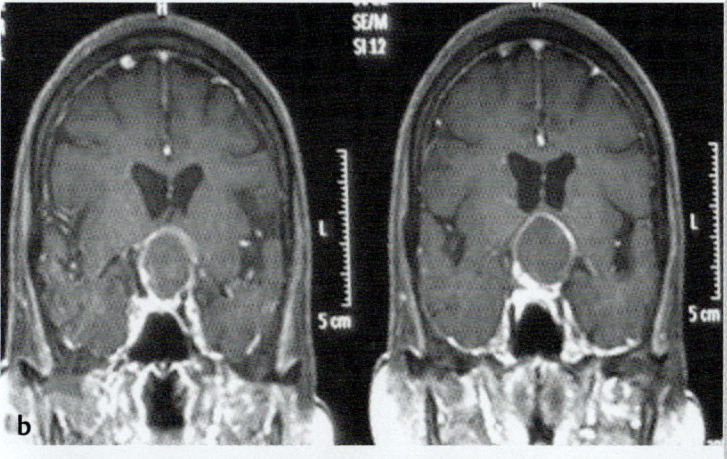

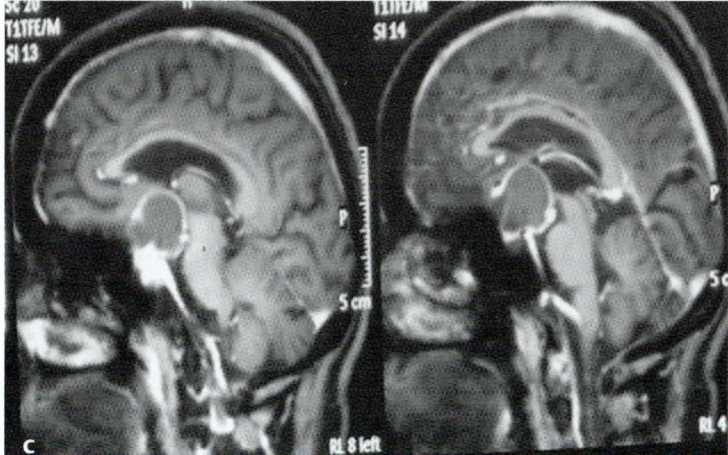

Fig. 11.22 (a–c) Post-contrast axial, coronal, and sagittal MR images of the recurrent craniopharyngioma. Although the sella component of the tumour is very limited, there is no lateral extension of the tumour.

Intra-Operative Images (Figs. 11.23–11.25)

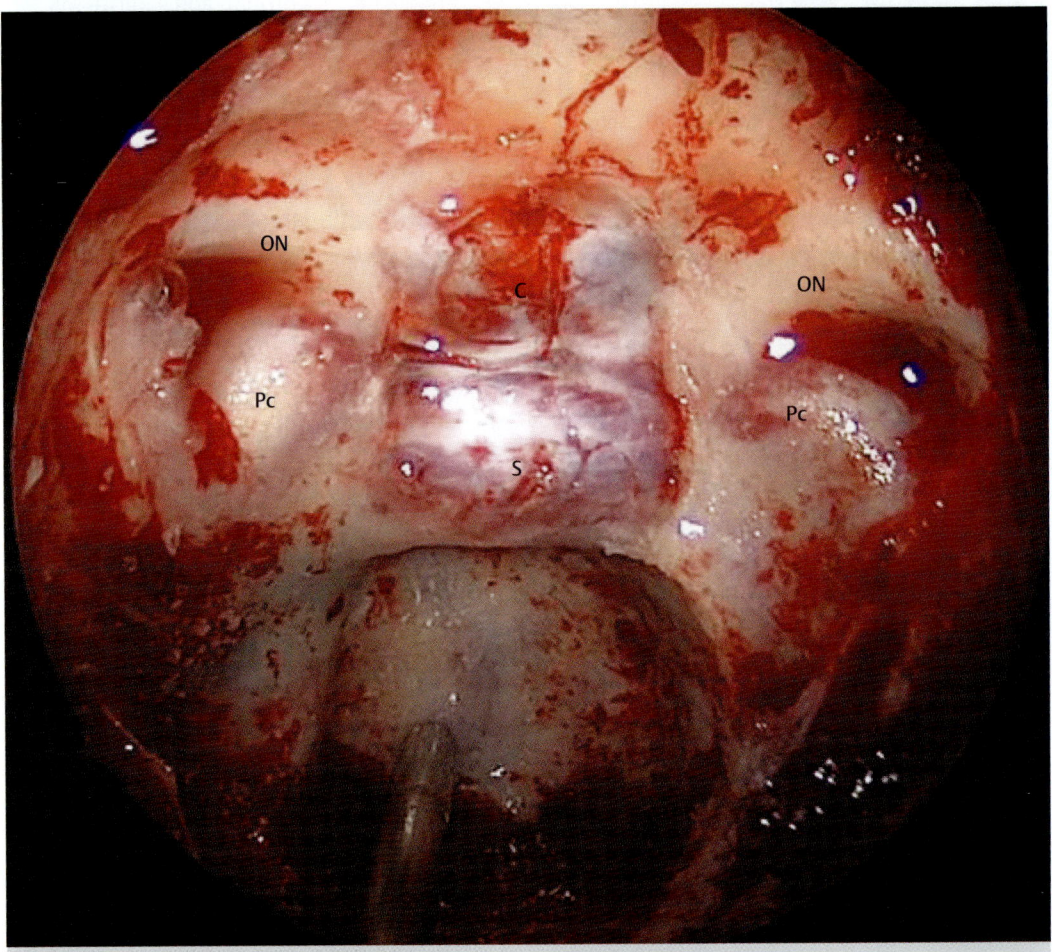

Fig. 11.23 Exposure of the sella (S) and the craniopharyngioma (C) after drilling of the tuberculum. ON, optic nerve; Pc, paraclinoid carotid.

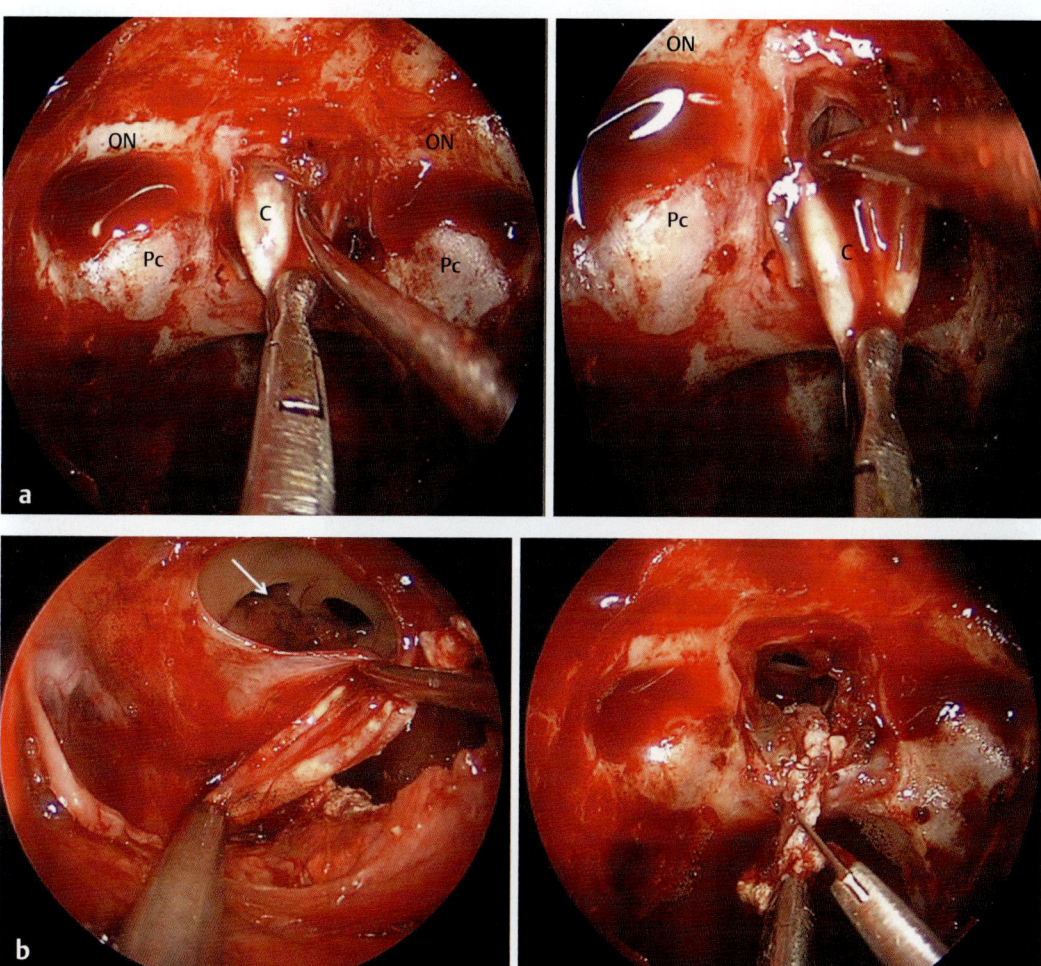

Fig. 11.24 **(a)** Extracapsular excision of the craniopharyngiomas **(C)** by doing sharp dissection using dural scissors. **(b)** The choroid plexus and the third ventricles (*white arrow*) are also visualised during the last bit of the tumour removal. ON, optic nerve; Pc, paraclinoid carotid.

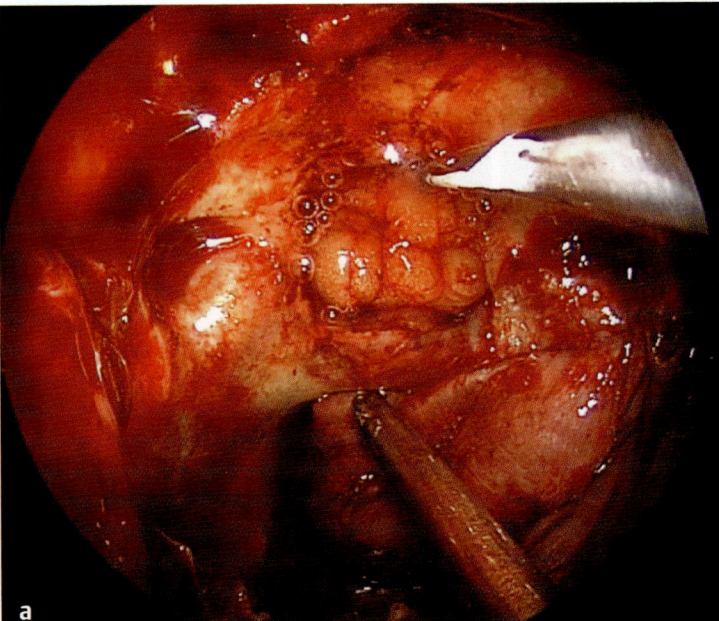

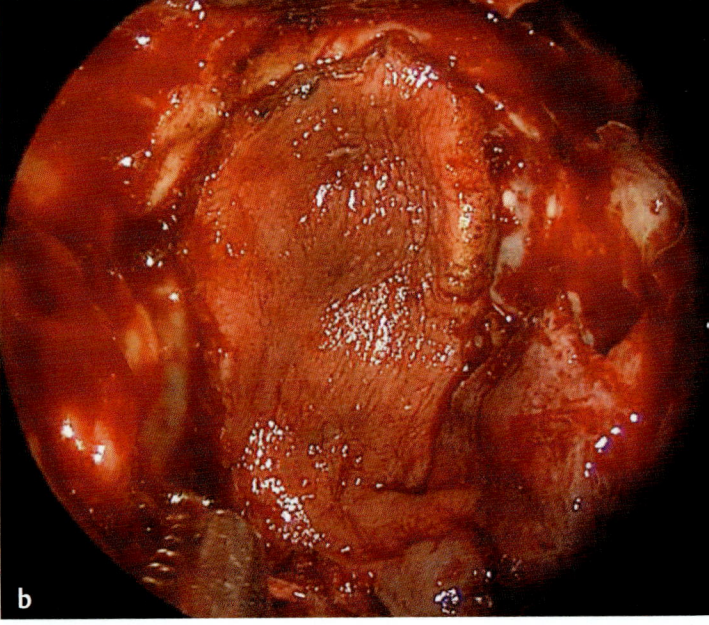

Fig. 11.25
Reconstruction of the tubercular defect using **(a)** inlay fat harvested from the lateral thigh and **(b)** overlay left-sided pedicled nasoseptal Hadad flap.

Post-Operative Scans 2017 (Fig. 11.26)

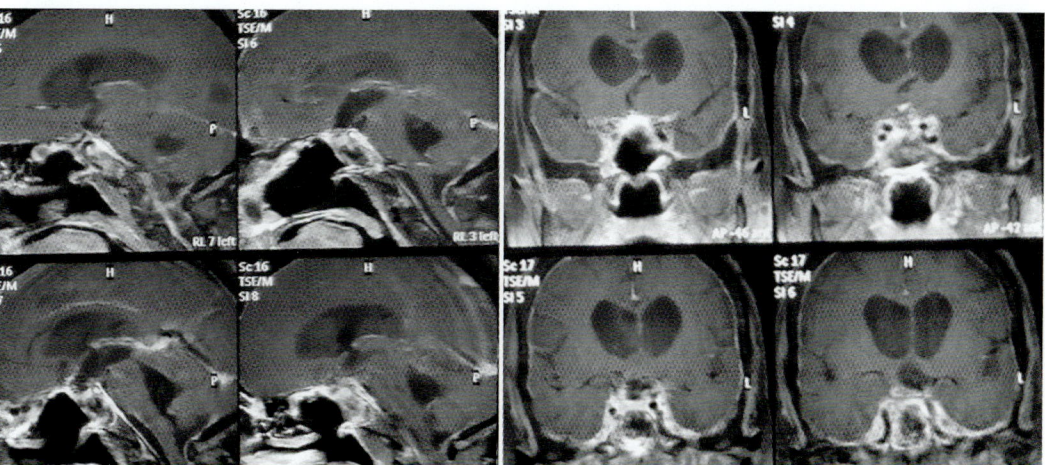

Fig. 11.26 Post-operative MR images in sagittal and coronal planes following endonasal transtubercular approach, demonstrating complete removal of the tumour.

Index